The Heart of YOGA

■ ■ ■ ■ ■ ■ ■ ■ ■ ■

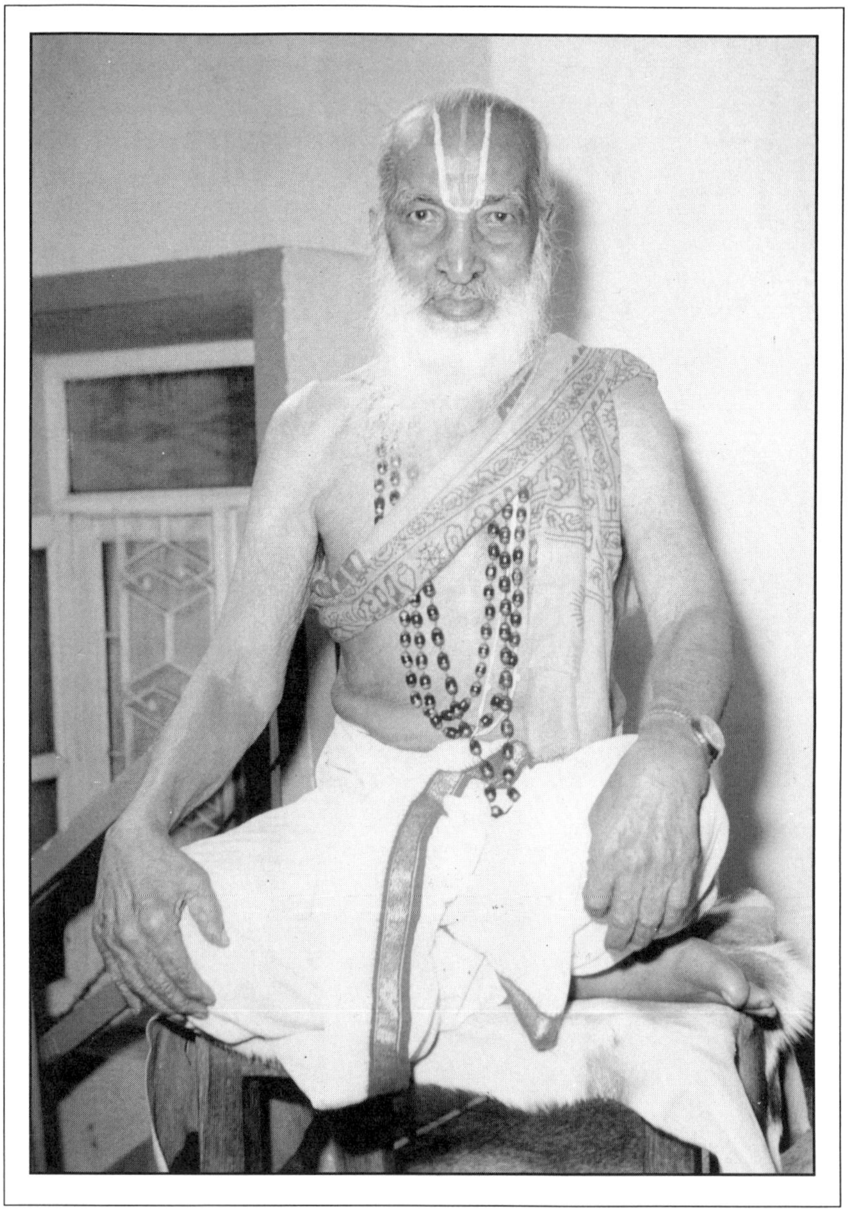

Śrī T. Krishnamacharya

The Heart of YOGA

DEVELOPING A PERSONAL PRACTICE

by T. K. V. Desikachar

INNER TRADITIONS INTERNATIONAL
Rochester, Vermont

Inner Traditions International
One Park Street
Rochester, Vermont 05767

All royalties from *The Heart of Yoga* go to the Krishnamacharya Yoga Mandiram, Madras. KYM is a registered charitable trust.

LIBRARY OF CONGRESS CATALOGING-IN-PUBLICATION DATA
Desikachar, T. K. V.
The heart of yoga : developing a personal practice / T. K. V. Desikachar.
p. cm.
ISBN 0-89281-533-7
1. Yoga, Hatha. I. Title.
RA781.7.D47 1995
613.7'046–dc20 95–31143
CIP

Printed and bound in the United States

10 9 8 7 6 5 4 3 2 1

Text design and layout by Kathryn Miles

This book was typeset in Times with Bodega Sans as the display typeface.

Distributed to the book trade in Canada by Publishers Group West (PGW), Toronto, Ontario

Distributed to the book trade in the United Kingdom by Deep Books, London

Distributed to the book trade in Australia by Millennium Books, Newtown, N.S.W.

Distributed to the book trade in New Zealand by Tandem Press, Auckland

I dedicate *The Heart of Yoga* to J. Krishnamurthi, who taught me how to be a good yoga student.

I am very grateful to my many friends who helped create *The Heart of Yoga*, especially to Indra Devi, Vanda Scaravelli, and Mark Whitwell.

CONTENTS

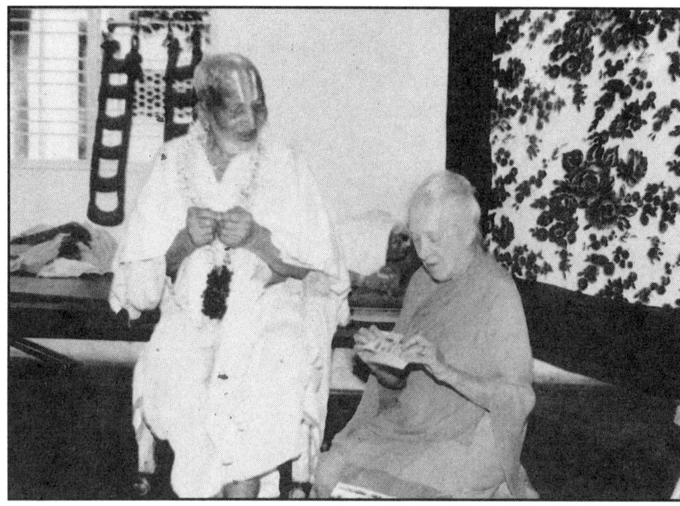

Krishnamacharya with Indra Devi at his centennial celebration.

A BLESSING

This book, written by Śrī Desikachar, is an invaluable source of information regarding the theory and practice of yoga. It is a must for students and teachers alike. Śrī Desikachar, himself a teacher par excellence, follows the yoga lineage of his father Śrī Krishnamacharya, one of the best yoga teachers of his time. It was my good fortune to be accepted by Śrī Krishnamacharya into his class, where I was not only the lone foreigner, but was also the only woman.

May this book serve as a guide and inspiration for all of the generations of yoga enthusiasts to come.

—With blessings, light, and love
from the heart of Indra Devi

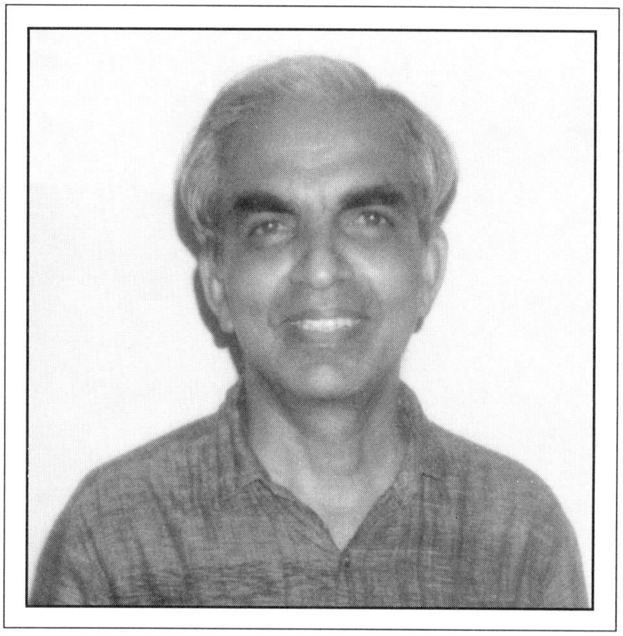

T. K. V. Desikachar

FOREWORD

I am grateful to have the opportunity to write about Śrī Desikachar, an exceptional yoga teacher, and it is with great pleasure that I write these few words to underline the importance of Śrī Desikachar's teaching.

What a nice person Desikachar is! One feels attracted to him—to be with him is a pleasure. His simplicity is one of the exceptional characteristics of his personality. He does not pretend in any way. In today's world it is refreshing to meet someone who knows so much and yet is so modest. Humility, from which simplicity follows, is a very precious quality. Desikachar is one of those few people who truly lives this quality.

The years Desikachar spent at university attaining his engineering degree have not been an impediment. On the contrary, once I asked what helped him most in the work he does now and he replied, "My engineering studies." It is likely that such training stimulated his sparkling intelligence, which later gave him the ability to transmit his teaching with clarity and precision. When Desikachar speaks he expresses himself in a natural and easy way, in a language that each one of us can understand and follow. He walks toward you with a light step, and his delightful smile lets you know that his heart is open.

I received a precious gift one day when he chanted for me and my friends. His clear sounds had a delicate and yet powerful flow, following the rhythm that arose from his lovely voice. The enchanting atmosphere created by the vibrations of that sound filled the room and remained a long time after he left.

Desikachar helps us realize that what is essential in the practice of yoga is the breath because each pose, each movement, originates from there. This balanced union brings harmony and order to our bodies and minds.

The way he can communicate these very special yoga teachings is extraordinary. He has great respect for the subject and for the person to whom he is conveying his knowledge. He does not push you into it, but very gently leads you to the door that eventually, and unexpectedly, may open to let you in.

—Vanda Scaravelli
Florence, Italy

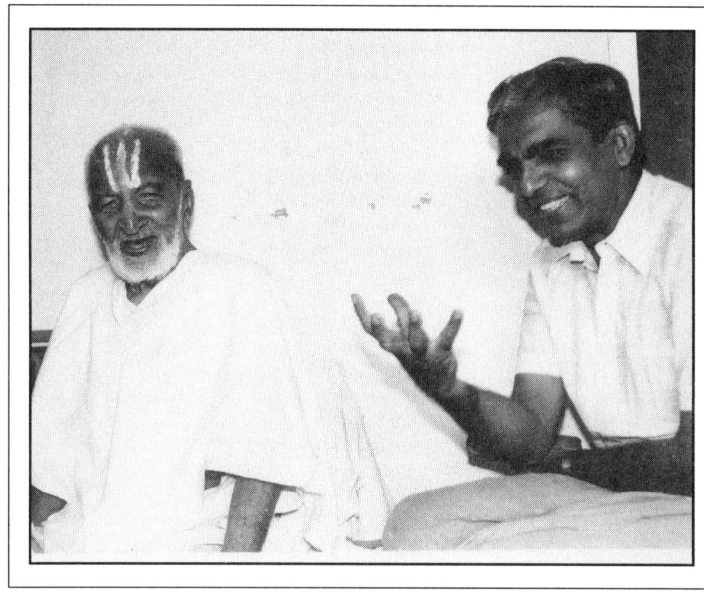

Śrī T. Krishnamacharya at age 100 and his son, T. K. V. Desikachar.

INTRODUCTION

Yoga is both a systematized body of knowledge and a practice. There are many reasons why a person might choose to practice yoga; in broad terms, the purpose of yoga is to reduce disturbance and return an individual to his or her inherent peace and power. To be successful in this endeavor, yoga must be adapted and practiced according to the needs, capacities, and aspirations of each student. Yoga is not a standardized practice. The emphasis on personal shaping of the yoga practice is a hallmark of Professor Krishnamacharya's yoga guidance. *The Heart of Yoga* summarizes Krishnamacharya's principles of yoga understanding and explains the method of adapting a practice to individual needs.

Desikachar's depth of knowledge, which he claims to be only a fraction of his father's understanding, informs his unique ability to converse about yoga. His teachings and his sensitivity to an individual's needs are always communicated in the context of sincere friendship and humor. Vanda Scaravelli wrote: "Desikachar is a serious, profound and special yoga teacher as well as an agreeable person to be with, one can laugh and have fun with him."[1] This is also my experience and it is my hope that these qualities of Desikachar's will come through in this book.

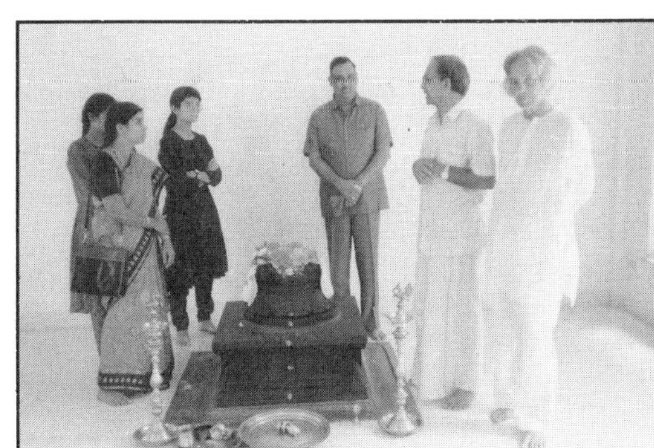

U. G. Krishnamurthi (right) with Desikachar and friends in the Sannadhi, "the Presence," a small temple in Desikachar's residence where Krishnamacharya is remembered.

Desikachar is a beautiful mix of the traditional and the contemporary man. He is absolutely devoted to his father, Krishnamacharya, who profoundly represents that which is ancient, deep, and true of India. Yet Desikachar received a Western-style education, earning a degree in engineering, and has been inspired by his radical contemporaries J. Krishnamurthi and U. G. Krishnamurthi, his friends of many years. Desikachar's background enables him to communicate the ancient understanding of yoga in a context that the Western mind can easily comprehend.

Like his father, Desikachar is a family man living in Madras. He spends most of his time in India, occasionally traveling to Western countries as a guest of his students. Many have had the good fortune of studying yoga privately with

1. Vanda Scaravelli, *Awakening the Spine.* London: HarperCollins, 1991.

Desikachar, which is the traditional way. His manner of teaching is utterly personal and caring, defining a yoga practice that takes into account each person's requirements. There is always good humor and a spirited communication of well-being. Over the years Desikachar's consistent, happy, and energetic disposition has led me to wonder if he may be a liberated man, that is, if he might have attained the goal of yoga. However, in my understanding it is a question of no relevance to such a person, and Desikachar never comments on it.

The one prevailing theme in Desikachar's teaching is that anyone who wants to can practice an authentic yoga, a yoga that is uniquely suited to his or her needs and interests, and experience its many benefits. Krishnamacharya claimed that anyone who can breathe and use his or her fingers can practice yoga. Taking into account the health, age, and cultural background of each person, there is always an appropriate practice that can be developed so that real yoga can occur. Desikachar is able to communicate with people from vastly different backgrounds and with different perspectives on spiritual life and make yoga useful for them. Students from the East and the West have expressed their appreciation of Krishnamacharya and his yoga.

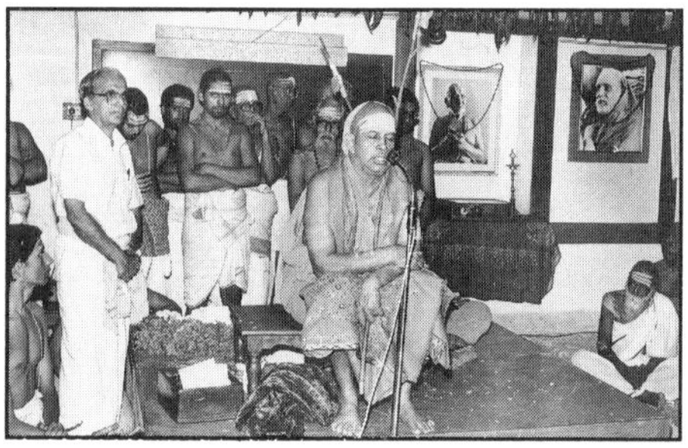

Desikachar with His Holiness Shankaracharya Jayendra Saraswathi Swami and his attendants on their visit to the Krishnamacharya Yoga Mandiram, 1993.

Some of Desikachar's students have been well-known teachers in their own fields, such as J. Krishnamurthi and Shankaracharya Jayendra Saraswathi Swami. Such teachers, who have influenced millions of people, have valued yoga highly as being helpful to body and mind. There could not be greater extremes between the teaching points of view of the iconoclast J. Krishnamurthi and the orthodox Shankaracharya, teacher to millions in the Hindu world, yet Desikachar has been at ease teaching both. This underscores the unique nature of Krishnamacharya's yoga—there is something in it for everyone. This is the application of yoga in the broadest sense.

Krishnamacharya studied for decades, first with his family and then more formally at universities. Finally he found his own teacher, Śrī Ramamohan Brahmachari, with whom he lived and studied in the Tibetan Himalayas for eight years. Krishnamacharya synthesized a vast amount of religious and yoga understanding. Desikachar, in turn, studied daily with his father from 1960 until 1989, when Krishnamacharya passed away at the age of 101 years. Together they summarized and clarified the ancient understanding and practice of yoga so that all people of all ages, regardless of their cultural or religious background, can learn and benefit from yoga teachings.

Krishnamacharya and Desikachar point out that yoga understanding developed in an ancient culture in which the notion of religion did not imply one social group against others, as it does today, causing much confusion among spiritual aspirants. Dharma or religion simply meant a virtuous way of life, and yoga was developed as a means of acknowledging or returning to the source of life. Because Krishnamacharya provided a context within which yoga can be practiced in conjuction with religious teachings, students have been able to

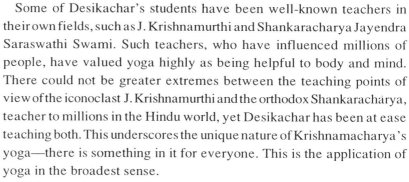

deepen their understanding and appreciation of their chosen tradition. I have seen the lives of people who were already involved in a religious practice become much fuller and happier having taken on the practice of yoga. The personal application of an appropriate yoga results in changes that are consistent with the purposes of all religious traditions, including Christianity. It offers a practical means by which other teachings may be quickened and realized.

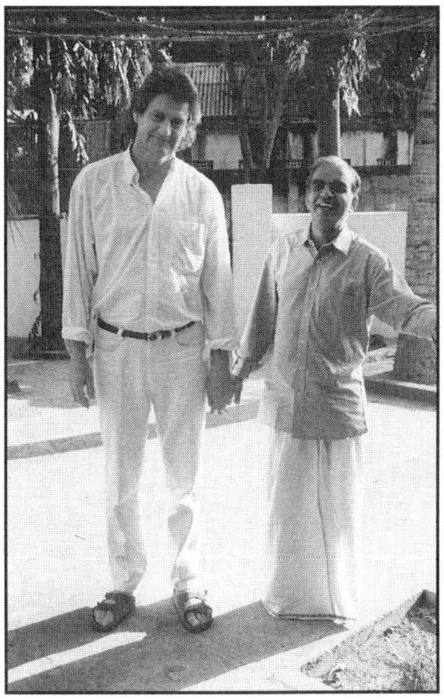

Desikachar with Mark Whitwell.

Of course, to practice yoga without reference to religious ideas is also valid. The precise summary of yoga understanding provided by Patañjali's *Yoga Sūtra* does not require a belief in religious concepts such as God, nor does it deny such thinking. Specifically, the Patañjali *Yoga Sūtra* concerns the attainment of a stable mind and healthy body so that personal goals may be achieved. Such attainment is quite independent of cultural background and religious inclination.

Krishnamacharya considered Patañjali's *Yoga Sūtra*, the reference text that underpins yoga, to be the most outstanding reference text for the guidance of yoga practice. The *Yoga Sūtra*, with Desikachar's commentary, is included as part 3 of this book. References are made to relevant sūtras throughout parts 1 and 2. Desikachar studied the *Yoga Sūtra* many times with his father, so we can take his commentary as an accurate representation of Krishnamacharya's understanding of Patañjali.

Desikachar emphasizes that the teacher/student relationship is of great importance in the study of yoga. This relationship is one of friendship and mutual trust. By the mere act of coming to a teacher, the student has already placed trust in the teacher that there is something to be gained. It is the teacher's responsibility not to exploit that trust; the teacher is entrusted to teach only according to the student's needs for personal freedom and well-being. The teachings should always be relevant to the student and allow for his or her growth and changing requirements. The teacher should have no psychological investment in being a teacher, and the teaching context should be free of attachment and steeped in a sense of natural friendship.

The problem with institutionalized yoga or textbook instruction is that the reality of a person's life situation is not taken into account. Without discrediting organizations that are obviously helpful to many aspiring yoga students, standardized or forced practices may not help in the study of yoga, and may in fact cause disturbance. The key to right teaching is in the adaptation of yoga to the individual, not the individual to yoga. Often organizations emphasize some aspects of yoga such as meditation or postures or high philosophical understanding without a realistic practice. Krishnamacharya taught that the whole spectrum of yoga practice must be carefully adapted to the individual's situation. Nothing can be forced.

As my capacity to practice and understand yoga developed over the years, Desikachar introduced new concepts and taught familiar things in different ways. He taught only what was relevant to me. Each person's situation determines the practices that are offered in the context of a supportive teacher/student friendship. In this way a student is led to an understanding of yoga that cannot be gotten directly from a teacher or a book, but is instead discovered by the student as his or her own realization. We are creatures of the universe, and the nature of the universe can be discovered in our own being as our inherent condition. A teacher cannot tell us about this so much as show us the path to our own understandings by way of this special guidance.

Feelings of gratitude and love may naturally develop as yoga realization progressively or suddenly unfolds. In yoga this is called *bhakti* or devotion, the natural feeling of gratitude to the teacher. Desikachar reports that he learned the nature of the teacher/student relationship when he taught great people. J. Krishnamurthi, for example, always demonstrated to Desikachar respect and gratitude for what he received, even though he too was a teacher.

Krishnamacharya taught that the eight limbs or aspects of yoga are not attained in linear progression; rather, the eight limbs are met simultaneously. Yoga distinguishes *sadhana*, "that which we can practice," and *siddhi*, "that which is given." There are aspects of yoga that we can intentionally practice and others that occur naturally as a result of doing this practice. The practices are physical postures and breathing exercises; all other aspects of yoga occur as a result of these practices. People who practice postures and breathing exercises report that the mind becomes more clear and less random in thought, and energy levels increase. There is a corresponding feeling of continuity between sense of self, environment, and others that some describe as a feeling of oneness.

By means of linking breath to the body in moving and stationary postures, the mind is connected with the body. We are brought into existence by the power of the universe. This power sustains the body and all its functions, including thinking and sense perception. When we attend to the process of linking breath with the whole body, the mind and the senses merge with the power of the universe. We might call this power *consciousness* and its active principle *energy*, or in yoga terms *puruṣa* and *prāṇa*. Through yoga, mind and senses become the communication mechanism of consciousness and energy rather than having apparently random and sometimes disturbing lives of their own.

When mind and senses are linked to consciousness, the objects of their perception are also joined with conciousness. At times there is sudden insight and brightness of perception, as clarity progressively develops and connectedness is recognized. Consciousness is felt to be the source of everything, and situations and objects are perceived from a radically new point of view. There is a sense of free participation in relationships and circumstances. With a clear mind we see things as they are, unclouded by assumptions or misapprehensions.

The habits of mind are strong, however. Yoga teaches that our obstructions need to be acknowledged and taken into account. A good yoga teacher helps the student develop a program that, practiced regularly, allows this joining of mind and senses to their source, to that which is most fundamental to existence.

Posture, breathing, meditation, and all the tools of yoga may be used, including elements of a person's familiar cultural or religious understanding. Whatever assists the student's development can be artfully adapted and modified as changes occur.

It fascinates me that the change in people who practice yoga is not the result of philosophical consideration or the study of spiritual ideas. Merely by following the careful instruction of connecting breath to the body in appropriate ways, as Krishnamacharya taught, and practicing on a daily basis, something shifts: insights come; the ability to focus on tasks and achieve goals develops; new ways of handling difficult emotions and situations are recognized; feelings of stillness, peace, certainty, happiness, love, or connectedness spontaneously occur; there is often a general improvement in life circumstances. The social and personal recommendations of *yama* and *niyama* seem to be more easily adopted as a result of yoga practice, when previously they were ideals that the student struggled with. Sometimes particular creative or relationship skills spontaneously arise to enrich a person's life.

These changes come not through arduous sessions or study of spiritual ideas but through a practice that may initially be twenty to thirty minutes long, placed appropriately in a person's daily routine. All eight limbs of yoga develop concurrently as a result of doing an appropriate practice of posture and breathing under the guidance of a knowledgeable teacher.

Krishnamacharya understood the yoga process and the art of adapting a practice to each person's needs. He taught that by beginning at the beginning, by developing awareness in the whole body and its instruments of perception—the mind and senses—yoga provides the means by which ordinary men and women can realize their potential. Through practice with body and breath, the student develops the ability to merge with the object of perception, to be with perceptions rather than against them and merely reacting to one's experience. Then an awareness of the profound context in which everything is happening may spontaneously develop. Hence, Desikachar instructs, "Yoga is relationship and relationship is peace." Krishnamacharya was certain that a yoga practice, rightly adapted to the individual, enabled one to discover the inherent connection to spirit, the source of body and mind. He taught that spirit, the context of life, is realized via the body, breath, and perception, in that order.

There is here an implied criticism of spiritual practices that attempt to bypass the body, breath, and ordinary experiences of life. Indeed, religious idealism that focuses on philosophical inspiration or an alternative reality to our present state can cause a conflict in the devotee by virtue of the stark difference between the proposed ideal and the actual experiences of life. In some cases the ideal itself can become an obstacle to clear perception. One must find a practical means of starting with present reality in order to feel the context, to recognize what is already true of body, breath, and perceptions. This inquiry requires no philosophy or speculation. For this reason Desikachar will often say, "In your life please emphasize the means, not the goal."

Krishnamacharya taught that we cannot practice meditation; all we can do is make the conditions right in body and mind so that meditation—the merging with our natural state—may spontaneously occur and understanding come. In other words, we should not willfully struggle to reach a goal or obtain a preconceived ideal. He also taught that the way to realize the great understanding of *advaita* (nondualism) is through yoga practice. Mere philosophizing or contemplation Krishnamacharya regarded as futile because it turns a great understanding into an idea, a separate object. His many years of assiduous study of the great philosophical systems of India convinced Krishnamacharya that yoga was required for a person to actualize the ideas that the great teachings proposed. His commitment to yoga developed from a clear understanding of India's entire religious and philosophical tradition. Advaita Vedānta is the dominant religious and philosophical influence of Krishnamacharya's society. He was fond of entering into debate with the Advaitins who did not practice yoga, insisting that their dualistic habits of mind could not be changed without an artful yoga. It is yoga that joins the two to become one, leading the perceiver to merge with the perceived.

Much of Krishnamacharya's teaching was counter to the prevailing views of Indian society. His stance that women had the right to practice yoga and participate fully in religious and social life was very controversial in the conventional society of his time. He defended his position by referring to Sanskrit texts indicating that women were educated and practiced yoga in ancient times. He held the view that women, as the nurturers of the community, had a special requirement and right to practice yoga, and he emphasized the benefits of yoga for pregnancy. He also predicted that women would have the greater part in spreading yoga throughout the world. This prediction is perhaps already proving to be true.

Krishnamacharya's explanation of *kuṇḍalinī* was also at odds with popular views. He taught that there were not two energies in the body, those being prāṇa and kuṇḍalinī, but that there was only one. Again he referred to Sanskrit texts to explain that, accurately translated, *kuṇḍalinī* means "obstruction." Yoga practice helps to remove obstuction so that prāṇa can move in all areas of the body, particularly through the central channel, or *nāḍī*, known as *suṣumṇā*.

Further, he explained that the goal of yoga was *vairāgya*, meaning "peace" in terms of detachment or freedom in the midst of all experience. As evidenced by the life of Professor Krishnamacharya, this is not a passionless state of detachment. On the contrary, all experience is integrated and forms a coherent whole in the context of this freedom. One acts with full energy and clear intention in the midst of life experiences. Krishnamacharya argued that without the elimination of attachments, which are the fundamental cause of unhappiness or obstruction, concepts such as kuṇḍalinī or tantra are not relevant to yoga. It is only when obstruction is removed that energy moves in the body and mind becomes connected to consciousness. Then the phenomenon described in the traditions of kuṇḍalinī and tantra may occur but are of no consequence. In other words, the goal of yoga is peace, not power. The practices that attempt to develop power without peace can be destructive. Hence there are constant warnings that one should not practice yoga techniques without the continual guidance of a competent teacher, even in the final stages of spiritual maturity. Peace cannot be attained through power, yet power is a result of peace. In peace—in recognizing one's inherent connection to the universe and all its possibilities—lies true power.

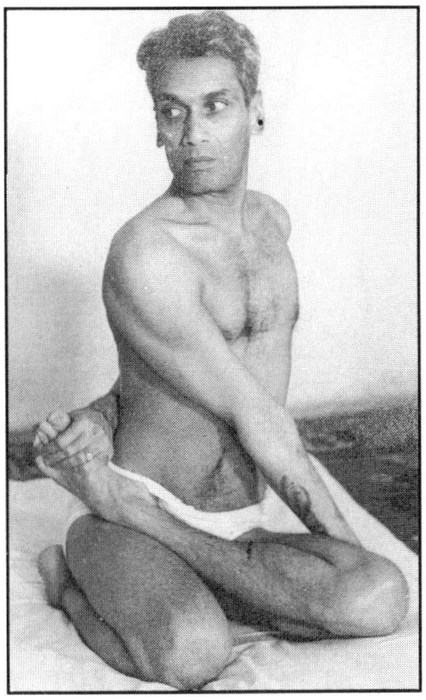

Krishnamacharya's student, the mahārājah of Kolhapur, demonstrating bharadvājāsana, 1940.

Krishnamacharya recommended that the best way to remove obstruction is through the careful consideration of one's circumstances and responses to life with a trusted teacher. Yoga practice may help to give clarity as to what needs to be changed, but at a certain point no amount of yoga or spiritual transmission can substitute for taking action to eliminate attachments to unhappy circumstances or habits of response that are creating obstructions in the body and mind. Yoga and the teaching relationship is a catalyst or agent of change, allowing change to occur naturally when the person is ready. Krishnamacharya made clear that detachment or freedom could not develop without trust in oneself, in one's teacher, and in yoga practice. He often said "You cannot have vairāgya without bhakti."

Although Krishnamacharya was deeply respectful of the beliefs and devotional feelings of others, he did not compromise his commitment to understanding the process of human development and communicating his perception of truth. He maintained that everything he communicated was taught to him by his guru and authenticated by ancient yoga texts; his fluency in Sanskrit enabled him to translate traditional texts accurately and interpret their meaning. In accordance with the tradition of yoga, he acknowledged that understanding is passed from teacher to teacher. Yoga knowledge is not attributable to any individual exclusively, but is the communication of a Greater Power or Absolute Source.

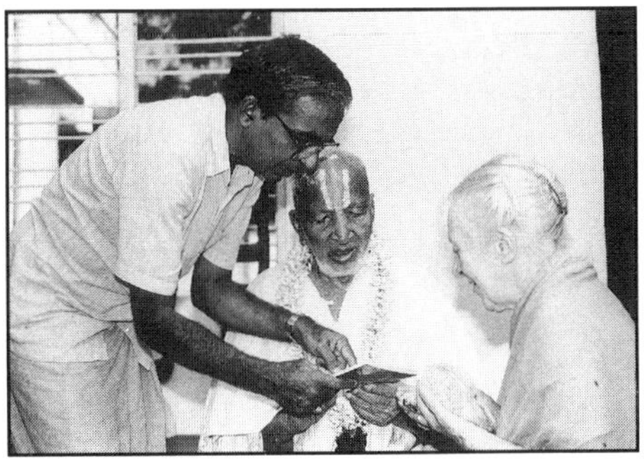

Desikachar, Krishnamacharya, and Indra Devi at Krishnamacharya's centennial celebration, 1988.

Krishnamacharya gave a vast amount of information to many people according to their individual needs. From this and other teaching sources standardized approaches to yoga have been derived that seem to be quite different from each other, confusing students and teachers alike. In my view, it is not useful to think of different styles of yoga: this is simply yoga, which comes from a vast and ancient source. The only authentic yoga is the one that works for each person according to circumstances and needs, and there are many possibilities.

Śrī Krishnamacharya is responsible for much of the yoga being taught in the world today. As early as the 1930s young men such as B. K. S. Iyengar (his brother-in-law) and Pattabhi Jois, who would go on to become famous teachers and popularize yoga throughout the world, studied with him. Krishnamacharya's first Western student, Indra Devi, has devoted her life to presenting yoga to the West, carrying the torch for her teacher with great love. All the while, Desikachar lived and studied with Krishnamacharya, and in the course of those thirty years, Desikachar learned how to practice and teach yoga effectively. He now represents the full breadth of his father's yoga teaching.

We owe much gratitude to Krishnamacharya and his worthy son Desikachar for bringing yoga into a modern context and making it useful in our time and place.

In ancient times yoga teachings were expressed in writing as a dialogue between teacher and student. In many places throughout *The Heart of Yoga*, we use this form to communicate some of Desikachar's teaching concepts and his early background.

MARK WHITWELL: Is a teacher necessary to learn yoga, or can we learn from reading your books?

DESIKACHAR: Mark, you have been through a long journey. You met me after you learned yoga through books—good books—and you're a bright man. Your own experience shows that without a good teacher you'd be in trouble. Why? Because a yoga teacher does not deal with his students in the same way as an engineer deals with a piece of straw or metal, systematizing everything as we do in construction projects. With human beings we are working with something very different, something that cannot be systematized or defined. Each student comes to the teacher with unique experiences and an individual mind. It is difficult enough to understand this mind *with* a teacher. Without a teacher it is even more difficult. Yoga concerns the mind, and since mind is unpredictable, since mind is not easily definable, it becomes necessary to seek somebody who knows a little more than you do. I have no doubts about this.

Q: How do I find a good teacher who is right for me?

A: You must be very lucky. You may have a teacher who is not the teacher for you in the long run. To find your teacher you must be lucky—I know that. The feelings of trust and certainty and natural friendship will be there for you to enjoy.

Q: You would then certainly appreciate that relationship, if you knew that you were lucky.

A: Yes.

Q: There are so many teachers—some well known and others not so well known—and their teachings diverge in important ways. It sometimes seems confusing.

A: The confusion is not because there are so many teachers. The confusion comes when we expect standard answers, or when we are looking for something that is preconceived. Then when one teacher seems to contradict another, we are confused. A good teacher is one who will not give you an answer but allows you to find the answer in yourself. A teacher is a guide; he will show you the answer that is inside you. And there *is* a right answer.

Q: From a traditional point of view, could you describe the relationship to the teacher?

A: I always emphasize that there should be a negotiable relationship between a teacher and a student. It is as if the student has to climb the mountain for the first time but does not have any shoes and does not know the way up the mountain. The teacher must help the student up the mountain; he cannot force him or her up. The best relationship between the student and the teacher is one that is established through the compassion and understanding of the teacher. Here the responsibility rests with the teacher.

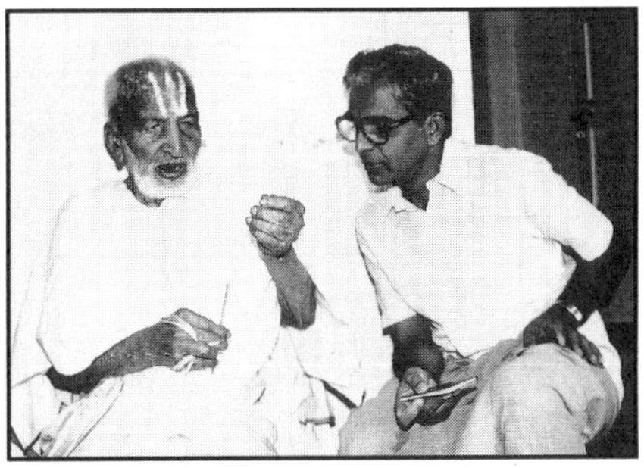

Father and son.

Q: Can you tell us something about your relationship with your teacher?

A: My father was my teacher and he was a very lovely person. He had an immense amount of training and knowledge. We were fifty years apart in age, so there was a great difference between us. His education and background were very different from mine, but what I remember most is that he always came to my level in working with me. I am a Western-educated person and he was a traditional teacher. He saw that I was different so he adapted his teachings to me. I took that as a great example of what we can do as teachers for others.

The fact that I was his son never interfered in the relationship, even though the relationship between a father and a son is different from the relationship between a teacher and a student. We were living in the same house with all our family members and others. I was a slow learner and would do stupid things, yet he never gave me an indication that I was lacking. He would only say words in support of me, such as, "You do not have the background I have," and he would patiently persevere with me.

Q: Was the father/son relationship there also?

A: When he was a teacher, he was a teacher. He would expect me to be on time. If he asked me to sit I would sit. That is the Indian tradition. He had the ability to separate the teacher relationship from the father relationship. I also spent a lot of time as his son, doing the natural things that a father and son do together.

Q: So you enjoyed both relationships?

A: I had the benefit of both.

Q: It seems paradoxical that you have been the yoga teacher to several great spiritual teachers such as J. Krishnamurthi and the Shankaracharya. Could you tell us how these teaching relationships have influenced you?

A: I must say that I have been very lucky to have met these people. Somehow they have the ability to accept me as a teacher. This is an extraordinary situation, as each of them is a very important person in his own way. Millions of people read their books and venerate them. They taught me that great people can be so simple, and that simplicity is an important quality in life. Another part of my learning was to be able to regard these great teachers as students. They demonstrated the attitude—the humility, dignity, and gratitude—of the student. My attitude toward my own teacher definitely grew through the example of these great people. I am extremely grateful to them.

Q: Were they able to come to you with the attitude of the student, even though they were great teachers in their own right?

A: I remember when I would go to Krishnamurthi and teach him, he would always be on time, he would make sure that I sat before he would sit, he would make sure that there was always a carpet for me to sit upon—the best carpet—and he was always picking the best flower to give me.

Q: And were you much younger than him?

A: Yes, I was much younger, yet he always showed the dignity and gratitude of a serious student. That taught me a lot.

Q: It seems a little paradoxical that such a wise person as J. Krishnamurthi decided that he needed yoga.

A: The teachings of my father are special. Where a human being wants to be healthy, physically and mentally free from illness, this yoga is very useful. People such as Krishnamurthi believed in yoga. Krishnamurthi practiced yoga to keep himself fit and feeling vital in his older age. Some thought he was too old for yoga but we adapted the yoga for his age and medical condition and he always enjoyed it. This is what is special about my father's teaching. His teaching of yoga is not meant to make a person go to the moon or do the best and most complicated gymnastics. It is to provide what a person requires. There is something in this teaching for everyone.

Q: Does this exclude the highest realization of yoga that we may call enlightenment?

A: As I said, it provides something for everyone. Whatever is required for growth can be provided. I know some people who gave up their religion and returned to it in a renewed way once they had begun this yoga.

Q: Many of today's spiritual organizations teach some form of yoga as part of their recommended path. But many of these yoga practices seem to be quite different from your father's recommendations, or they seem to emphasize certain aspects.

A: What finally matters is what a person perceives. If somebody is happier through what these great organizations provide, then membership is right for that person. I have good friends who have greatly benefited from belonging to such organizations. They are not my students but they have learned to practice yoga in my father's way. Their lives in these organizations have become much richer and brighter through practicing yoga.

Q: Can someone stay loyal to their chosen teacher and learn a yoga practice in the Krishnamacharya way?

A: Yes. Take the case of somebody like the Shankaracharya. He is the teacher par excellence for the Hindus. They have their own philosophy and their own religious practices, but these things did not prevent the Shankaracharya from doing yoga. The Hindus asked us to teach them yoga and we did. They are not loyal to my father. They practice as a practical requirement of the human system and they are loyal to their own tradition. There is something good about my father's teaching: it is possible not to interfere in a person's spiritual and cultural life and yet still do yoga to encourage his or her development.

Q: There is a wide variety of yoga practices taught, and talk of many different kinds of yoga. Why is this?

A: Because yoga is not fixed. Yoga is creation. I know the way that you teach will be different from the way I teach, and the way I teach is different from the way my father taught. We all have different experiences, different backgrounds, different perspectives on yoga and why it is important for us. So it is not a surprise that different people find different things through the same yoga teaching. Even in our own yoga institution different teachers will teach in different ways according to their own perspective and priorities and interests in yoga. The *Yoga Sutra* says that each person gets different things from the same teaching based on his or her own perspective. There is nothing wrong with this. This is how it is.

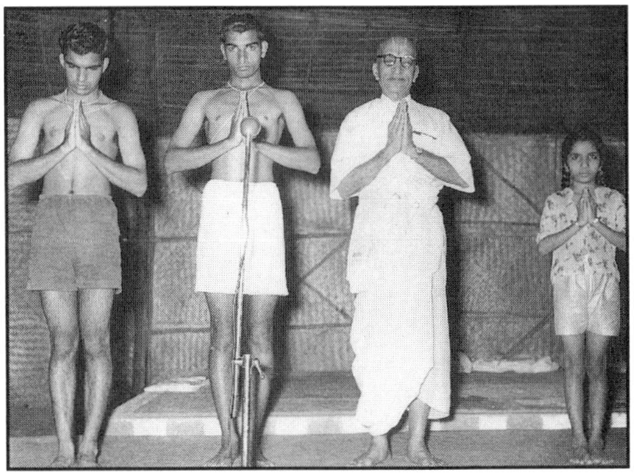

Krishnamacharya and his children at a public lecture.

Q: It seems a little unusual however that several teachers, all of whom were students of your father, have very different methods of teaching.

A: Well, here there are two questions: How long was their association with my father? And how much did they have to be on their own when they were called upon to teach? My association with my father was very long. I observed him teaching others at different stages of his life from 1960 to almost the end of his life. He was teaching different people in different ways according to their needs, their age, their health, and so on. This taught me a lot of things. Further, for those thirty years I was exposed to many aspects of his teaching. I had the real thing day after day, so I could absorb much of his teaching and at the same time I could always go back to him with questions and case studies. In that way he would help me with my teaching. Take your own case, for example. If you had some health problem, I could easily go and ask my father for help. So I had an enormous exposure that others who are now teaching were not able to enjoy. When called upon they found other ways of teaching, which is fine.

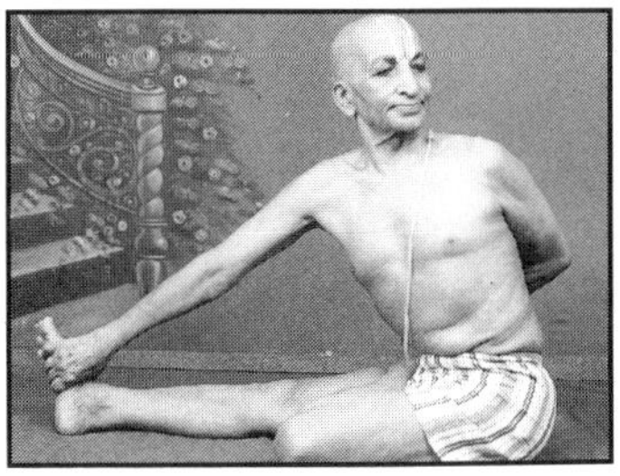

Krishnamacharya at 79.

Q: It seems that your father had a vast knowledge of yoga and religious traditions. He spent nearly three decades in the early part of this century in various traditional institutions and later with his teacher in Tibet. A great amount of information has been summarized and made useful for our modern context.

A: Yes, his background is wide. His own family is unique in the sense that his ancestors were all practicing yoga. So his first lessons in yoga were from his family — his father and his grandmother. He was fluent in Sanskrit at a very young age, so he could learn very quickly as he got older. He was lucky to go to Banaras and learn from the best teachers of the Indian traditions. There he also came to know of his yoga master in Tibet. So his learning started very early and went on and on. I would say today that the condensed aspect of what he knew represents only one millionth of what he could have passed on if he had lived much longer. We have lost a lot because of his passing and we have lost a lot because more students did not stay with him and learn all that they could. What I represent is insignificant compared to the totality of my father's understanding in many areas, not just in yoga but anything in the Indian tradition, including healing and subjects like astrology and Āyurveda.

Q: So with this vast amount of knowledge he was able to understand each person's requirement in yoga.

A: Yes. My father went to Bengal and studied Āyurvedic medicine, the Indian system of healing. He knew a lot about the soul through his understanding of Āyurveda and the Upaniṣads. He knew a lot about how to improvise yoga through his guru's teaching. He knew a lot about spirituality and devotion because he was also a very religious person. He was a person who represented India in total and he could draw on his vast knowledge to help anyone who wished to do yoga. He could also do extraordinary things like stop the heartbeat and breath for long periods of time. He always told me, however, that he would teach me only what would be useful for mankind.

Q: I'd like to discuss the results brought about by the yoga practice. The yamas and niyamas appear to be very sensible and are desirable attitudes in life. Yet many people say that it is virtually impossible to change and to be more aligned to the yama and niyama recommendations. They complain that we humans never seem to live up to them.

A: Frankly, these qualities are potentials, and one person may have much more than another person. Yoga is something like a catalyst that brings out the best in us. If somebody has the predisposition to be a very sociable person, yoga will act as a catalyst to bring this out. In others this predisposition may not be there to the same extent. I know some people who are practicing much yoga, including diet changes and meditative practices, yet they remain very unfeeling people, even cruel. Some are even yoga teachers themselves. There are other people who do a few simple things in yoga and much change occurs. So yoga is a catalyst, what is called *nimitta* in Sanskrit. Its presence brings out certain changes, things that are latent and not yet obvious. However, it can only bring out what is already there. A good teacher can bring out these qualities, no matter how small the potential. If they do not exist, however, nothing can bring them out.

Q: Do the qualities of yama and niyama simply come as a result of doing a yoga practice, rather than struggling to change?

A: Struggling is antithetical to yama and niyama. If the potential is there, then yoga will be a catalyst toward growth. Simply struggling will not produce a change.

Q: Some people say that physical yoga is not necessary or is even a distraction for spiritual understanding. What do you think?

A: As long as I am healthy I might say these things. As long as I am healthy and as long as I do not have weakness, as long as I don't have any suffering I may say this. The moment there is suffering it is a different story. I recall a person who was a champion in speaking about death. He used to give conferences about being free of the fear of death; he became very popular and traveled the world giving lectures. Then with his business and all his traveling he started to get chest pains and stress symptoms. He grew panicky and had to go to the doctor every day to have an EKG test. His doctor recommended that he do some yoga. "You must relax, you must go home and do some breathing exercises. It will be good for you." And so he came to me. When he spoke about the fear of death he was a happy person, but when he worked too much and became ill his body gave way, and then he had trouble. So as long as there is no illness and there is no suffering in body or mind, there is nothing to worry about. But the body and mind are not constant; they are always changing. Yoga can help with the changes. Wait and see.

Q: So often it is ill health that will motivate a person to do yoga. Is it possible that people could feel the motivation to practice yoga without ill health?

A: What is health? What is sickness? Why do people come to you? So many people come to you. They don't go to a doctor, they go to a yoga teacher. Something is not well inside them. That is what brings them to you. Their own potential is limited, so they come to you hoping for some help. The classic example for the role of yoga is in ancient society, where it was used to prevent ill health and keep the community well. Just so, in our sick society, that is the place for yoga. Many Indians who come to us are sick; they have not solved problems through medication so they come to us, like Westerners come to you. Something is missing. They are looking for something. That is sickness. Sickness is not just a physical thing. Dissatisfaction with life and the inability to express potential are sicknesses. Look at your student who wrote the poems. She was a poet before she did yoga but she didn't know it. Thanks to you she became a poet. It is a kind of sickness not to realize our potentials. Or I may be an artist already, I may love to create sculptures, but nobody is interested in my art. That is disturbing. Yoga may help me to relax from this disturbance.

Q: Is it possible to overcome ill health, whether physical or emotional, without the use of āsana or prāṇāyāma?

A: Yes, when people are too sick to do āsana or prāṇāyāma then we can find other solutions. Very simple breathing, the use of sound, listening, or quiet meditation can be helpful.

Recently I met a person who owns a very big business and works extremely long hours because he is responsible for the success of an international company. He said, "I can't remember names, I can't remember telephone numbers or figures. I don't know why at my age of forty-two I am forgetting even my own telephone number. I sleep well, I eat well, I have no problem with my family, so why is this happening to me?" I spoke to him for forty-five minutes. Relationship is very important in yoga teaching. He needed to talk about these confidential matters with somebody he could trust. After five or ten minutes he began to feel better because he talked to someone for the first time.

There is always the need to talk through problems with someone you can trust. A good yoga teacher who has the care and the time fits this role very well. That is why we value private relationship, one to one. My father insisted on this. Teach them privately, he said, because yoga is *tapas* [practice]. One has to be alone. You are talking to God through your teacher. In fact, you are talking to yourself through your teacher. This is what is called *svādhyāya*. That is yoga—to look at yourself, to know yourself.

I told the businessman to do some breathing. "Please take some breaths, sir," I said. "Breathing is not your business. Breathing is not your family. Breathing is not your body. Breathing is breathing. Just breathe and see what happens. How can you breathe when you work so many hours? You're here, then you're in London, then you're in Africa. Please find fifteen minutes to follow your breath." And I showed him some simple exercises using the breath.

Breathing in this way means you care for yourself, you give some time to your own system to rejuvenate, and consciously you do it. This is not yoga, this is not meditation, this is just breathing. You are breathing twenty-four hours a day, but *you* are not breathing. Some power is breathing for you. Be with that, know that.

Q: You've said many times that we can't intentionally meditate, but we can make the conditions right so that meditation will occur.

A: That is because you cannot begin with nothing. You can do something like breathing so that you can consciously and intentionally be with yourself. All the principles of meditation are in āsana and prāṇāyāma when they are done properly. People search for meditation; here you don't have to do that. You allow for meditation to simply occur through right posture and breathing. Once you are attentive to posture and breathing everything opens up and meditation may occur.

Q: There is much interest these days in understanding nondualism. Some teachers say that is all that is needed. What is the difference between the way your father taught and Advaita Vedānta?

A: My father said about advaita, and I quote, "The word *advaita* has two parts, *a-* and *dvaita*." So to realize advaita we should first realize dvaita. It is a very interesting idea. In other words, to realize advaita, nondualism, one must first realize dvaita, dualism. We must start with the reality of our situation. Most of us are in dualism, and we have to accept duality and start from duality before it can become one, before we can know nonduality. Imagine: if there were only one, then there would not be the word or the concept of advaita. The concept of advaita itself implies two. Yoga makes this clear. There are two in the beginning—at least that is the habit of the human mind. Yoga links the two and through this link the two become one. That is advaita. So yoga is the step toward advaita. The two must be recognized, then brought together, otherwise even the advaita idea becomes an object. The moment I say I am an Advaitin, I am making the word *advaita* into an object and I create division in myself. Yoga is the method and the approach to make this great realization a reality. That is why the greatest teacher of Advaita Vedanta, the first Shankaracharya, emphasized yoga in many of his books. Many people don't know that the Shankaracharya, the great master of Advaita Vedanta, commented on the *Yoga Sūtra*, explaining the importance of yoga and emphasizing the importance of such things as *nāda* [sound] and *bandha* [a body lock]. He spoke of yoga as an important means for reaching that goal called advaita.

Q: My own experience is that your teaching and your father's teaching clarify all the different spiritual teachings that influence our lives, from very radical points of view to the more traditional yoga teachers. I find that I am able to make sense out of those other communications by being able to understand them in the context of your yoga understanding.

A: Yes, I have never felt in the wrong place. I have known many great teachers of many different traditions, and I have never felt strange in their presence. I think this is a tribute to my father's teaching. I have never felt myself to be against somebody. I know these people are often at odds among themselves, but I have never felt so. I felt so peaceful in the great cathedrals in Paris, yet I am not a Christian. I was with J. Krishnamurthi. I was with U. G. Krishnamurthi. I have been with great theosophists, with great *ācāryas* [teachers]. I have friends who are devoted Muslims and others who are Christians. My own experience has taught me that my father's teaching is universal; it helps us make sense of all religious traditions and spiritual points of view and practice. It helps us understand how everything fits and what is the right practice for us. I think this is the best testimony for yoga.

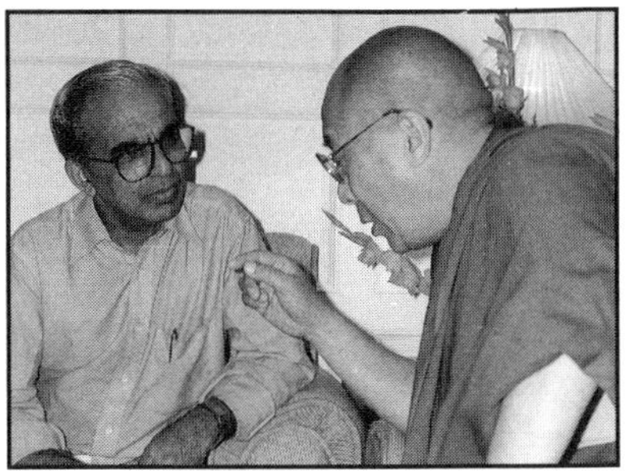

Desikachar and His Holiness, the Dalai Lama.

Q: Recently you went to Tibet, to the place where your father spent eight years with his teacher. You commented on how the Tibetan tradition was similar to your father's tradition and how much you appreciated that tradition of Buddhism in Tibet.

A: Yes, we could communicate very well with the lamas, and we found their spirit and enthusiasm for practice was similar to our own. There are some differences, but I think these differences are very superficial. You know, in my office I have a photograph of my father and a statue of the Buddha. I look at them both. We feel that the Buddha was a great yogi.

Q: Can yoga be taught in a class situation or should it always be one-on-one with the teacher?

A: Many things can be taught in a class situation. Often the group support for people who share the same interests or difficulties can be very helpful, as in the group for patients of bypass surgery that we teach here at the *mandiram*. However, as my father said, we are not magicians, and it is not easy to handle many people at the same time. In yoga, the purpose is to bring some change, and the teacher is the reference point. You always remember what the teacher told you—not what you read in the book or what he spoke in the class, but what he told *you*. You need the teacher, you need the intimacy. Yoga is intimate. There is no yoga between one and a million; yoga is between two—the teacher and the student. In the Upaniṣads it is beautifully stated: In education the first requirement is the teacher, the second is the student. What should happen between them is learning. How it should happen is through the constant teaching of that which will be relevant to the student. That is education.

Q: Sometimes yoga is described as being a long and arduous task toward achieving a goal. What do you think?

A: It depends on what the goal is. Most often, people are doing yoga for some simple reason, and they progress into more involved, step-by-step practices. Each step can be enjoyable, fitted to the reality of where each person is now. As my father said, if you go step by step, there will be no problems. Enjoy each step. Trying to leap many steps at once can be a problem.

Q: Can anyone practice yoga?

A: Anybody who wants to can practice yoga. Anybody can breathe; therefore anybody can practice yoga. But no one can practice every kind of yoga. It has to be the right yoga for the person. The student and teacher meet and decide on a program that is acceptable and suitable to the person.

Q: All over the world there are many teachers who are known to be gurus. Many are from India, and others are not. There is a popular understanding now of the word *guru*. From the yoga tradition, what is a guru?

A: A guru is not one who has a following. A guru is one who can show me the way. Suppose I'm in the forest and somehow I've lost my way. Then I meet somebody and ask, "Can you please show me the way home?" That person might say, "Yes, you go this way." I say, "Thank you," and I go my way. That is a guru.

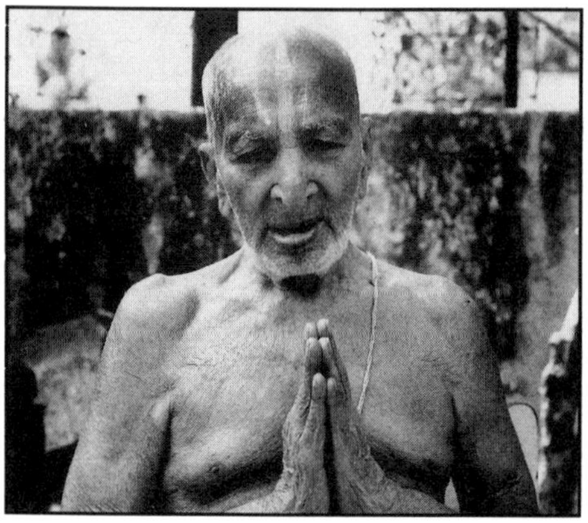

Krishnamacharya at 100 years.

There is an image in the world today that the guru has a following and his students follow him like the Pied Piper. That is not good. The true guru shows you the way. You go your way and then you're on your own, because you know your place and you are grateful. I can always thank my guru naturally and enjoy the relationship, but I do not have to follow him around, because then I am not in my own place. Following the guru's destination is another way of losing yourself. The yoga concept of *svadharma* means "your own dharma" or "your own way." If you try to do somebody else's dharma, trouble happens. The guru helps you find your own dharma.

Q: Was your father a guru?

A: He never said so, but many people think so.

Q: Why did he never say that of himself?

A: That's a delicate question, but since he is my father, I can tell you. The guru is not one who says, "I am the guru." There are great stories in the Upaniṣads of the guru who rejected the very idea of teaching. One of the qualities of a person who is clear, who is wise, is not to need to say "I am clear, I am wise." There is no need to say this. The person knows the way and he or she shows the way. It is simple. Humility is one of the qualities of a clear person—there is nothing to prove to anybody. My father was like this.

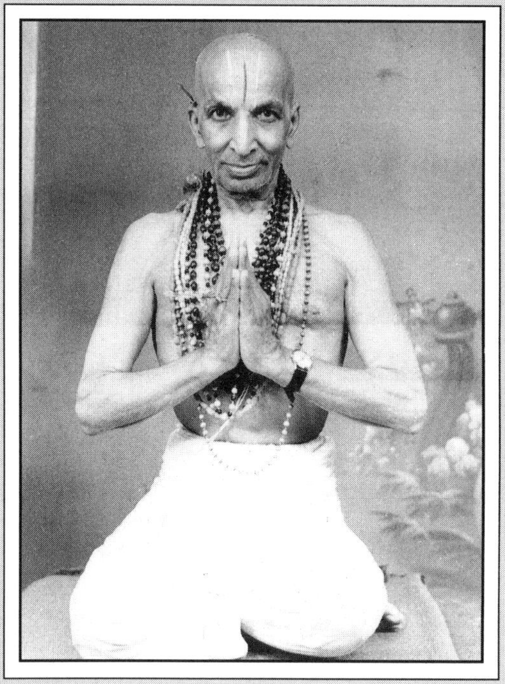

Krishnamacharya, 1966.

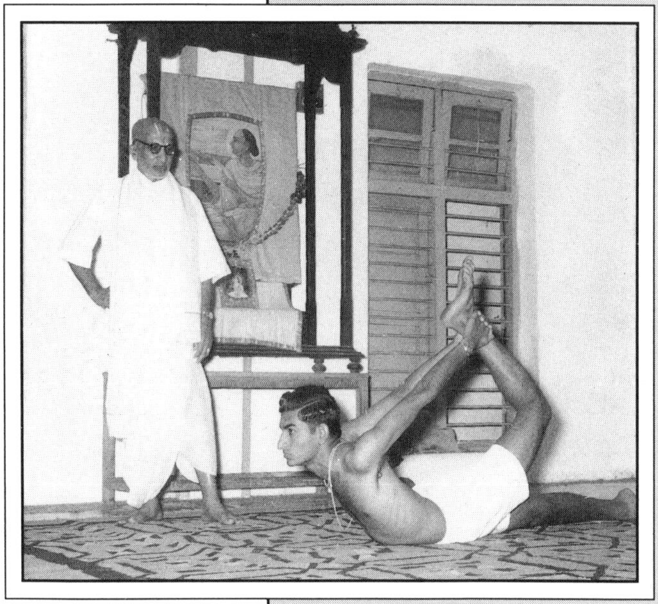

Center: Krishnamacharya with his son Shribhasyam in eka pāda dhanurāsana.

Bottom: Krishnamacharya with student in trikonāsana.

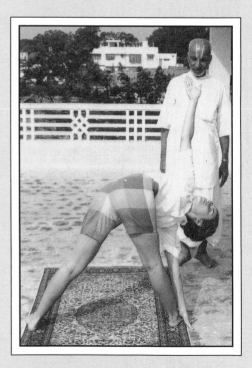

Part I
The Practice of Yoga

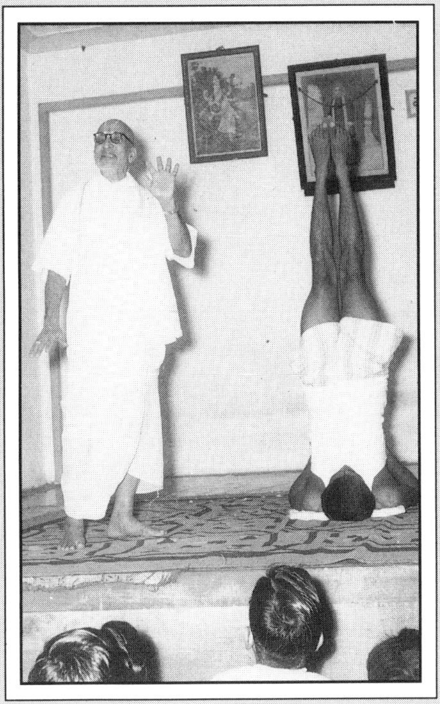

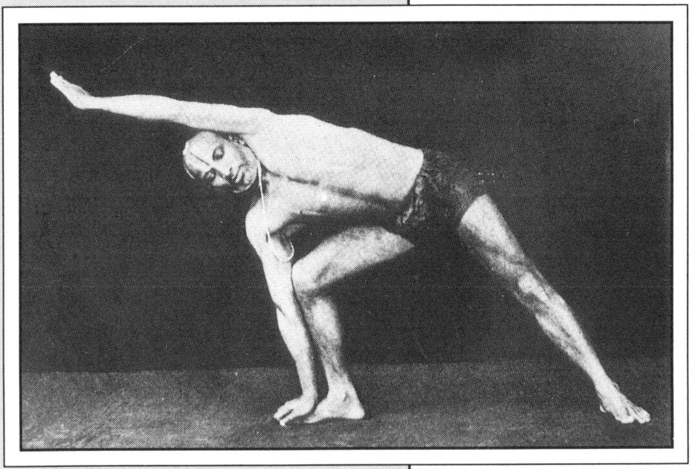

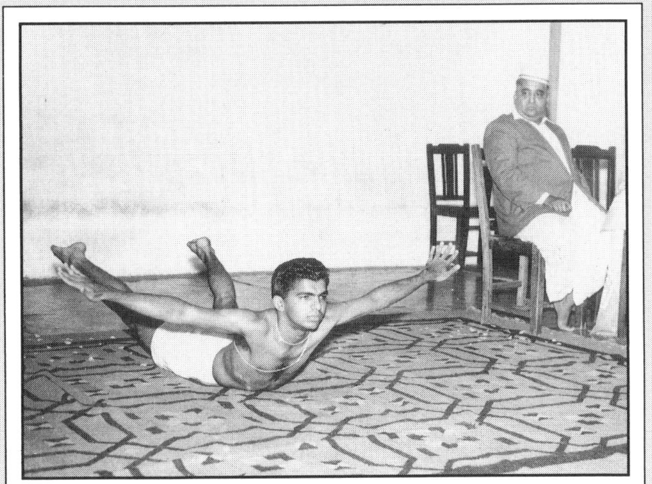

Top: Krishnamacharya lecturing while a student demonstrates śīrṣāsana.

Center: Krishnamacharya at age 46 demonstrating utthita pārśva koṇāsana.

Bottom: A young Desikachar demonstrates vimanāsana.

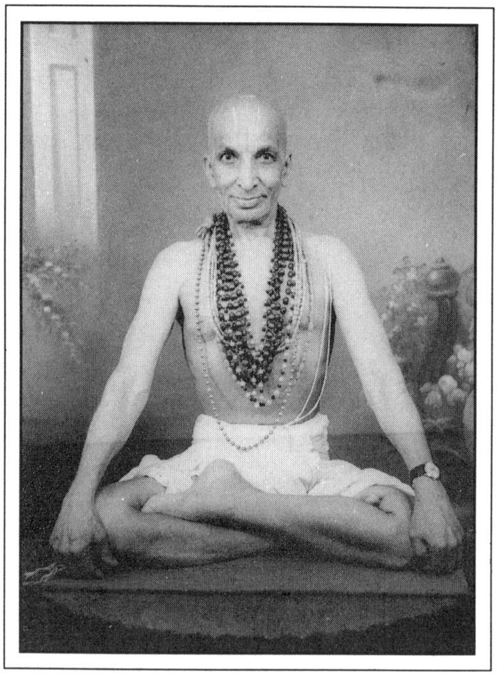

Krishnamacharya in siddhāsana.

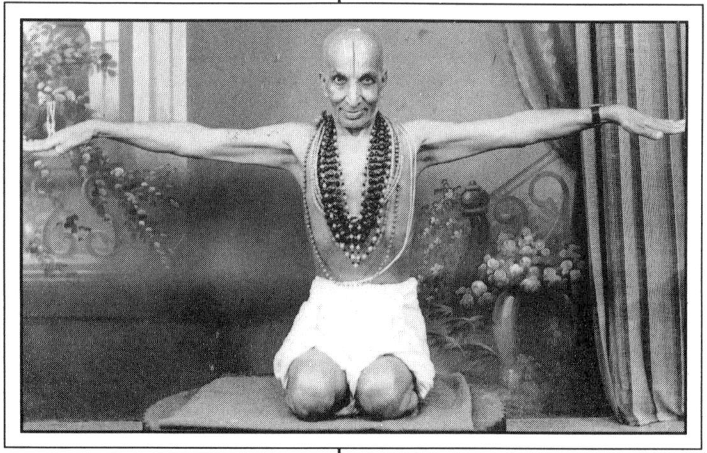

Krishnamacharya demonstrating a variation of vajrāsana.

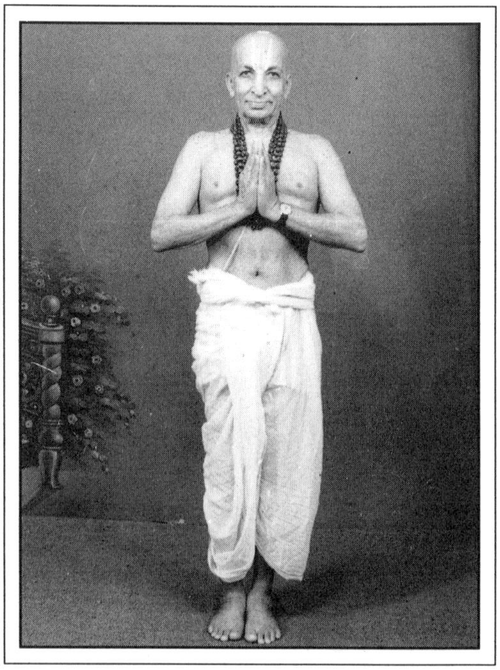

Krishnamacharya in samasthiti.

1

Yoga: Concept and Meaning

To begin, I should like to share some thoughts that might help us understand the many different meanings of the word *yoga*. Yoga is one of the six fundamental systems of Indian thought collectively known as *darśana*; the other five darśana are *nyāya*, *vaiśeṣika*, *sāṃkhya*, *mīmāṃsā*, and *vedānta*.[1] The word *darśana* is derived from the Sanskrit root *dṛś*, which translates as "to see." *Darśana* therefore means "sight," "view," "point of view," or even "a certain way of seeing." But beyond these lie another meaning; to understand this one we must conjure an image of a mirror with which we can look inside ourselves. And in fact all the great texts introduce us to ways of seeing that create opportunities for us to recognize ourselves better. We look deeper inside ourselves as we come to terms with the teachings. As one of the six darśanas, yoga has its origins in the Vedas, the oldest written record of Indian culture. It was systematized as a special darśana by the great Indian sage Patañjali in the *Yoga Sūtra*. Although this work was followed by many other important texts on yoga, Patañjali's *Yoga Sūtra* is certainly the most significant.

Many different interpretations of the word yoga have been handed down over the centuries. One of these is "to come together," "to unite." Another meaning of the word *yoga* is "to tie the strands of the mind together." These two definitions may at first glance seem very different, but really they are speaking about the same thing. While "coming together" gives us a physical interpretation of the word *yoga*, an example of tying the strands of the mind together is the directing of our thoughts toward the yoga session before we take on an actual practice. Once those mental strands come together to form an intention, we are ready to begin the physical work.

A further meaning of the word *yoga* is "to attain what was previously unattainable." The starting point for this thought is that there is something that we are today unable to do; when we find the means for bringing that desire into

[1] For a guide to the pronunciation of Sanskrit, see pages 147–48

action, that step is yoga. In fact, every change is yoga. For example, when we find a way to bend the body forward and touch our toes, or learn the meaning of the word *yoga* with the help of a text, or gain more understanding of ourselves or others through a discussion, we have reached a point where we have never been before. Each of these movements and changes is yoga.

Another aspect of yoga has to do with our actions. *Yoga* therefore also means acting in such a way that all of our attention is directed toward the activity in which we are currently engaged. Suppose for example that while I am writing, one part of my mind is thinking about what I want to say while another part is thinking about something entirely different. The more I am focused on my writing, the greater my attentiveness to my action in this moment. The exact opposite might also occur: I might begin writing with great attention, but as I continue to write my attention begins to waver. I might begin to think about the plans I have for the day tomorrow, or what is cooking for dinner. It then appears as if I am acting with attentiveness, but really I am paying little attention to the task at hand. I am functioning, but I am not present. Yoga attempts to create a state in which we are always present—really present—in every action, in every moment.

The advantage of attentiveness is that we perform each task better and at the same time are conscious of our actions. The possibility of making mistakes becomes correspondingly smaller the more our attention develops. When we are attentive to our actions we are not prisoners to our habits; we do not need to do something today simply because we did it yesterday. Instead there is the possibility of considering our actions fresh and so avoiding thoughtless repetition.

Another classic definition of *yoga* is "to be one with the divine." It does not matter what name we use for the divine—God, Allah, Īśvara, or whatever—anything that brings us closer to understanding that there is a power higher and greater than ourselves is yoga. When we feel in harmony with that higher power, that too is yoga.

So we see that there are many possible ways of understanding the meaning of the word *yoga*. Yoga has its roots in Indian thought, but its content is universal because it is about the means by which we can make the changes we desire in our lives. The actual practice of yoga takes each person in a different direction. It is not necessary to subscribe to any particular ideas of God in order to follow the yoga path. The practice of yoga only requires us to act and to be attentive to our actions. Each of us is required to pay careful attention to the direction we are taking so that we know where we are going and how we are going to get there; this careful observation will enable us to discover something new. Whether this discovery leads to a better understanding of God, to greater contentment, or to a new goal is a completely personal matter. When we begin discussing *āsanas*, the physical exercises of yoga, we shall see how the various ideas implicit in the meaning of the word *yoga* can be incorporated into our practice.

Where and how does the practice of yoga begin? Should we always begin on the physical level? I would say that where we begin depends on our personal interests. There are many ways of practicing yoga, and gradually the interest in one path will lead to another. So it could be that we begin by studying the *Yoga Sūtra* or by meditating. Or we may instead begin with practicing āsanas and so start to understand yoga through the experience of the body. We can also begin with prāṇāyāma, feeling the breath as the movement of our inner being. There are no prescriptions regarding where and how our practice should begin.

Books or yoga classes often give the impression that there are prerequisites for the study of yoga. We may be told that we should not smoke, or that we should be vegetarian, or that we should give away all our worldly goods. Such ways of behaving are admirable only if they originate within us—and they may as a result of yoga—but not if they are imposed from outside. For instance, many people who smoke give up the habit once they begin a yoga practice. As result of their practice they no longer want to smoke; they do not give up smoking in order to practice yoga. We begin where we are and how we are, and whatever happens, happens.

When we begin studying yoga—whether by way of āsanas, prāṇāyāma, meditation, or studying the *Yoga Sūtra*—the way in which we learn is the same. The more we progress, the more we become aware of the holistic nature of our being, realizing that we are made of body, breath, mind, and more. Many people who start studying yoga by practicing āsanas continue to learn more poses until the only meaning of yoga for them lies in physical exercise. We can liken this to a man who strengthens only one arm and lets the other one become weak. Similarly, there are people who intellectualize the idea of yoga; they write wonderful books and speak brilliantly about complicated ideas such as *prakṛti* and *ātman*, but when they are writing or speaking they cannot sit erect for even a few minutes. So let us not forget, we can begin practicing yoga from any starting point, but if we are to be complete human beings we must incorporate all aspects of ourselves, and do so step by step. In the *Yoga Sūtra*, Patañjali emphasizes all aspects of human life, including our relationships with others, our behavior, our health, our breathing, and our meditation path.

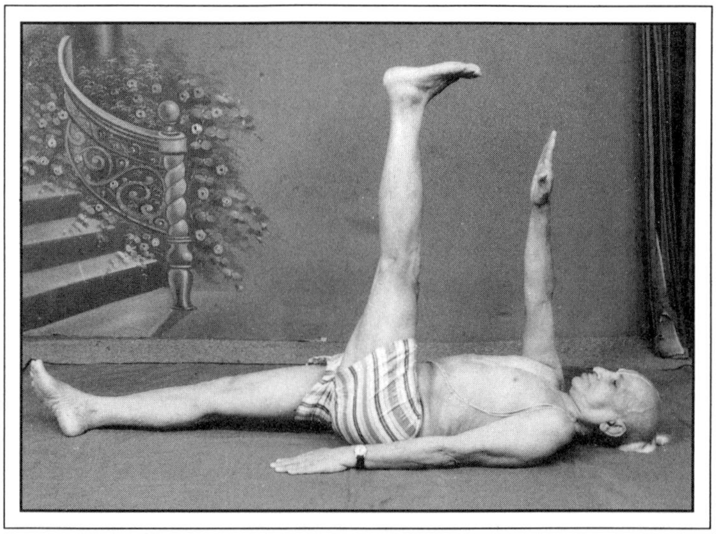

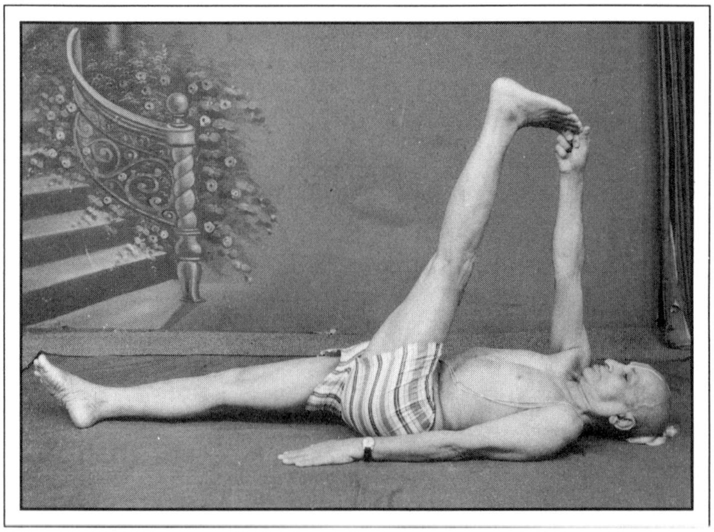

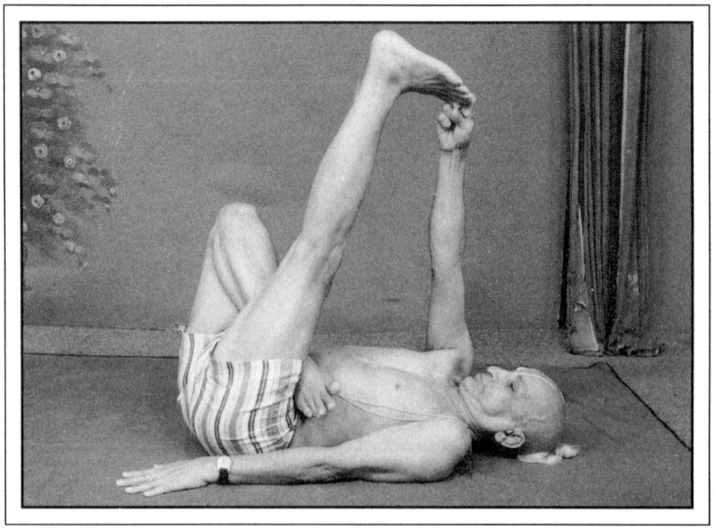

Krishnamacharya demonstrating eka pāda ūrdhva prāsārita pādāsana variations.

2

The Foundations of Yoga Practice

To explain yoga I shall refer to the ideas expressed in Patañjali's *Yoga Sūtra*, the guide to yogic practice that I prefer to any other text on yoga. In a certain way the *Yoga Sūtra* is more universal than any other text because it focuses on the mind—what its qualities are and how we can influence it. As defined in the *Yoga Sūtra*, yoga is the ability to direct the mind without distraction or interruption. No one can deny that such a process is beneficial to all people for living a focused and productive life. Other yoga texts talk about God, consciousness, and other such concepts that are not necessarily accepted by or consisent with various philosophies and religions. If I understand yoga as a path that is accessible to every human being, then it seems perfectly natural that my discussion be based on the *Yoga Sūtra* precisely because questions about the qualities of mind are universal ones. Speaking in terms of God or a Supreme Being often disturbs people, regardless of whether they accept or reject the notion. Patañjali's *Yoga Sūtra* is exceptionally open, which is in part what makes it so profound. The notion of God is neither rejected nor forced on anyone. For this reason I think the *Yoga Sūtra* makes yoga more comprehensible than any other text.

Perception and Action

An important concept from Patañjali's *Yoga Sūtra* has to do with the way we perceive things, and it explains why we are always getting into difficulties in life. If we know how we create such problems, we can also learn how to free ourselves of them.

How does our perception work? We often determine that we have seen a situation "correctly" and act according to that perception. In reality, however, we have deceived ourselves, and our actions may thus bring misfortune to ourselves or others. Just as difficult is the situation in which we doubt our understanding of a situation when it is actually correct, and for that reason we take no action, even though doing so would be beneficial.

The *Yoga Sūtra* uses the term *avidyā* to describe these two ends of the spectrum of experience. Avidyā literally means "incorrect comprehension," describing a false perception or a misapprehension. Avidyā confuses the gross with the subtle. The opposite of avidyā is *vidyā*, "correct understanding."[1]

Now what is this avidyā that is so deeply rooted in us? Avidyā can be understood as the accumulated result of our many unconscious actions, the actions and ways of perceiving that we have been mechanically carrying out for years. As a result of these unconscious responses, the mind becomes more and more dependent on habits until we accept the actions of yesterday as the norms of today. Such habituation in our action and perception is called *saṃskāra*. These habits cover the mind with avidyā, as if obscuring the clarity of consciousness with a filmy layer.

If we are sure we do not clearly understand a given situation, generally speaking we do not act decisively. But if we are clear in our understanding we will act and it will go well for us. Such an action stems from a deep level of perception. In contrast, avidyā is distinguished by superficial perception. I think I see something correctly, so I take a particular action and then later have to admit that I was mistaken and that my actions have not proved beneficial. So we have two levels of perception: One is deep within us and free of this film of avidyā, the other is superficial and obscured by avidyā. Just as our eye is transparent and clear and should not itself be tinted if it is to see colors accurately, so should our perception be like a crystal-clear mirror. The goal of yoga is to reduce the film of avidyā in order to act correctly.

The Branches of Avidyā

We seldom have an immediate and direct sense that our perception is wrong or clouded. Avidyā seldom is expressed as avidyā itself. Indeed, one of the characteristics of avidyā is that it remains hidden from us. Easier to identify are the characteristics of avidyā's branches. If we notice that these are alive in us, then we can recognize the presence of avidyā.

The first branch of avidyā is what we often call the ego. It pushes us into thoughts such as "I have to be better than other people," "I am the greatest," "I know that I'm right." This branch is called *asmitā* in the *Yoga Sūtra*.

The second branch of avidyā expresses itself in making demands. This branch is called *rāga*. We want something today because it was pleasant yesterday, not because we really need it today. Yesterday I had a glass of fruit juice that tasted delicious and gave me the energy I needed. Today something in me says: "I want another glass of this sweet juice," even though I do not really need it today and it may not even be good for me. We want things we do not have. What we do have is not enough and we want more of it. We want to keep what we are asked to give away. This is rāga.

1. *Yoga Sūtra* 2.3–5.

Dveṣa, the third branch of avidyā, is in a certain way the opposite of rāga. Dveṣa expresses itself by rejecting things. We have a difficult experience and are afraid of repeating it, so we reject the people, the thoughts, and the settings that relate to that experience, assuming they will bring us pain again. Dveṣa also causes us to reject those things with which we are not familiar, even though we have no history with them, negative or positive. These forms of rejection are the expressions of dveṣa.

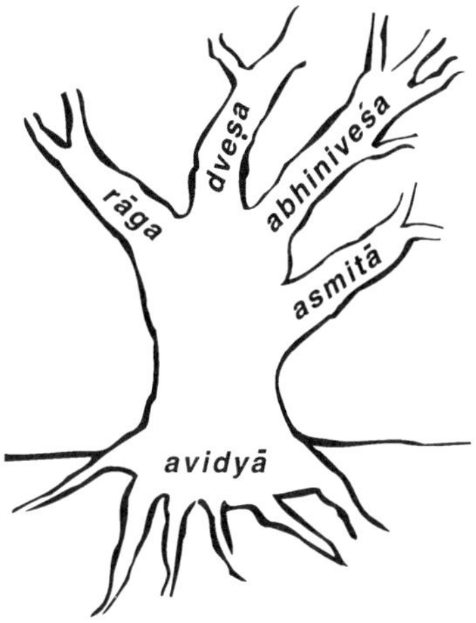

Figure 1: Avidyā is the root cause of the obstacles that prevent us from recognizing things as they really are. The obstacles are asmitā (ego), rāga (attachment), dveṣa (refusal), and abhiniveśa (fear).

Finally, there is *abhiniveśa*, fear. This is perhaps the most secret aspect of avidya and its expression is found on many levels of our everyday life. We feel uncertain. We have doubts about our position in life. We are afraid that people will judge us negatively. We feel uncertain when our lifestyle is upset. We do not want to grow old. All these feelings are expressions of abhiniveśā, the fourth branch of avidyā.

These four branches of avidyā, singly or together, cloud our perceptions. Through them avidyā is constantly active in our subconscious mind and as a result of this activity we end up feeling dissatisfied. For example, if āsanas are being practiced in a class, we have a tendency to compare ourselves with others. We notice that someone is more limber than we are, and that comparison creates dissatisfaction. Yet the practice of āsanas is not a sporting contest. Just because one person can bend forward further than another does not necessarily mean that she is more advanced in her yoga practice. Such comparisons lead to a satisfaction that relies on a feeling of superiority, or to a dissatisfaction that stems from a sense of inferiority. Such dissatisfaction often weighs so heavily upon us that it constantly haunts us and will not leave us alone. In both cases the origin of our feelings remains hidden from us.

Let me give you another example of the persistence of avidyā. Suppose I make a mistake in a discussion regarding the *Yoga Sūtra*. Normally I would admit to the mistake and apologize. This time when my friend says that my opinions on this great text are wrong, I feel a pain deep inside myself. I feel sick. Perhaps, under the influence of asmitā, I try to prove that my friend is wrong and I am right. Or abhiniveśa may impell me to withdraw from the situation altogether. Either way, I reject that which challenges me instead of accepting the criticism and learning from the situation.

As long as the branches of avidyā are expanding there is a great chance that we will make false moves because we do not weigh things carefully and make sound judgments. When we perceive that problems have somehow arisen, we can assume that avidyā was instrumental in their making. Yoga decreases the effects of avidyā so that true understanding can take place.

We notice avidyā more by its absence than its presence. When we see something correctly there is a profound peace inside us—we feel no tension, no unrest, no agitation. For instance, when I am conscious of speaking slowly I sense that there is a spring from which quietness comes, and vidyā, clear understanding, is within me. But if I am not certain about what I am saying, I tend to speak too fast. I use unnecessary words and I might break off my sentences. So when our understanding is clear we feel quietness and calmness deep within us.

Constancy and Change

If we subscribe to yogic concepts, then everything that we see, experience, and feel is not illusion; it is true and real. Everything is real, including dreams, ideas, and fantasies. Even avidyā itself is real. This concept is called *satvāda.*

Although in yoga everything we see and experience is true and real, all form and all content are in a constant state of flux. This concept of continual change is known as *pariṇāmavāda.* The way we see things today does not have to be the way we saw them yesterday. That is because the situations, our relationship to them, and we ourselves have all changed in the interim. This notion of constant change suggests that we do not have to be discouraged by the existence of avidyā. If things go badly, they can always change for the better. Of course, they could always get worse too! We never know what may happen in life, and that is why it is important to be attentive. Whether things get better or worse depends to a considerable extent on our own actions. The recommendation of a regular yoga practice follows the principle that through practice we can learn to stay present in every moment, and thereby achieve much that we were previously incapable of.

Yoga subscribes to the notion that deep within us there is something that is also very real but, unlike everything else, is not subject to change. We call this wellspring *puruṣa* or *draṣṭṛ,* meaning "that which sees" or "that which can see correctly." When we are swimming in a river and cannot see the bank, it is difficult to notice the current. We are moving so much with the river that we may scarcely see its flow. But if we go to the bank where we have firm ground it is much easier to see how the river is flowing.

Puruṣa denotes the position from which we can see; it is the power in us that enables us to perceive with accuracy. The practice of yoga encourages this unhampered seeing to simply happen. As long as our mind is covered by avidyā, our perceptions are clouded. It is when we feel quietness deep within us that we know we truly understand, and it is this kind of understanding that can have a strong, positive effect on our lives by leading us to right action. This true understanding, which results from decreasing avidyā, does not usually occur spontaneously. The body and mind are used to certain patterns of perception, and these tend to change gradually through yoga practice. It is said in the *Yoga Sūtra* that people alternately experience waves of clarity and cloudiness when first beginning a yoga practice. That is, we go through periods of clarity followed by times in which our mind and perception are quite lacking in clarity.[2] Over time there will be less cloudiness and more clarity. Recognizing this shift is a way to measure our progress.

2. *Yoga Sūtra* 3.9.

One may ask, is it an expression of asmitā (the ego) when someone begins yoga because he or she wants to be better? Such a question may lead us to important discoveries about the meaning of avidyā. We are subject to avidyā, and when we notice that—directly or indirectly—it becomes clear to us that we have to do something about it. Sometimes our first step is the need to become better or feel more accomplished. It is no different from someone saying, "I am poor, but I'd like to become rich," or "I'd like to become a doctor." I doubt that there is anyone who really does not want to improve himself, and even if our first step springs from the desire to become better and is therefore rooted in the ego, it is still a right step because it takes us on to the first rung of the yoga ladder. Furthermore, we do not stay permanently committed to this initial goal of self-improvement. According to the *Yoga Sūtra*, the recognition and conquest of avidyā and its effects is the only ladder by which we can climb upward. The goal of wanting to make something better may be the first rung on the ladder. And it is indeed true that by practicing yoga we gradually improve our ability to concentrate and to be independent. We improve our health, our relationships, and everything we do. If we could begin above this first rung, this desire for self-betterment, then perhaps we would not need yoga.

How can we climb this ladder? In Patañjali's *Yoga Sūtra,* three things are recommended to help us do this. The first is *tapas.* Tapas comes from the root word *tap*, to "heat" or "cleanse." Tapas is a means by which we can keep ourselves healthy and cleanse ourselves inwardly. Tapas is often described as penance, mortification, and a strict diet. But its meaning in the *Yoga Sūtra* is the practice of āsanas and prāṇāyāma, that is, the physical and breathing exercises of yoga. These exercises help get rid of blocks and impurities in our system as well as giving us other benefits. By practicing āsanas and prāṇāyāṃa we are able to influence our whole system. It is the same principle as heating gold in order to purify it.

The second means by which we can discover the state of yoga is *svādhyāya. Sva* means "self" and *adhyāya* translates as "study or investigation." With the help of svādhyāya we get to know ourselves. Who are we? What are we? What is our relationship to the world? It is not enough to keep ourselves healthy. We should know who we are and how we relate to other people. That is not easy, for we do not have such a clear mirror for our minds as we do for our bodies. But we can see a reflection of our mind as we read and study certain texts, as we discuss them and reflect upon them. That is especially so with great works such as the *Yoga Sūtra*, the Bible, the *Mahābhārata*, and the Koran. By studying texts like these we can see ourselves.

The third possible way suggested in the *Yoga Sūtra* to approach the state of yoga is *īśvarapraṇidhānā*. Usually this term is interpreted as "love of God," but it also means a certain quality of action. Practicing prāṇāyāma and āsanas, keeping oneself healthy, and reflecting on oneself do not constitute all our actions. We also have to pursue our career, gain qualifications, and do everything else that is part of normal life. All these things should be done as well as possible. Yet we can never be sure of the fruit of our actions. That is why it is better to become slightly detached from our expectations and to pay more attention to the actions themselves.

Altogether, these three ways of being—health, inquiry, and quality of action—cover the entire spectrum of human endeavor. If we are healthy, know more about ourselves, and improve the quality of our actions, it is likely that we will make fewer mistakes. It is recommmended that we work in these three distinct areas in order to reduce avidyā. Together they are known as *kriyā yoga*, the yoga of action. *Kriyā* comes from the word *kṛ*, meaning "to do." Yoga is not passive. We have to participate in life. To do this well we can work on ourselves.

I have already explained that yoga is a state in which two things are joined into one. I also said that yoga means attentiveness in action, which is necessary if we want to achieve a point or a posture that was previously unattainable. The yoga of action, kriyā yoga, is the means by which we achieve yoga as a state of being. Although it is only one part of yoga, kriyā yoga is the practical branch of yoga that can lead to a change for the better in all aspects of our life.

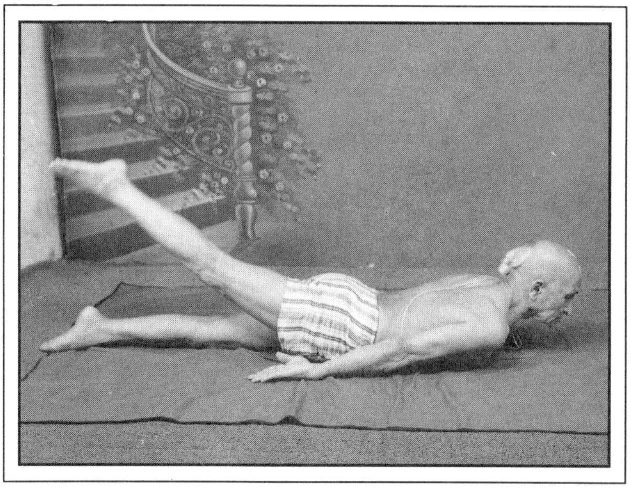

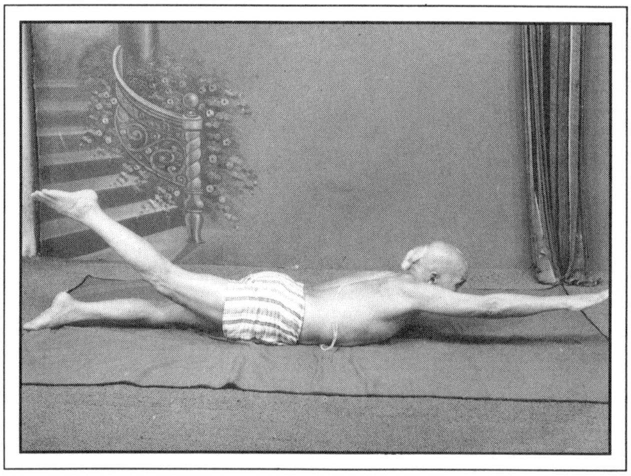

Krishnamacharya in śalabhāsana variations.

3

The Principles of Āsana Practice

The practice of yoga gives us the chance to experience the many different meanings of the word *yoga*. We have already described yoga as a movement from one point to another, higher one that was previously beyond our reach. It doesn't matter whether this shift comes about through practicing āsanas, through study and reading, or through meditation—it is still yoga.

In our practice we concentrate on the body, the breath, and the mind. Our senses are included as part of the mind. Although it theoretically appears possible for body, breath, and mind to work independent of one another, the purpose of yoga is to unify their actions. It is primarily the physical aspect of our practice that people see as yoga. They will rarely notice how we breathe, how we feel the breath, and how we coordinate our breathing with our physical movement; they tend to only see our flexibility and suppleness. Some may want to know how many āsanas we have mastered or how many minutes we can stay in a headstand.

Much more important than these outer manifestations is the way we *feel* the postures and the breath. The principles that follow are ages old, developed by many generations of great yoga teachers. These principles describe in detail the āsanas and the breath and, above all, how they relate to each other. They also establish guidelines for prāṇāyāma, the breathing techniques that will be described in a later chapter.

What is an āsana? *Āsana* translates as "posture." The word is derived from the Sanskrit root *as* which means "to stay," "to be," "to sit," or "to be established in a particular position." Patañjali's *Yoga Sūtra* describes an āsana as having two important qualities: *sthira* and *sukha*.[1] Sthira is steadiness and alertness. Sukha refers to the ability to remain comfortable in a posture. Both qualities should be present to the same degree when practicing any posture. Neither

[1]. *Yoga Sūtra* 2.46.

sukha nor sthira are present when we sit with crossed legs for a photograph if we have to stretch them out again immediately afterward because they are hurting. Even if we achieve the steadiness and alertness of sthira there must also be the comfort and lightness of sukha, and both must be present for a certain length of time. Without both these qualities there is no āsana. This principle of yoga is fulfilled only when we have practiced a particular āsana for a certain period of time and feel alert and unstressed as we practice it. The following precepts only serve to ensure that every āsana is practiced with both sthira and sukha.

Beginning from Where We Are

When we go into a posture or carry out a movement that feels tense, it is difficult to notice anything else besides that tension. Perhaps when we sit in a cross-legged position our only thought is for the pain in our strained ankles. In doing this we are not really in the āsana we are striving for—we are obviously not yet ready for this particular position. Rather, we should first practice something easier. This simple idea is the foundation for our whole yoga practice. Practicing the postures progressively, we gradually achieve more steadiness, alertness, and overall comfort.

If we want to make this principle of āsana practice a reality, we have to accept ourselves just as we are. If we have a stiff back we have to acknowledge this fact. It may be that we are very supple but our breath is very short, or perhaps our breathing is all right but our body gives us certain problems. It is also possible to feel comfortable in an āsana while the mind is somewhere completely different. That is not āsana either. It is only possible to find the qualities that are essential to āsana if we recognize our own starting point and learn to accept it.

Joining Breath with Movement

Yoga is as much a practice involving breath as it is involving the body. The quality of our breath is extremely important because it expresses our inner feelings. If we are in pain it shows in our breathing. If we are distracted we lose control of our breathing. The breath is the link between the inner and outer body. It is only by bringing body, breath, and mind into unison that we realize the true quality of an āsana.

Recognizing our personal starting point begins with the exploration of the body, including the breath.[2] For this we use simple breathing exercises, such as making the inhalation as long as possible. In this way we can observe whether it is the chest or the abdomen that expands and whether the back stretches with the breath. To explore the present state of the body, we use dynamic movements of the arms, legs, and trunk. For instance, we direct a group of yoga beginners in raising and lowering their arms. Then we ask, "Did the arm movement primarily stretch your back, or did it stretch another part of

2. We call this process svādhyāya, one of the three aspects of kriyā yoga, the yoga of action. Svādhyāya refers to everything that contributes to the exploration of myself. See chapter 2, and *Yoga Sūtra* 2.1.

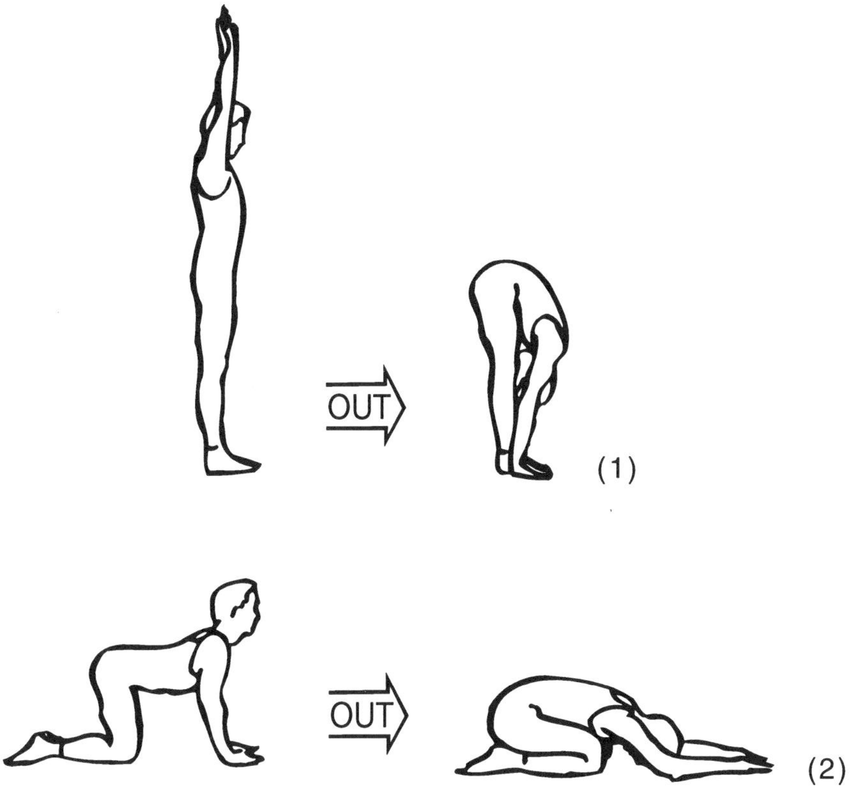

Figure 2: Natural breathing in the forward bend, shown in (1) uttānāsana (standing forward bend) and (2) a variation of cakravākāsana (cat pose).

your body more?" Some will say the movement stretched the back; others will have noticed extension predominantly in the shoulders.

The reason why people have differing experiences in this situation is because some large movements are initiated in various ways by various people. Those who have a stiff back find that all the effort for initiating movement at the arms comes from the shoulders, whereas those who are more supple will notice that the initiation happens at the scapulae, closer to the spine.

Observing the body in this way is the first step toward changing uncomfortable or inefficient habits of movement and posture that cause stiffness and ultimately hinder the flow of vital energy through the body. This kind of investigation requires a teacher who can lead the students on their journey of discovery. If a teacher cannot do this, the students are not only in danger of misunderstanding yoga but may also get discouraged.

The first step of our yoga practice is to consciously link breath and body. We do this by allowing every movement to be led by the breath as we practice the āsanas. The correct linking of breath and movement is the basis for the whole āsana practice. The simple exercise of raising the arms on an inhale and lowering them on an exhale helps us find the rhythm of combined breath and movement.

Figure 3: Natural breathing in the backward bend, shown in (1) dvipāda pītham and (2) bhujaṅgāsana.

Normally we are not conscious of our breathing. It is an automatic process and we do it without will or volition. For breath and movement to be coordinated, our mind must attentively follow their union. When we do this, inhalation and exhalation are no longer automatic but become a conscious process. Finding the natural link between breath and movement is the most important aspect of āsana practice. It requires determining whether it is the inhalation or the exhalation that is amplified or made easier by a certain movement, and then making sure that that breath is the one we combine with the movement on which we are focusing.

Continuing with our example of the arm movement described above, the natural breath rhythm would show an ease in inhaling as we raise our arms and an ease in exhaling when we lower them. Also, the length of the inhalation and exhalation would determine how quickly we raise and lower our arms. In practicing this simple movement we can learn one of the basic principles of yoga—that is, to become fully involved with our actions.

The consciously directed breath supports and strengthens the natural coordination of breath and movement. For instance, on a natural exhalation the ribs sink while the diaphragm rises and the front of the belly moves back toward the spine. The same movement happens internally in every forward bend; that is, the ribs sink and the belly is pushed back toward the spine. So in order to amplify the natural breath, we breathe out in all exercises where a forward bend is the primary movement of the body. The examples in figure 2 show the breath cycle connected to the movement of the forward bend.

In performing backward-bending postures such as dvipāda pītham (table pose) or bhujaṅgāsana (cobra pose), the movement of the ribs raises the chest and causes the spine to bend backward. By deliberately combining the backward bend with an inhalation, as shown in figure 3, you make the movement easier and more effective. (In contrast with forward bends, which are only done on the exhalation, in certain backward bends we have the freedom to breathe out or in. This will be discussed later.)

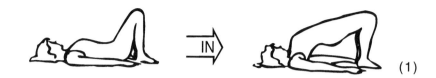

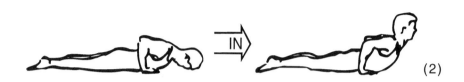

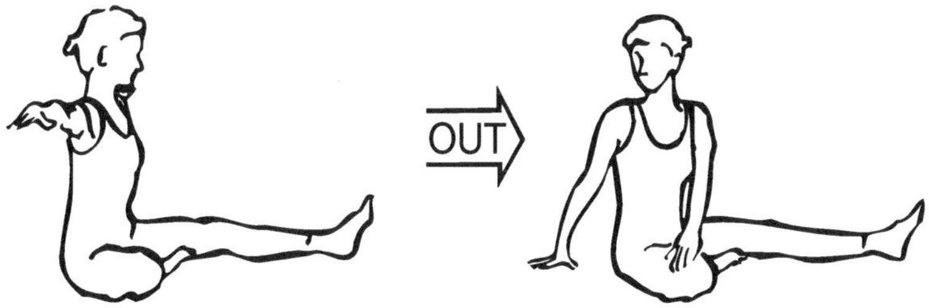

Figure 4: Beginning matsyendrāsana (half spinal twist) with an exhale follows the natural breath rhythm.

Twists are also closely linked with a specific breathing pattern. As the spine and ribs rotate, the space between them is reduced and the abdominal area is slightly compressed; the diaphragm meanwhile moves upward. So if we combine the beginning of the twist with an exhalation, as shown in figure 4, we are following the natural pattern of breathing.

The rules for linking breath and movement are basically simple: when we contract the body we exhale and when we expand the body we inhale. Exceptions are made only when we want to create a particular effect in the āsana by altering the natural breathing pattern. As I have stated before, we do not simply inhale and exhale without attention, but instead we make sure that the breathing initiates the movement. The length of the breath will determine the speed of the movement. This integration of breath and movement in time becomes quite natural.

There are various ways of encouraging the conscious awareness of breath and movement, thereby avoiding mindless repetition. One good method for this is to introduce a short pause at the end of every movement. After raising the arms as we breathe in, for example, we can pause momentarily. Then after we have lowered our arms with the exhale, we can pause for another moment. Pausing at the end of each movement helps us remain conscious of both the movement and the breath. Losing this attention causes our practice to become mechanical, and then we are no longer doing yoga.

The Fullness of Breath

While one goal is to direct the breath quite consciously during our āsana practice, we are also aiming at making our breathing—both the inhalation and the exhalation—fuller and deeper than it normally is.

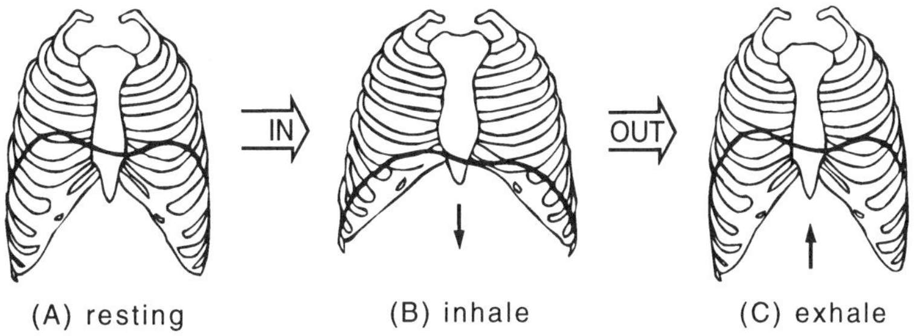

Figure 5: Movement of the diaphragm and rib cage through a breath cycle.

The movement of the diaphragm during a breath cycle is shown in figure 5. From the rest position (A), the diaphragm moves downward on inhalation (B). After the lungs have been filled, the diaphragm moves back to the rest position (C). In the process a deep inhalation expands the rib cage (B) by making the ribs rise, thus moving the diaphragm down and slightly straightening the spine in this region. On a deep exhalation the opposite occurs: the front of the belly moves toward the spine, the diaphragm rises, and the spine settles back into its starting position.

People often breathe only in the abdomen, without expanding the chest. Others hardly use the diaphragm at all, restricting their breathing to the upper chest. Very tense people or asthmatics can sometimes hardly move the abdomen or chest at all when they breathe. The technique for gaining a fuller breath consists of consciously expanding the chest and abdomen on inhalation and consciously contracting the abdomen on exhalation. This simple breathing technique described below, together with the integration of breath and movement, is a means for bringing greater depth to the quality of our yoga practice.

I suggest that when we inhale we first fill the chest and then fill the abdomen, and as we exhale we release the abdomen first and then finally empty the upper lobes of the lungs in the chest region.[3] This is contrary to the way of breathing taught in many yoga classes. The technique I am suggesting has the great advantage of stretching the spine and straightening the back. The moment we start to breathe in, the ribs rise and the spine, to which they are attached, is extended upward and slightly straightened. When using the other technique of breathing first into the abdomen and then into the chest, the abdomen expands so much that it inhibits the expansion of the chest and consequently the spine is not extended enough. As well, the abdominal organs are pressed down rather than the diaphragm being given room to move freely by the rising action of the chest. Because we are interested in breathing that assists the movements of the body and does not hinder the extension of the spine, this chest-to-abdomen breath is best to use. Experiment with both methods and feel the difference.

3. Interestingly enough, this understanding of the direction of the breath, which has a long tradition in yoga and is mentioned in the very oldest texts, coincides with the findings of the latest research on the neurophysiological and mechanical basis of breathing. See *Respiratory Physiology: The Essentials* by John B. West, M. D., Ph. D. (Baltimore: Williams & Wilkins, 1990.)

The Breath Is the Intelligence of the Body

Let's explore further the possibility of *feeling* the breath as it moves in and out. By doing this, the quality of our breathing while we are practicing āsanas gradually improves.

When practicing an āsana our attention should be directed toward the central point of the movement of breath. For instance, the main action when we breathe in moves from the upper chest to the navel; when we breathe out the action is mostly in the abdomen. Our attention is on these movements. Consciously following the breath is a form of meditation in which we try to become completely one with the movement. This is the same attention to action that we discussed earlier. Whoever masters this can direct his attention toward any sort of activity.

In order to produce a fine, smooth feeling when we breathe, we narrow the flow of breath in the throat, producing a gentle breathing sound. It is as if there were a valve in the throat that we close slightly in order to control the breath. The measure for this control is our sound, which becomes very gentle and ultimately should not require any effort or create any feeling of tension. After this technique is mastered, the sound is present during both inhalation and exhalation. This technique, *known as ujjāyī,* allows us to hear as well as feel the breath as it becomes deeper and longer.

The practice of this technique has two advantages. First, we are closer to the flow of our breath and in this way can remain more alert during āsana practice. Second, the sound tells us when we have to stop or change an āsana. If we do not succeed in maintaining a gentle, even, quiet sound, then we have gone beyond our limits in the practice. The quality of breath is therefore the clearest indication of the quality of our āsana practice.

Another technique for invigorating and deepening our practice is to lengthen the natural pause between the exhalation and inhalation and between the inhalation and exhalation. After breathing out we hold the breath and stop moving; we do the same after breathing in. The length of time we hold the breath is critical; if the breath is held too long, whether following inhalation or exhalation, the body will rebel.

In order to introduce this practice safely, we make quite sure that holding the breath does not disturb the inhalation or exhalation in any way. For example, while we are practicing an āsana in the usual way we may perhaps breathe in comfortably for five seconds, then breathe out for five seconds. We might then try holding the breath for five seconds following the exhalation. On the next inhalation we might notice that we need to draw the breath in more rapidly than before. That is a clear indication that we are not yet ready for this breath-retention technique. If holding the breath is too demanding, inhaling or exhaling or both will be negatively affected. Be certain you are ready for this technique before using it. Remember that yoga is a practice of observing yourself without judgment.

However beautifully we carry out an āsana, however flexible our body may be, if we do not achieve the integration of body, breath, and mind we can hardly claim that what we are doing is yoga. What is yoga after all? It is something that we experience inside, deep within our being. Yoga is not an external experience. In yoga we try in every action to be as attentive as possible to everything we do. Yoga is different from dance or theatre. In yoga we are not creating something for others to look at. As we perform the various āsanas we observe what we are doing and how we are doing it. We do it only for ourselves. We are both observer and what is observed at the same time. If we do not pay attention to ourselves in our practice, then we cannot call it yoga.

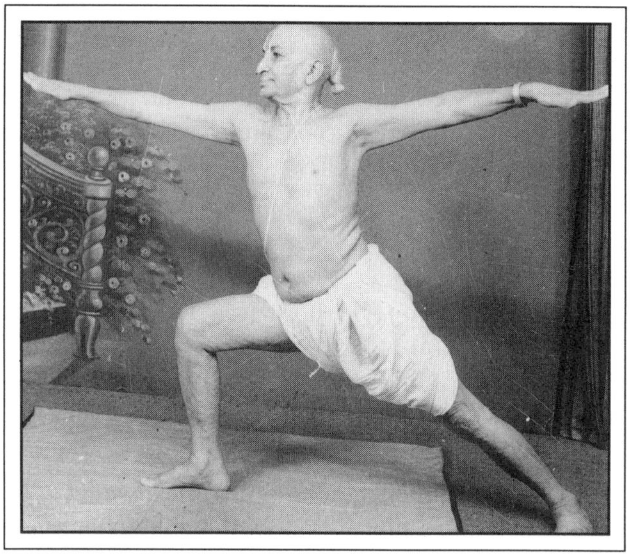

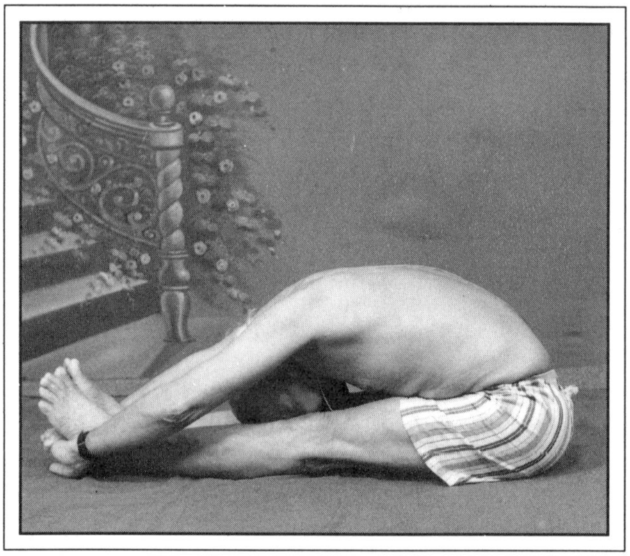

The principles of bṛmhaṇa and laṅghana are illustrated here by Krishnamacharya, age 79, in vīrabhadrāsana (above) and in paścimatānāsana.

4

The Careful Construction of a Yoga Practice

How can we realize the qualities of sthira and sukha—the steady alertness and the lightness and comfort of being—necessary for a good yoga practice? The *Yoga Sūtra* refers to a beautiful image from Indian mythology to illustrate the concept of *sthirasukha*. The story tells of Ananta, the king of snakes, floating on the ocean, his long snake body coiled to form a comfortable couch on which the god Viṣṇu lies. The snake's thousand heads reach up and out like a protective umbrella over Viṣṇu. On the umbrella rests our earth.

The snake's body is soft and gentle enough (sukha) to serve as a couch for a god and at the same time is firm and steady enough (sthira) to support the whole earth. We should endeavor to bring those same qualities of gentleness and steadiness to our āsana practice, all the while making sure that we exert progressively less effort in developing them.

In order to attain sthira and sukha, our yoga practice has to be sensible and well structured. When we practice āsanas there is a starting point where we begin, just the same as for anything else in life. The starting point for this practice is the condition of our entire being at that present moment. It therefore helps to know as much as possible about our whole constitution so that we can advance step by step, developing our practice in accordance with our abilities.

Developing a yoga practice according to the ideas expressed in the *Yoga Sūtra* is an action referred to as *viṅyāsa krama*. *Krama* is the step, *nyāsa* means "to place," and the prefix *vi-* translates as "in a special way." The concept of viṅyāsa krama tells us that it is not enough to simply take a step; that step needs to take us in the right direction and be made in the right way.

Viṅyāsa krama thus decribes a correctly organized course of yoga practice. It is a fundamental concept in yoga having to do with constructing a gradual and intelligent course for our practice, and is important to employ irrespective of whether we are dealing with āsana practice, prāṇāyāma, or some other aspect of yoga. We start our practice where we are and look toward a certain goal. Then we choose the steps that will lead us toward realizing that goal and will then gradually bring us back into our everyday life. But our daily practice does not return us to the exact place we started. The practice has changed us.

A famous yogi of old named Vamana is reputed to have said that without viṅyāsa the āsanas of yoga cannot be mastered. The concept of viṅyāsa krama is useful as a guide for carrying out not only our yoga practice but also all the tasks of our everyday life.

To realize the qualities of sthira and sukha in your āsana practice you must first gain an understanding of the steps necessary for preparing your body, your breath, and your attention for the āsana you have chosen to practice. You must also consider whether there is an immediate or long-term danger of problems arising from the practice of this āsana and, if so, determine the poses necessary to bring balance to the breath and body.

Counterposes

Yoga teaches us that every action has two effects, one positive and one negative. That is why it is so important to be attentive to our actions—we must be able to recognize which effects are positive and which are negative so that we can then emphasize the positive and try to neutralize the negative. In following this principle in our āsana practice, we use postures to balance the possibly negative effects of certain strenuous āsanas. We call these neutralizing postures counterposes or *pratikriyāsana*.[1]

Let's take the headstand as an example. Many people say that they would not make it through the day if they didn't practice śīrṣāsana, the headstand. First thing in the morning or in the evening before going to bed they do a headstand for ten minutes, and they feel very good doing it. They do not prepare in any way for the āsana; they simply stand on their head and then they break off their practice. What they often do not notice for a long time to come is the negative effect hidden in this position. Although doing a headstand is good because it reverses the usual effects of gravity on the body, while in the headstand the weight of the whole body is carried by the neck. Our narrow neck, which is designed to carry only the weight of the head, now has to support the whole body. Consequently, after practicing the headstand it is very important to offset any possible negative effects by doing an appropriate balancing exercise. If we do not, we may experience feelings of dizziness, the neck may over time become chronically stiff or, worse still, the vertebrae in the neck may deteriorate or become misaligned, jamming the nerves between them, a situation that leads to overwhelming pain. Unfortunately this occurs

1. *Prati* means "against; counter"; *kṛ* translates as "to do."

quite frequently for those who are not studious in using counterposes to balance the effects of the headstand.

It is brought home to me again and again how much damage can be caused by practicing in this way. Proper āsana practice is not just a matter of advancing step by step to a certain goal; we also have to come back into a position from which we can comfortably resume our everyday activities without experiencing any harmful effects from our practice.

Writing about the necessity of counterposes reminds me of an interesting story. I have two brothers. When we were children we had a very tall coconut palm in our garden. My older brother kept telling me and my other brother that he knew how to climb tall trees like this one, so we challenged him to show us. I can still remember how we taunted him, chanting, "Climb up, climb up!" In the end he did climb the tree. Going up was fairly easy, but when he wanted to come down he did not know how to do so without falling. There was nobody around who could help him, so he was stuck in the tree for quite a while.

So it is with our āsana practice: It is not enough to climb the tree; we must be able to get down too. When we do a headstand, we should be able to come back into a normal position without any problems. It is important to balance the headstand with a counterpose such as the shoulderstand (sarvāṅgāsana) in order to relieve the pressure on the neck.

For any one āsana there may be various counterposes possible, depending on where the tension is felt. Whenever we feel excessive tension in any area of the body after a posture, we must try to alleviate it with a counterpose; that is, the simplest āsana that relieves the tension. The counterpose for a powerful forward bend is a gentle back bend. Conversely, a powerful back bend will be followed by a simple forward bend. Again, the reason for practicing counterposes is to return the body to its normal condition and to ensure that no tensions are carried on into the next posture or into our everyday business.

Observing the principle of dual effects and thereby determining the sequence of āsanas in your session is one way of bringing viṅyāsa krama into your practice. The step-by-step awareness of viṅyāsa krama should also be a part of the practice of an individual āsana, and the development of our practice over time.

Designing a Session

Now we are going to look at how to build the sequence of an āsana session. The way we develop our session will depend on our immediate needs, our long-term goals, and what activities are going to follow our practice. A course of āsanas designed to prepare the body for playing tennis will be different from one meant to help someone remain alert in a mentally taxing environment, and that will differ from a practice meant to help someone with chronic insomnia to relax deeply before going to bed.

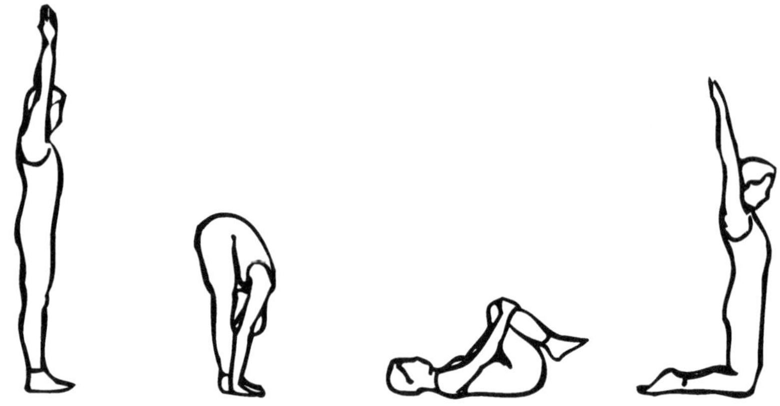

Figure 6: Āsanas to begin a practice: tadāsana (1), uttānāsana (2), apānāsana (3), and raised vajrāsana (4).

There are countless āsanas and, it seems, just as many books about them. How does one begin to make choices about which postures to practice? The list of possible āsanas are endless because the body's great flexibility allows almost limitless possibilities as far as posture goes. It is entirely up to the student, in light of both his lifestyles and goals, to determine whether it makes sense to practice many or only a few āsanas and to determine which ones are worthwhile. Different people require different āsanas. For instance, many of us are so stiff in the legs that we need to practice a lot of standing postures. On the other hand, dancers with flexible, well-formed legs are so supple that there is no reason for them to put a lot of effort into standing postures. There are a great many āsanas, but we do not need to practice all of them. It is much more important to find a direction for our practice and to draw up a sequence of āsanas that meets our own needs and through which we can discover the qualities that are to be found in āsana practice. A teacher is an important resource for helping make these choices.

Our point of departure for practice will be different every day. That may be difficult to put into effect in the beginning, but the more we get into the practice of an authentic yoga, the more we will understand how to observe ourselves and find our own starting point each time. The situation from which we begin our practice is constantly changing. Let's say I hurt my knee yesterday and therefore cannot sit cross-legged in the morning. I would then do exercises to help me to loosen my knee. It is important to examine our condition before starting and continually throughout our practice. If we bend forward from a standing position, for instance, we will feel whether our legs and back are stiff; these things are easy to discover when we begin to be attentive to the body. Once we begin to observe ourselves in this way and recognize our starting point, we are able to develop our practice for the greatest possible benefits.

Certain principles should be followed in determining how to begin a session. Before doing an āsana we should be sure that the body is ready for it. For instance, if we try to sit cross-legged first thing in the morning before observing our bodies or preparing our legs properly, we can very easily damage our knees. Gentle warm-up exercises will ease the body into readiness. It is not a good idea to start our practice with back bends or twists. We should begin each practice with the simplest poses—āsanas that bend the body forward naturally or those in which we raise our arms or legs are suitable. Beginning with the simplest postures, we gradually progress toward more difficult ones.

Some āsanas with which we can begin our practice are shown in figure 6. These include tadāsana (mountain pose), uttānāsana (forward bend), apānāsana (wind-relieving pose), and raised vajrāsana (thunderbolt pose). Figure 7 shows āsanas with which we should not begin our practice. These include śīrṣāsana (headstand), trikonāsana (triangle pose), dhanurāsana (bow pose), and halāsana (plow pose).

There are two ways of practicing an āsana. The *dynamic* practice repeats the movement into the āsana and out again in rhythm with the breath. In *static* practice we move into and out of the pose in the same way as with the dynamic practice, but instead of staying in continual movement with the breath, we hold the pose for a certain number of breath cycles, directing our attention toward the breath, certain areas of the body, or both, depending on the goals we have for performing that particular āsana. Dynamic movements allow the body to get used to the position gently and gradually. For this reason it is always better to practice an āsana dynamically first, before attempting to hold it.

There are other important benefits to be gained from the dynamic form of practice. For example, many āsanas cause great problems for beginners when they try to hold them in static practice for lengthy periods of time. As well, experienced practitioners of yoga often get caught in the habit of focusing their attention on fixing the posture somehow in static practice rather than really working in it and exploring its possiblities. A dynamic practice gives us greater possibilities for bringing breath to particular parts of the body and heightening the intensity of the effect. A dynamic performance of āsanas therefore not only helps to prepare for difficult static postures but also intensifies the practice of a particular āsana or gives it a special direction. For all these reasons, the

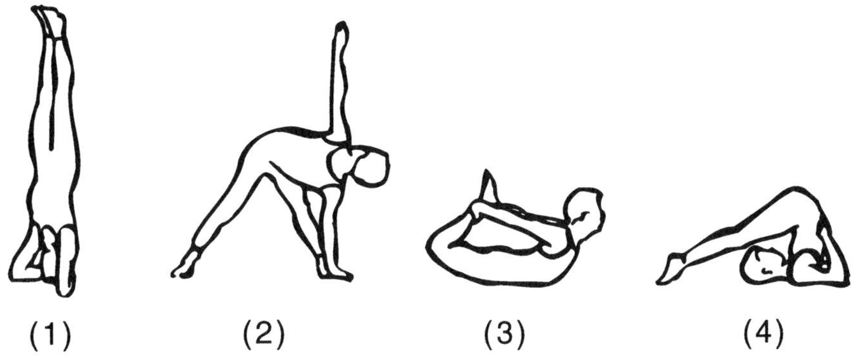

Figure 7:
Some āsanas are too demanding to begin a practice with. These include: śīrṣāsana (1), trikonāsana (2), dhanurāsana (3), and halāsana (4).

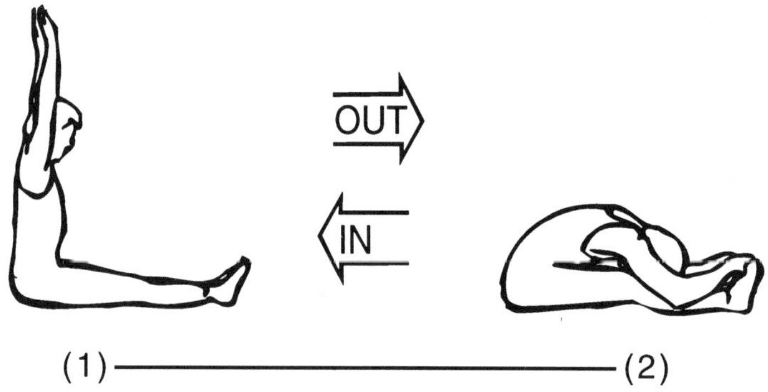

Figure 8: The dynamic practice of paścimatānāsana.

dynamic practice of āsanas should be an essential part of every yoga session, whether you are a beginner or a more advanced practitioner.

Figures 8 and 9 show dynamic practice sequences. In figure 8, paścimatānāsana (seated forward bend) is performed continuously, the student moving in a fluid manner from step 1 to step 2 and back to step 1, repeating this sequence several times on the rhythm of the breath. Only after preparing the body in this way is it sensible to go into the seated forward bend and hold the position while continuing to breathe. Over time we can gradually increase the number of breaths we take while holding the pose.

The sequence shown in figure 9 is more strenuous. In this practice of pārśva uttānāsana (a standing forward bend) we move from step 1 to step 2 on an inhale, and step 2 to step 3 on an exhale. Then we inhale to go back to step 2, exhale to step 3, and continue in this pattern (3, 2, 3, 2) for several cycles. We finally come back to step 1 on an exhale. Repeating the entire sequence (1, 2, 3, 2, 1) on each cycle would be a less strenuous way of practicing this posture dynamically.

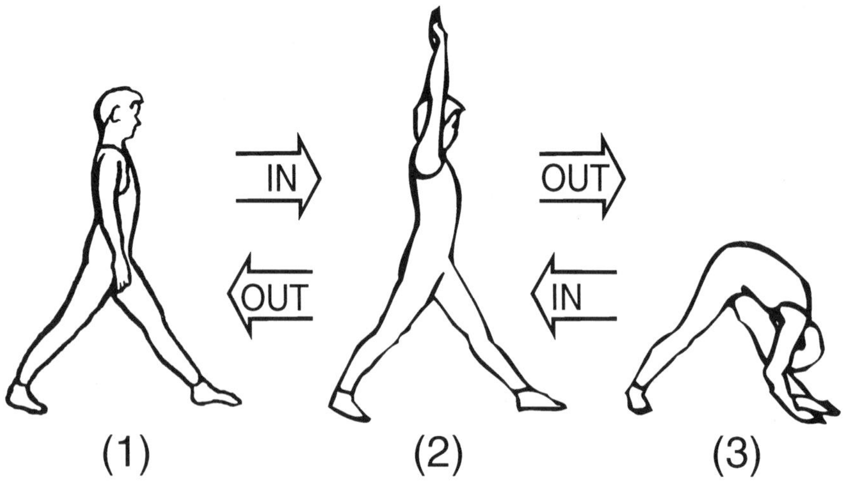

Figure 9: The dynamic practice of pārśva uttānāsana.

The number of repetitions in a dynamic practice session is a question of individual needs and requirements. In practicing the standing forward bend dynamically, the legs may become tired or we may experience back strain. Such symptoms are a sure sign that we have overstepped our limits, and they come too late to be reliable first indications that we have even reached our limit. It is the breath alone that can give us early enough warning that we have pushed ourselves too far. As I said before, as long as we can quietly follow our breath we will remain within the limits of our own physical abilities. The moment we have to draw a rapid breath through the nose or mouth without maintaining the gentle, even sound in the throat, we must stop practicing that sequence. (Asymmetrical poses must be done with the same number of breaths to each side, so account for this before finishing.) We will gradually build the stamina to increase the number of repetitions for any given pose.

If we want to hold an āsana within a sequence of postures, we can achieve more if we repeat it dynamically first. If we have set ourselves a particular āsana as a long-term goal, practicing dynamic variations will be the best help on the way to achieving that goal. Counterposes should be practiced dynamically whenever possible, to lessen the risk of creating new areas of tension in the body.

Examples of Appropriate Counterposes

The following few paragraphs will give you an idea of how the principle of balancing effects through the choice of counterposes is applied in our yoga practice.

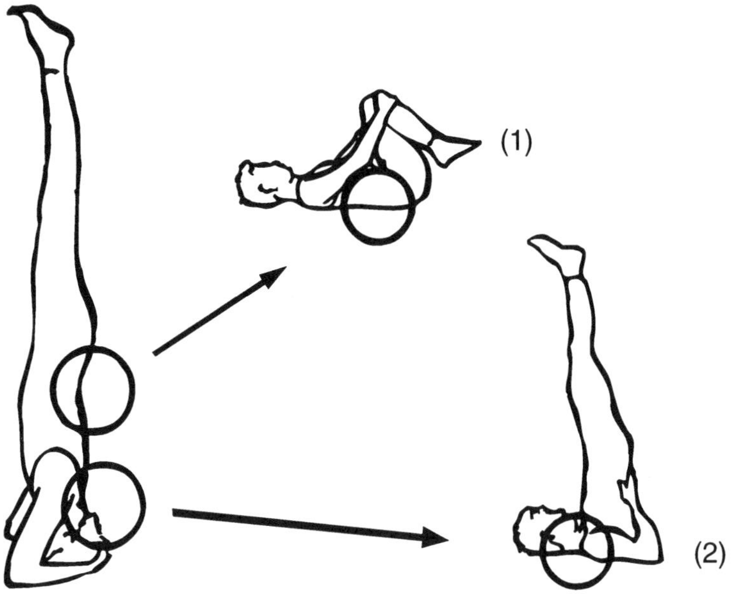

Figure 10: Possible counterposes for the headstand: apānāsana (1) and sarvāngāsana (2).

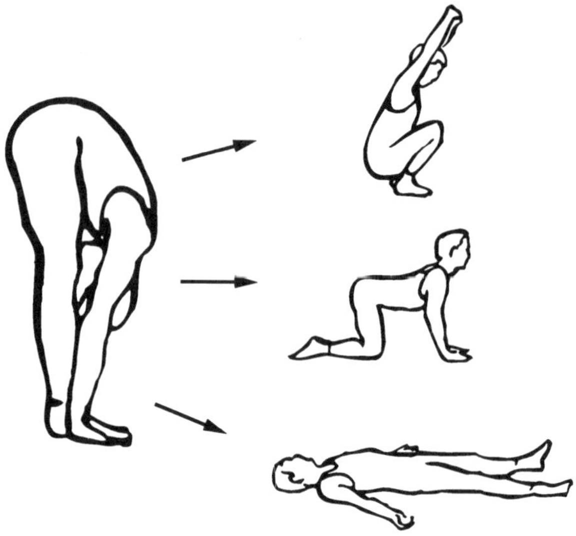

Figure 11: Possible counterposes for uttānāsana: utkaṭāsana (1), cakravākāsana (2), and śavāsana (3).

As I mentioned earlier, various counterposes will be necessary for countering the effects of the headstand (see figure 10). Those who have a sway back will want to follow śīrṣāsana with a counterpose for the lower back because the headstand can focus a lot of tension there. Apānāsana, the wind-relieving pose, (1) is suitable for this.

Practicing the headstand requires also practicing the shoulderstand (sarvāngāsana) (2), which relieves the pressure on the neck. Because the shoulderstand is itself a very demanding static pose, it too requires a counterpose such as the cobra (bhujaṅgāsana). Sequences such as this, in which poses and counterposes follow each other, play an important part in our practice.

Figure 11 shows possible counterposes for uttānāsana. Whenever we feel tension in the legs after practicing uttānāsana, utkaṭāsana, the squatting pose (1) may be useful. Cakravākāsana (2) may benefit a sore back resulting from uttānāsana, or it may well be enough to simply rest the back in śavāsana, the corpse pose (3). Figure 12 shows some āsanas and an example of a counterpose for each.

At this point it should be clear that a good yoga practice is not haphazard but instead follows certain principles. The principles that give our practice an intelligent structure are:

- begin where you are
- warm up and loosen the whole body at the start of a session
- before you perform an āsana, make sure you know and can perform an appropriate counterpose
- practice an āsana dynamically before holding it
- practice the counterpose immediately following the main āsana
- make sure the counterpose is simpler than the main āsana

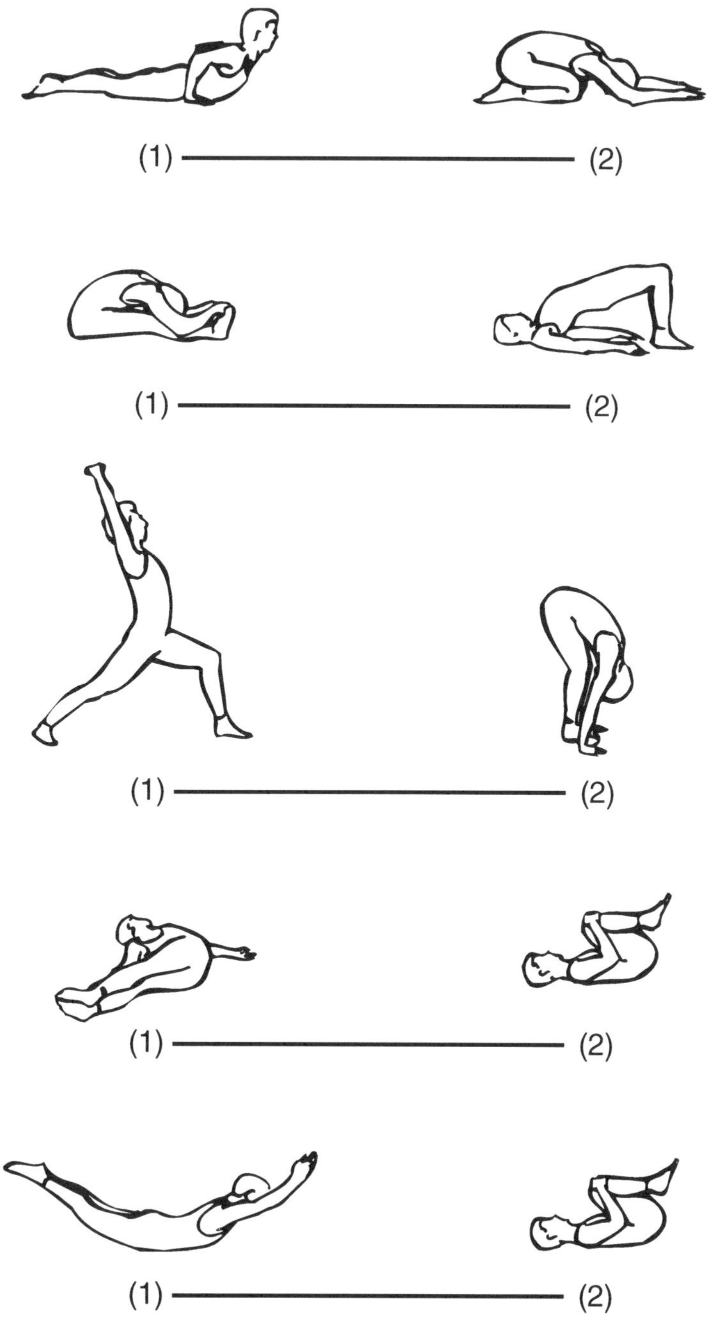

Figure 12:
Five main āsanas (1) and a counterpose for each (2).

Let me clarify these principles for you with two examples of simple āsana sequences. Whether the following sequence of āsanas is beneficial for a particular person depends on many factors, including the structure and flexibility of the spine and the flexibility of the legs and hips. Consider these sequences as examples only, knowing that your own carefully constructed practice will take into account your unique structure and your particular goals.

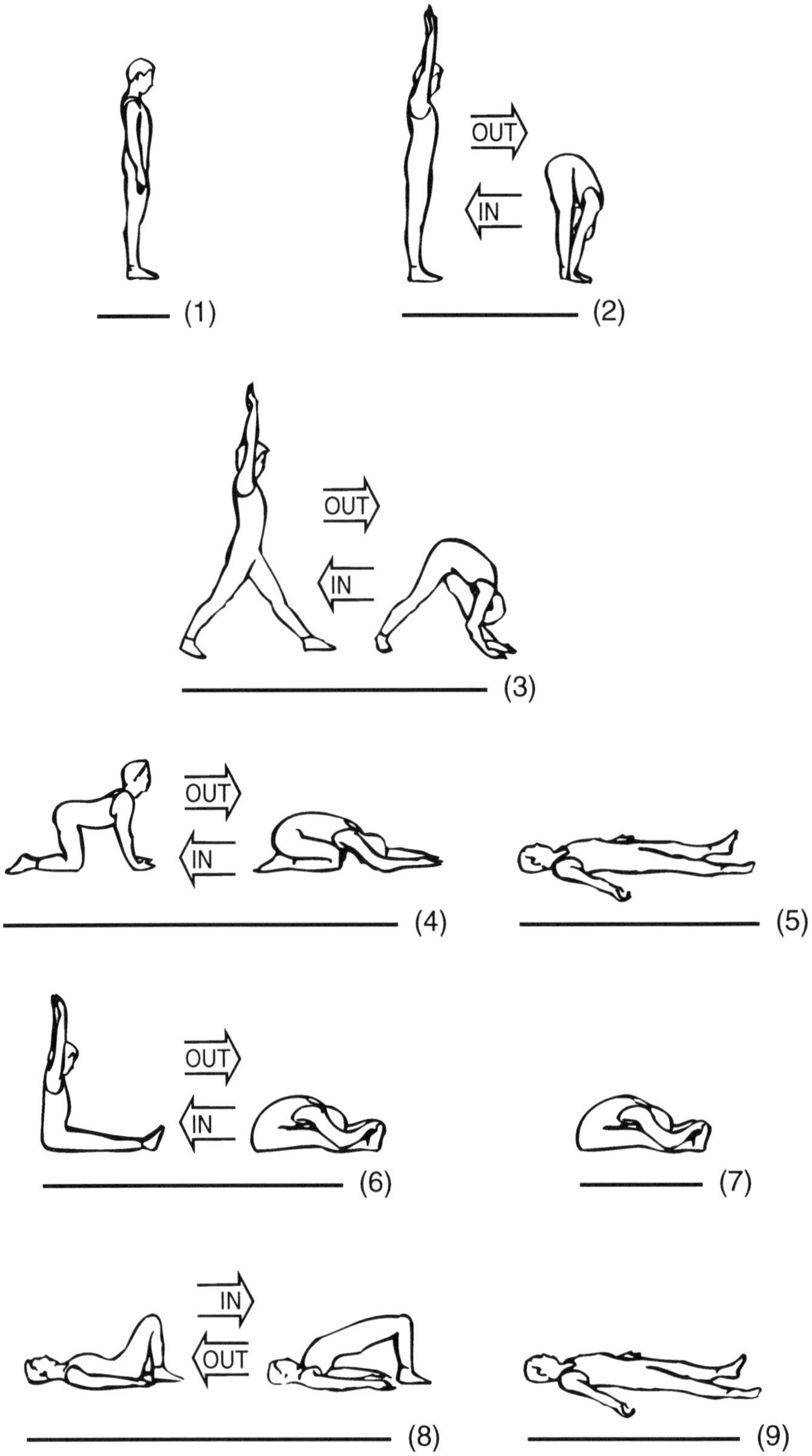

Figure 13: A sequence of warm-up exercises and counterposes for paśсimatānāsana.

Figure 13 shows a short sequence for approaching paśćimatānāsana, the seated forward bend. We start in samasthiti, the standing pose (1), to make contact with the body and breath. We then warm up by practicing uttānāsana (2) dynamically, repeating the sequence several times; this forward bend is the first preparation for paśćimatānāsana. We then practice pārśva uttānāsana (3), repeating the posture four times, beginning with holding for one breath, then two, then three, and finally four breaths. Then change sides and repeat. In this way we can gradually increase the stretch in the legs. As a counterpose for the work in the legs we then perform a dynamic version of cakravākāsana (4), so that we do not take any tension into the next posture. Then rest a while in śavāsana (5).

Now we are ready to practice the main āsana, paśćimatānāsana (6). We first practice it dynamically, in preparation for the static posture and as an aid for feeling the part the breath plays in this exercise: we stretch upward as we breathe in and bend forward as we breathe out. One possible way of working in the posture is to feel the movement of the inhalation in the back as we straighten it, then feel the movement of the belly toward the spine as we breathe out, bending forward without losing the extension. After practicing paśćimatānāsana dynamically, we stay in the pose for several breaths (7), paying attention to both body and breath.

Dvipāda pītham (8) can be used as a counterpose to the seated forward bend, in order to open the hips and compensate for the powerful forward bend. The practice of this āsana would finish with a long rest in śavāsana (9).

The next sequence of āsanas gives an example of a gentle practice for backward-bending postures. Without preparations and counterposes, back bends can lead to cramps, pain, and other problems. The sequence of āsanas shown in figure 14 gives good preparation and resolution exercises for the backward-bending pose śalabhāsana (locust pose).

All of the exercises in this sequence are practiced dynamically. The warm-up (1) is a simple exercise to link the breath with the movement. Yet the back is already being gently exercised, as moving the arms upward causes a slight movement in the spine. A variation of apānāsana (2) follows, to help loosen the lower back. Then the gentle back bend of the first exercise is repeated but in the slightly different form of lying with knees bent (3).

Dvipāda pītham (4) is a more powerful exercise. We must be very careful in this āsana to go just a little higher with each inhale. The back certainly has to work here, although it is assisted by the legs. Dvipāda pītham is followed by a short rest (5). A variation of cakravākāsana (6) can release tensions in the back that may have come with doing dvipāda pītham.

We prepare the back further with a simple variation of bhujaṅgāsana (7). Finally, we are ready to practice a simple variation of śalabhāsana (8). The back now has to support the legs as well as the trunk. It has been made ready by all the exercises preceding this one.

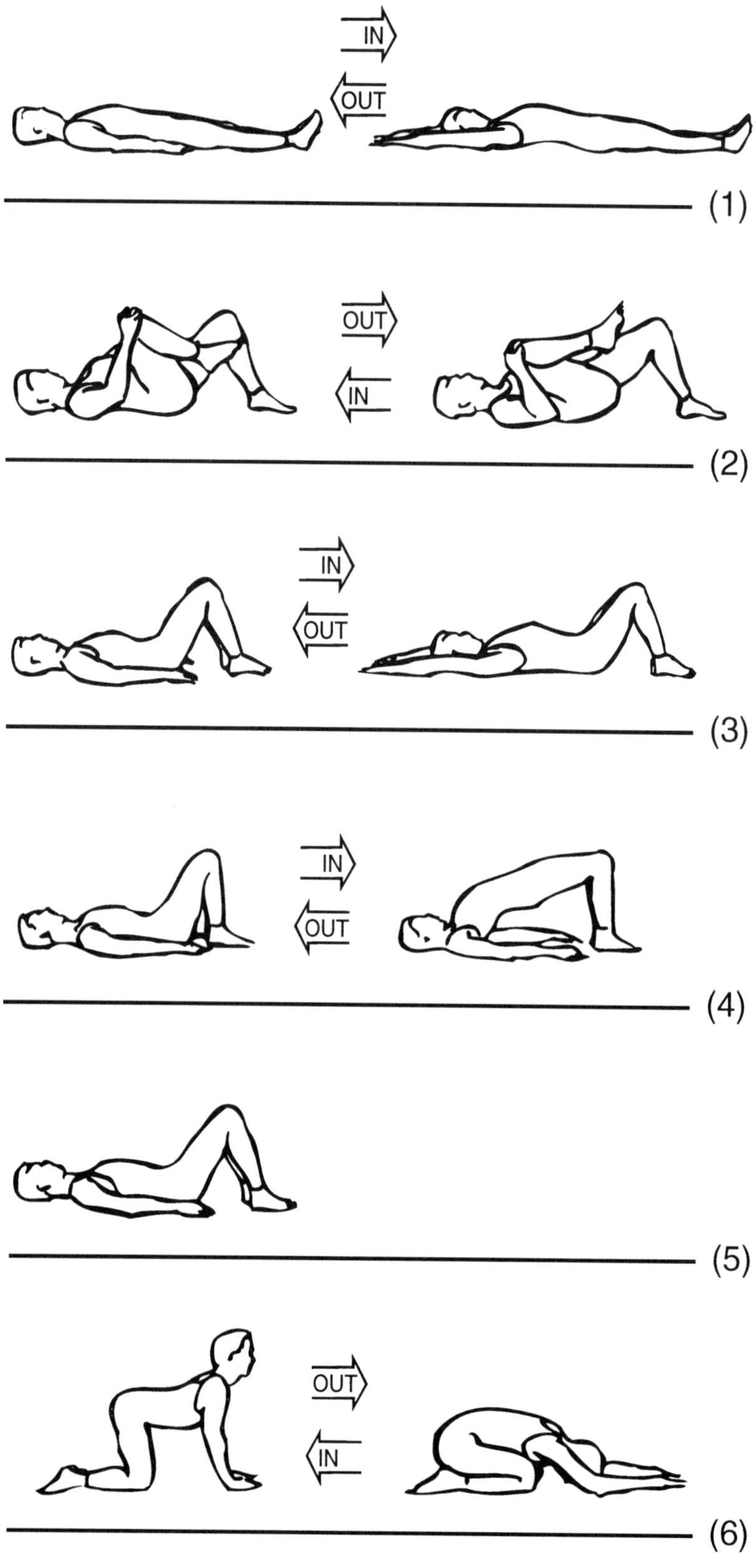

Figure 14a: A sequence of warm-up exercises and counterposes for śalabhāsana.

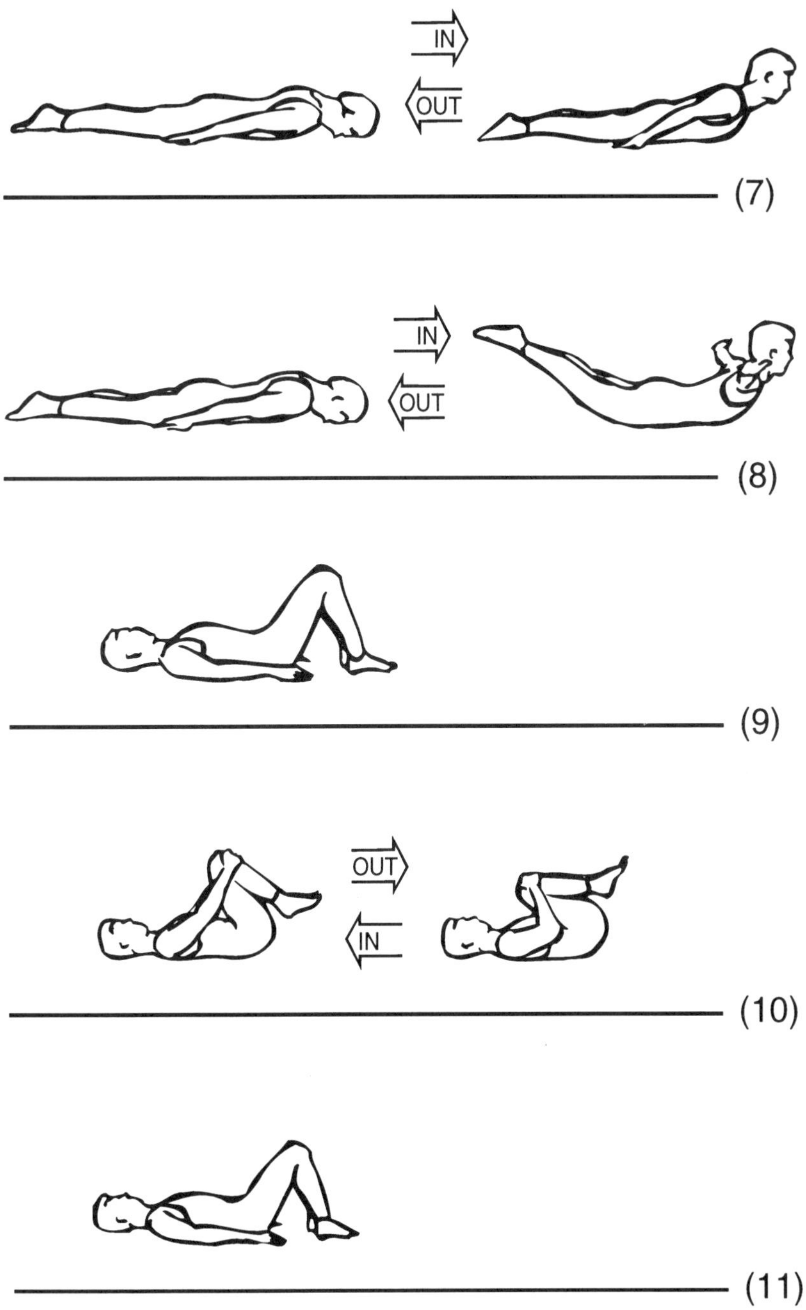

Figure 14b:
A sequence of warm-up exercises and counterposes for śalabhāsana.

After śalabhāsana we have another short rest, with knees bent and feet on the floor (9), to relieve the back. A pratikriyāsana or counterpose for śalabhāsana is apānāsana (10), which relaxes the lower back. The sequence ends with a rest (11).

The Breath

The inhalation and the exhalation can be emphasized in various ways in āsana practice. We can divide the breath into four parts:

- the inhalation
- the exhalation
- the retention after inhalation
- the retention after exhalation

We use breath retention in our āsana practice to intensify the effects of a posture. Let us suppose we are bothered by a feeling of heaviness in the abdominal region and have decided to practice the seated forward bend to help us feel lighter. We can practice the āsana in its simplest form, that is, dynamically, with a slow breath rhythm. Or we might also bend forward on the exhalation as usual, contracting the abdomen as we do, but instead of coming up again right away, we might stay in that position and hold the breath for a few seconds. Holding the breath after exhalation intensifies the effects of the āsana on the abdominal region. Conversely, holding the breath after inhalation in certain āsanas intensifies the effects in the chest region. As a working rule, the following principles apply in our yoga practice:

- an emphasis on long inhalation and holding the breath after inhalation intensifies the effects of the posture in the chest area
- an emphasis on long exhalation and holding the breath after exhalation intensifies the effects of the posture in the abdominal area
- the forward-bending poses lend themselves to holding the breath following exhalation, while the backward-bending poses lend themselves to holding the breath following inhalation

The practice of lengthening the exhalation or holding the breath after exhalation is called *laṅghana* in Sanskrit, meaning "to fast" or "to reduce." Laṅghana supports the elimination processes and has a cleansing effect on the body by enlivening the organs, especially the organs in the abdominal region. So, for example, if someone has a problem in the area below the diaphragm, it could benefit them to do a laṅghana practice.

The practice of lengthening the inhalation or holding the breath after inhalation is called *bṛmhaṇa*, which best translates as "to expand." Bṛmhaṇa practice has the effect of energizing and heating the body. A bṛmhaṇa element should be introduced into the practice of a student who lacks energy. The ability to lengthen the exhale should be achieved before introducing bṛmhaṇa, as too much fire without elimination can create disturbing patterns of energy. To receive that which is new (fresh energy), we must first release what is old and no longer benefits us.

Figure 15 shows the principles of laṅghana and bṛmhaṇa applied to āsanas. The warrior pose or vīrabhadrāsana (1) is, by its very nature, an āsana that works in a bṛmhana way. Practiced with a long inhalation, perhaps followed by a short breath retention, it will work even more profoundly in an expansive direction. The seated forward bend (2) is an āsana to which the principle of laṅghana naturally applies. Through a deliberate and slow exhalation, possibly followed by holding the breath, the effect of the āsana is intensified.

There is one very important rule to follow: if holding the breath reduces the duration of your next inhale or exhale, stop. You are not ready for this practice and can work up to it instead.

In terms of the circulatory system, the breath should never be held if there is a sudden increase in the pulse rate. Heartbeat and respiration are interdependent and if the breathing is poor, the pulse increases. There are psychological reasons for this rule too; many people are very nervous about their hearts and a rapid increase in their pulse rate might cause anxiety. The guiding principle is that holding the breath should never make us uneasy, but rather we should be able to quietly observe the quality of our breathing.

The principles of laṅghana and bṛmhaṇa can be used to good advantage only with appropriate knowledge and understanding. They must never be applied without careful consideration of particular circumstances. I shall go into this in more detail when we discuss prāṇāyāma.

About Resting

Now a few words on something else that is important in the way we plan our yoga practice: rest between āsanas. We must of course rest whenever we become out of breath or are no longer able to control our breath. But even if our breathing remains quiet and regular, certain parts of the body may become tired or perhaps sore and we must rest them as well. Also, if we have decided to practice an āsana twelve times and we feel exhausted after the sixth time, then we must stop immediately and go into stillness. There is one rule to follow regarding rest: if we need a rest, we take one.

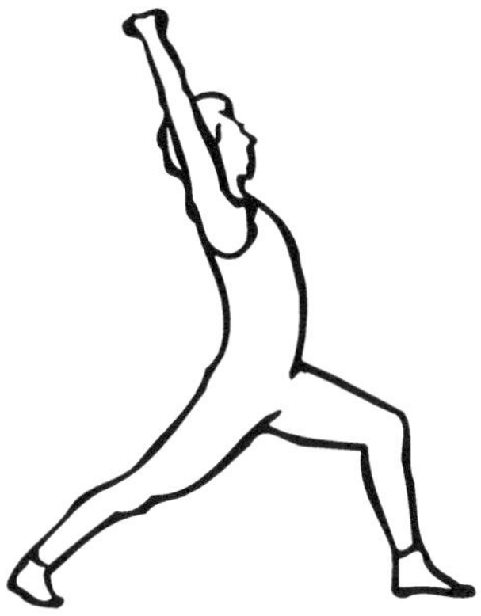

Figure 15: Bṛmhaṇa—expansive breath retention—in the warrior pose (1); laṅghana—contractive breath retention—in the seated forward bend (2).

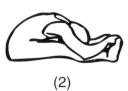

We also take a rest as a way of making a transition between one kind of āsana and another. For instance, it is essential to rest between an intense back bend such as a dhanurāsana and a powerful forward bend such as a paśicimatānāsana. We must give ourselves this rest even if we do not feel the need for it. The rest gives us the opportunity to feel the effects of the posture and allows the muscles time to return to their balanced tone. If we do not rest after doing dhanurāsana, as in our example, we may overwork the back in the following forward bend. To avoid this, we must rest and observe the reaction of our muscles and whole body.

Let me give you another example. Many people feel good while they are performing a headstand, but when they lie down afterward they notice a pressure in the chest. We know that when we stand on the head the weight of the abdomen is on the chest and compresses the ribs, though we might not feel pressure until we rest. The feeling in the chest is only the reaction of the ribs and will be relieved by resting before performing the counterpose. Generally one should rest between one intense pose and an equally demanding counterpose, such as with the headstand and the shoulderstand. However, if the counterpose is very simple you can go directly into it without a break.

A period of rest is also needed before practicing prāṇāyāma. In prāṇāyāma our attention is directed primarily toward the breath, while during āsana practice our breathing depends on the various physical exercises. Because the āsanas require us to pay attention to the body, it is good to rest afterward and prepare ourselves mentally for prāṇāyāma. How long we will rest before prāṇāyāma will depend on how many āsanas we have just practiced. If we have been doing āsanas for fifteen minutes, then two or three minutes of rest will do; if we have been practicing for an hour or more, we should rest for at least five minutes before going into prāṇāyāma.

While I have been giving you examples of sequences for the full practice of certain āsanas, including warm-ups and counterposes, it is important to recognize that a book can never match the qualities of a good teacher. The best way toward self-discovery and gaining greater insight into your own body and mind through yoga is to seek the advice of a teacher.

The practice of yoga is essentially a practice of self-examination. Āsanas and prāṇāyama can help us discover certain things about ourselves, but unfortunately we cannot always trust our own perceptions. Our habitual way of seeing things makes it difficult for us to look at them differently from experience to experience; our habitual way of seeing limits our self-understanding. Because a teacher's perception is not limited by our unique conditioning, he or she can often see what capacities lie hidden in us.

Books on yoga begin at different levels. A person with little experience in yoga would have a difficult time choosing the āsanas best suited to his or her condition. A good teacher is important for finding out which postures are most useful, and on which ones the student needs guidance. A teacher helps us in getting to know ourselves and inspires us to do the work toward greater self-discovery. A book can support the encouragement that comes from the teacher.

For the purpose of introducing Krishnamacharya's yoga teachings to a wide audience, I have chosen to write this book. The āsana sequences I describe of course do not take into account any one individual's personal needs. You must tailor these general sequences to suit your goals.

People often ask whether there is a general sequence of āsanas suitable for anyone to follow. Yes, we can think about the order of āsanas in a general way. To simplify things, let's ignore the fact that yoga practice must be geared to a particular person and his or her individual needs, and therefore can never follow a general plan absolutely. Let us for the time being forget about the fact that certain āsanas require particular preparation or counterposes for certain people or that a sequence of āsanas has to allow for rests now and then. We have already discussed these thoroughly. Let us shift the focus of our attention to the way we can group the āsanas according to the position of the body relative to the earth and to the basic movement of the spine.

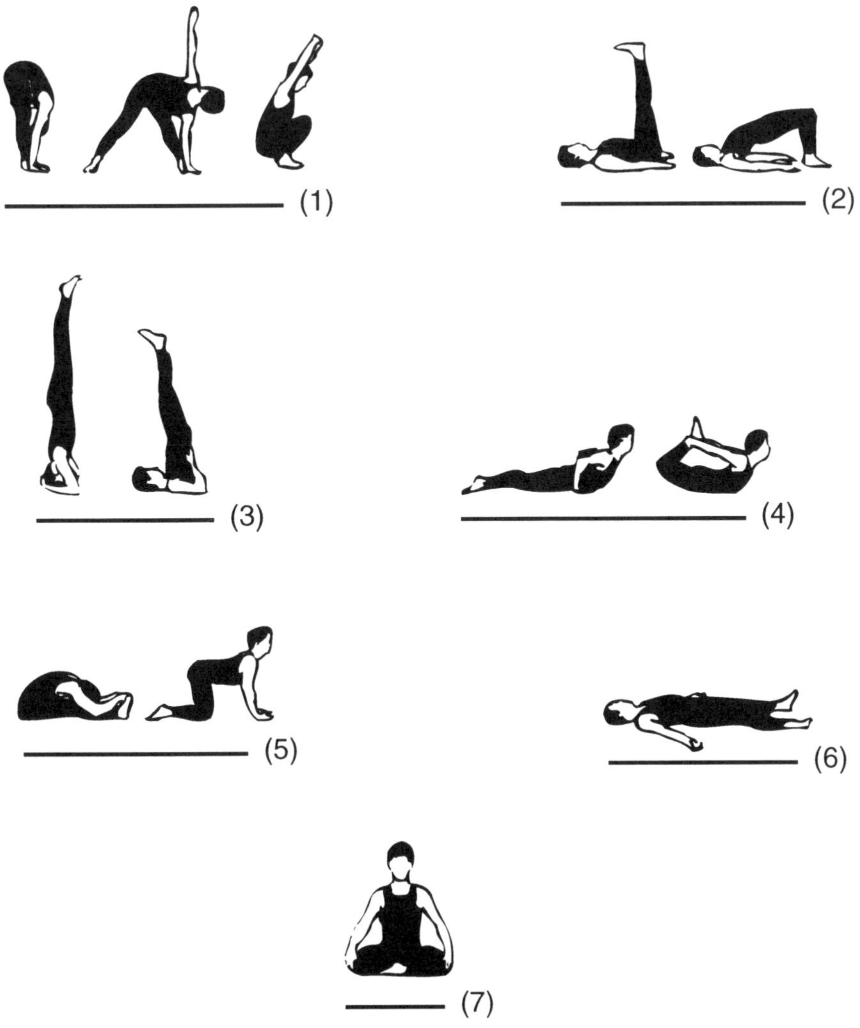

Figure 16: For general purposes the āsanas can be practiced in the following sequence: standing exercises to warm up with (1); exercises lying on the back (2); inverted postures (3); exercises lying on the belly (4); exercises in a sitting or kneeling position (5); a rest lying on the back (6), and breathing exercises, which are normally done in a sitting position (7). This outline does not consider any preparation for strenuous āsanas or the counterposes and rests required.

We can divide the āsanas into standing postures, those performed lying on the back, inverted postures, those performed lying on the stomach (back bends), and finally, sitting and kneeling postures. Which of these āsanas should we choose and what order might be sensible?

Figure 16 illustrates some postures suggested in this general sequence. At the start of our practice we need exercises that warm us up, make us supple, and use the whole body. Standing āsanas are best for this. They are suitable for loosening up all the joints, including the ankles, knees, hips, spine, shoulders, neck and, to a certain extent, the wrists as well. There are people who often have problems in the hips, knees, and ankles, and other people who for various reasons are not able to begin in a standing position. The majority of us, however, should spend five or ten minutes warming up with standing āsanas.

The exercises with which we begin our practice should also help us to experience and observe the state of our body and breath. The start of our practice should be designed so that we can find out about our physical and mental states in a simple and risk-free manner. Simple standing postures afford us this opportunity.

After doing the standing postures it is a good idea to lie on your back and practice āsanas in this position, which are also useful preparation for the inverted postures to come. The inverted postures help counter the effects of gravity on the body and are also very important for inner cleansing. Furthermore, the well-known inverted postures such as the headstand and the shoulderstand put us in positions that are completely opposite to our normal daily positioning. These postures allow us the opportunity to discover new and previously unknown aspects of ourselves.

After the inverted postures comes a group of āsanas performed lying on the belly—these are all back bends. Some of these āsanas are excellent counterposes for certain inverted postures; for example, the cobra harmonizes the effects of the shoulderstand and is often used as its counterpose.

This general sequence of āsanas can be concluded with some exercises in a sitting or kneeling position. Then, after an adequate rest, we can practice prāṇāyāma and other exercises that require an upright position. Appendix 2 shows four general practice sequences that can be tailored to fit individual needs.

Figure 17 shows a good sequence of āsanas practiced as minimum preparation for prāṇāyāma. Uttānāsana (1) can be practiced as a warm-up. To prepare the back and neck and to experience the quality of our breath, we could then practice dvipāda pītham (2). Cakravākāsana (3) opens the chest and back. A rest lying on the back (4) concludes the āsana practice. Then some of us might choose the simple cross-legged position (sukhāsana) (5) in which to practice prāṇāyāma. Others for whom this is uncomfortable might be better off sitting on a chair. Nothing is lost by sitting on a chair and the quality of breathing in prāṇāyāma is not adversely affected.

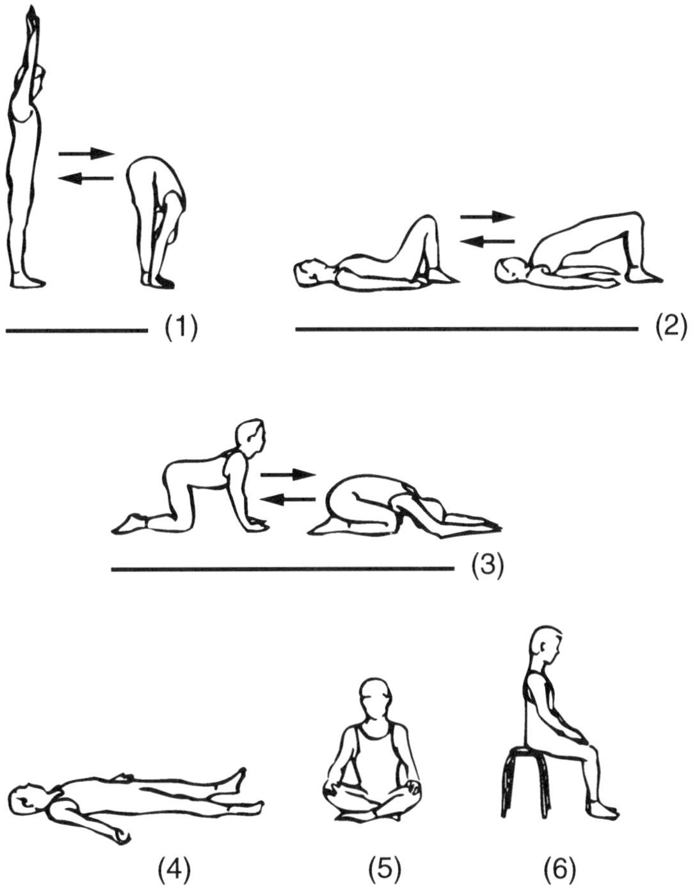

Figure 17: Āsanas in preparation for prāṇāyāma.

If we are planning to work with certain breathing patterns such as predetermined lengths of inhalation and exhalation or breath retention, then āsanas such as these have the added advantage of putting us in touch with our breath before we begin our prāṇāyāma practice.

Just as the practice of specific āsanas is dependent on the student's needs and goals, so is the time of day chosen for our practice dependent on what is possible. The one rule to follow in this respect is to wait two or three hours following a meal to begin yoga practice. Practicing on an empty stomach is best, so for those who have a flexible daily schedule, the best time for practice is before breakfast.

Our practice has to be developed daily, taking into account our free time, our goals, and our needs. We must always plan our practice as a unit, irrespective of whether the time available is short or long, so that the session is always made up of a balanced group of exercises. (If there is danger of being interrupted or running out of time during your practice, then it's better to plan a short sequence of āsanas.) Through adhering to the principle of viṅyāsa krama, we construct a gradual and intelligent course for our yoga practice that helps us meet our goals.

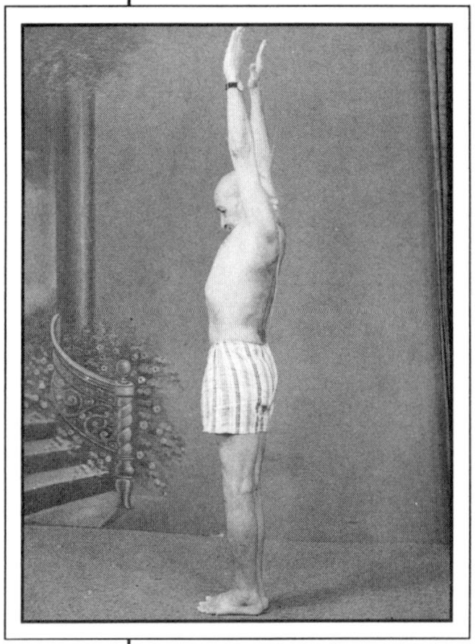

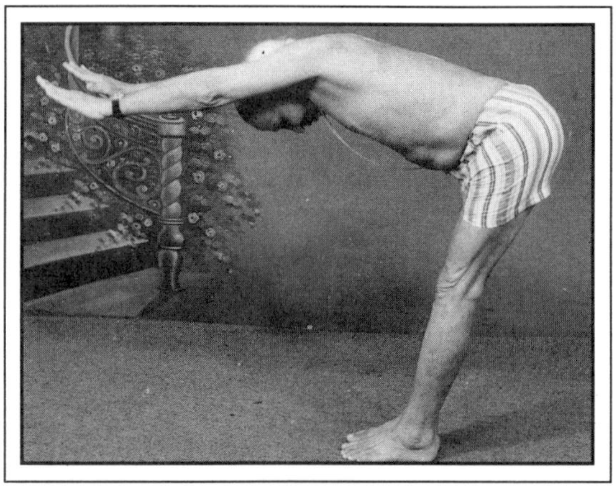

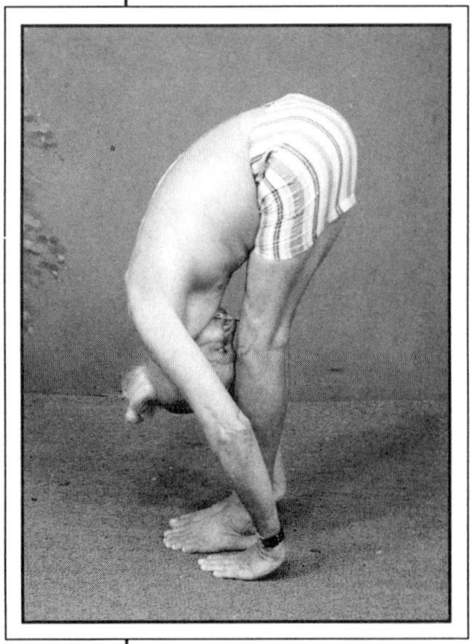

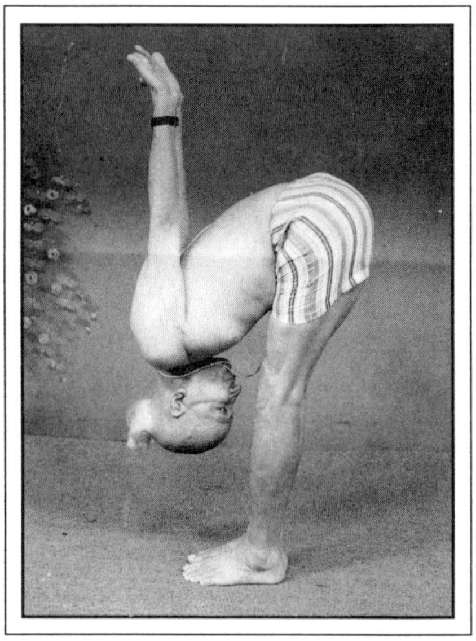

Krishnamacharya performing uttanāsana.

5

Āsana Variations

I have already stated that āsanas can be practiced in various ways. I should now like to discuss the possibilities for varying certain āsanas and discuss why you might do this.

One reason we work with āsana variations is to extend our physical capabilities. Most people begin a yoga practice with the expectation of achieving certain results. You might wish to strengthen your back, cure yourself of asthma, free yourself from pain, or simply feel more energetic. These particular goals are achieved by practicing the āsanas in various ways. For instance, someone with a stiff shoulder would adapt particular āsanas to address that lack of mobility. Someone dealing with asthma would perform āsana variations that focused on opening the chest and lengthening the breath cycle. Āsana variations help us achieve maximum gain with minimum effort by intelligently addressing our physical needs.

The other important reason for practicing āsana variations is to encourage attentiveness. If we practice the same āsanas over and over again for a long stretch of time, they can easily become mere routine, even if the choice of āsanas and breathing exercises is well planned and designed specifically for our condition and goals. Our attention to what we are doing steadily diminishes with this kind of unbroken repetition, and boredom sets in. Varying the āsanas renews attention and opens our senses to new experiences. Attention is the state of being in which we are fully present to what we are doing, enabling us to feel all that is happening in our bodies. Being in the state of open attention creates the opportunity for experiencing something we have never felt before. If we do not work with variations and instead repeat the same postures over and over again, we lose this opportunity for new experiences. Staying alert and constantly discovering new awarenesses are essential features of a correct āsana practice. The proper practice of āsanas requires our mind to be fully focused; this is automatically achieved by arousing interest and attentiveness through new experiences.

Ways of Varying an Āsana

Varying the Form

The simplest way to vary an āsana is to alter its form. Figure 18 shows several different variations of uttānāsana.

Figure 18: Three possible variations of uttānāsana.

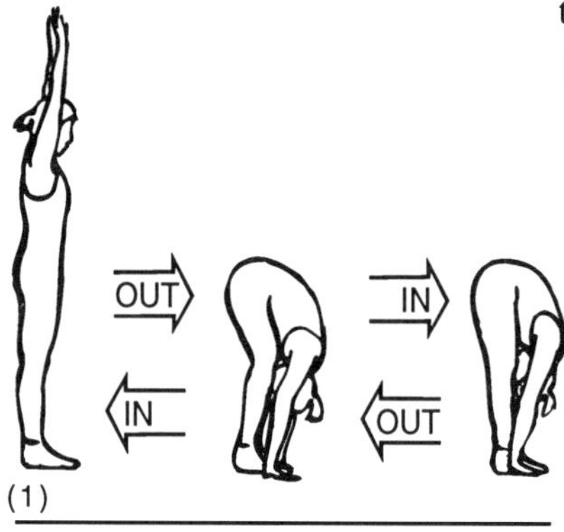

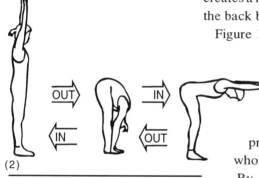

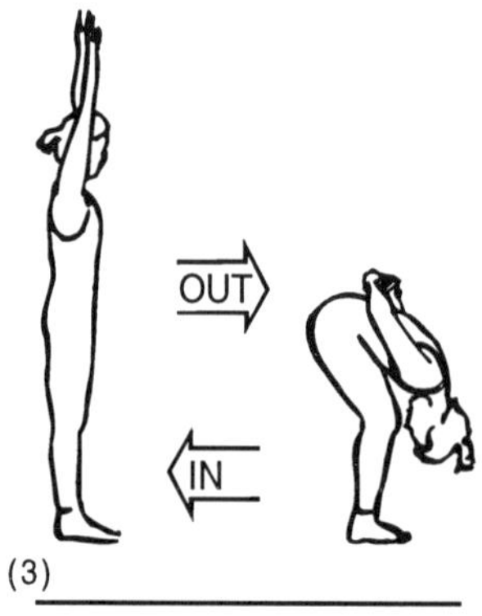

One possibility for varying uttānāsana after bending forward is to straighten the legs as you breathe in and then bend them slightly as you breathe out (1), making the legs work harder. The stretch in the legs can be made even more intense by placing some padding under the toes and ball of the foot. Practicing uttānāsana in this way puts a lot of strain on the lower back and is therefore considered risky for some people. Know your limitations before choosing such variations.

If we want to strengthen the back with the help of uttānāsana, we bend fully through the exhale, then come up halfway again as we breathe in (2). The legs remain slightly bent so that the whole back is worked only moderately.

In a third variation of uttānāsana we bend fully through the exhale, then clasp the hands behind the lower back and bend the legs (3). This variation creates a lot of movement in the lower back but reduces the risk of overworking the back by bending the legs.

Figure 19 shows several variations of śalabhāsana. For many people the classic form of śalabhāsana (1) is too demanding to be useful, yet because it is a very effective and efficient āsana, it is a fitting addition to most yoga practices. Adaptation of classic śalabhāsana can be chosen to meet the requirements and strength of each person. The important point in choosing variations is to practice within your capacity while keeping the breath linked to the whole body, regardless of whether the body is moving or stationary.

By varying the arm and leg movements in śalabhāsana, you can intensify or reduce the work in the back, the abdomen, and the chest. For example, by placing the hands at the base of the ribs (2) and inhaling into the back bend with alternating leg movements, the work in the lower back, abdomen, and chest will be reduced while encouraging a significant arch in the upper back. Raising both legs and the chest on the inhale (3) will deepen the effect in the lower back and abdomen while still allowing for a significant arch in the upper back and chest. Raising the opposite arm and leg (4) will strengthen, balance and integrate the two sides of the body. As we strengthen we can use the arms to intensify the effect in the lower and upper back. Raising the arms to shoulder height (5) strengthens the neck and shoulder muscles and encourages their integration with the muscles of the back. This variation should be practiced only when there is sufficient arch in the upper back.

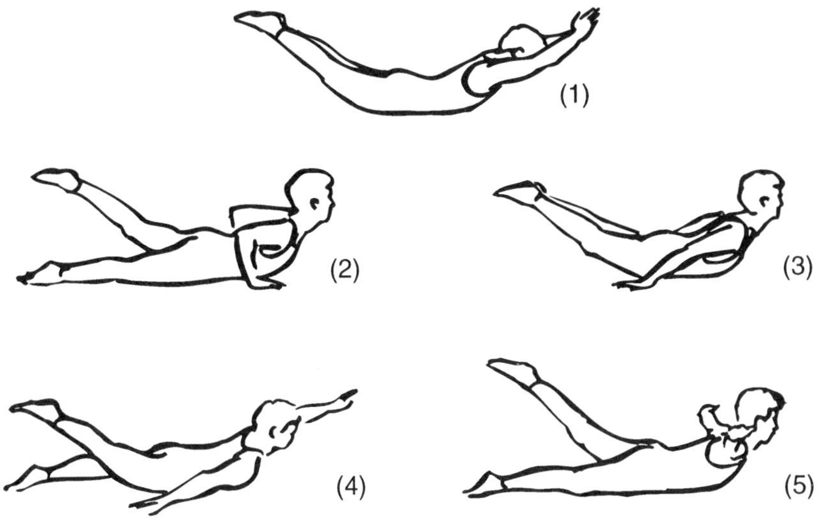

Figure 19: Variations of śalabhāsana.

In śalabhāsana, retaining the breath following the inhale is very strengthening. Śalabhāsana itself will facilitate a deep exhale and retention after exhale. Each variation in body and breath will change the effect and function of the āsana in specific ways. In all the variations shown here, the legs, arms, and forehead can return to the floor on the exhale. Or you may choose to exhale in the raised position, which will deeply work the abdominal region.

A person with stiff legs is not restricted from enjoying the benefits of the classic form of paścimatānāsana, shown in figure 20, step (1). For example, bending the knees on the exhale (3) will deepen the forward bend. Indra Devi, a very accomplished yogini and my father's first Western student, told me this is how my father first taught her paścimatānāsana, adapting the classic pose for her needs. Raising the seat (4) will also allow for a deeper bend. Variations of the arm positions such as are shown in examples 2 and 5 will work the upper back and shoulders while assisting to deepen the āsana. You should not, however, use the muscles in the arms to attempt to intensify the forward bend.

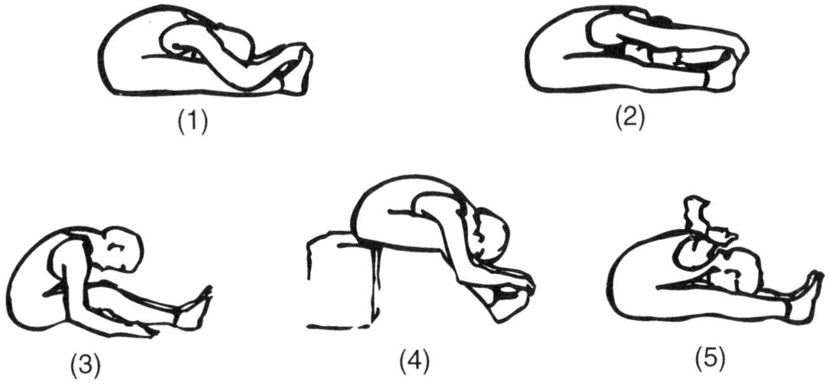

Figure 20: Variations of paścimatānāsana.

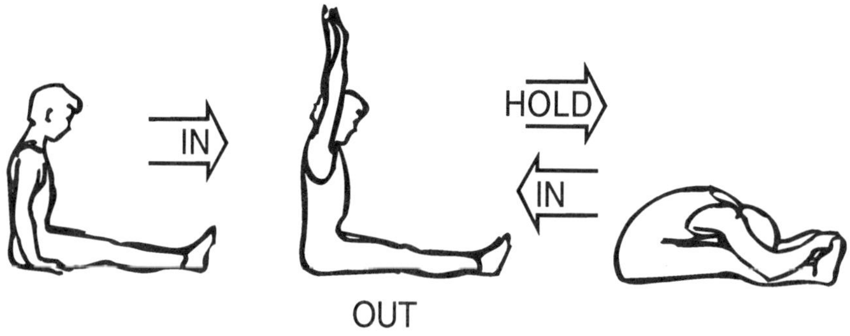

Figure 21: Varying the breath in paścimatānāsana.

This should instead occur without force, the movement linked to the exhaled breath. The forward bend can be intensified on the exhale and relaxed on the inhale so that the body's natural elasticity is enhanced with the breath.

There are a great many āsana variations such as these. Each time we practice a variation, the effect of the āsana, and consequently our attention, is directed toward different areas or needs. Āsana variations are not just for people with specific physical problems. They can help all yoga practitioners remain open to discovery.

Varying the Breath

Another way to vary an āsana is to alter the breathing. For example, instead of freely inhaling and exhaling we can direct the breath so that the inhalation and exhalation are of the same duration, or we might choose to hold the breath.

Normally we coordinate each movement with either an inhalation or an exhalation. Sometimes, however, it is useful to move while holding the breath. Remember: if we want to increase the effect of the āsana in the chest area, we concentrate on the inhalation; if we want to increase the effect on the abdomen and lower back, we concentrate on the exhale. So to vary the breath in paścimatānāsana, a pose that naturally works on the belly and lower back, we breathe in as we raise our arms, then hold this pose as we breathe out. Then without breathing in, we bend forward and pause (see figure 21). In this way we intensify the effect of the exhalation. Inhale to come back to the seated position, arms overhead. This sequence can be repeated as many times as an easy breath rhythm can be maintained.

Holding the breath after the inhale intensifies the effects through the chest area, and can be used to good advantage in such postures as bhujaṅgāsana.

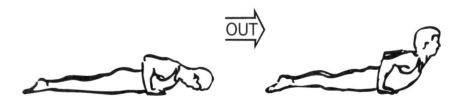

Figure 22: Varying the breath in bhujaṅgāsana.

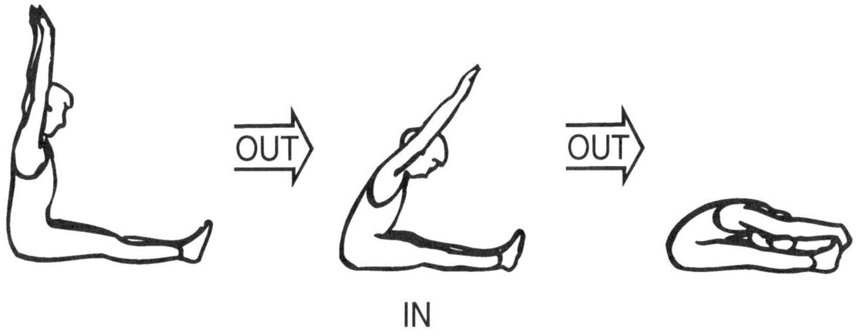

Figure 23: Practicing paśćimatānāsana in steps.

Another interesting variation to work with is reversing the normal breathing pattern. For example, in bhujaṅgāsana we would raise the upper body on the exhalation instead of on the inhalation (see figure 22). Many people use the belly more than the back muscles to push themselves up into bhujaṅgāsana. Breathing out contracts the abdomen and so doesn't allow it to be used in this way. Raising the upper body on the exhale will make the pose feel very different.

Once we know our own capacities for holding the breath with comfort, we can be imaginative with the way we use the breath. Suppose we want to focus our āsana practice to bring attention to the upper back. We would then choose postures such as bhujaṅgāsana or śalabhāsana that work this area, and at the same time focus on the inhalation in the breath cycle. We might practice making each inhalation longer than the one before. Or we might hold the breath after inhalation, which will increase the volume of air in the lungs and expand the chest.

Variations serve two purposes: to address a particular need and to create attentiveness. Holding the breath following the inhale or exhale can increase tension in the body. If you feel this happening, bring your awareness to the place where the tension is gathering. If the tension does not dissipate with awareness, slowly come out of the āsana.

Varying the Rhythm

Many āsanas can take on a new quality if we break them up into steps (krama). Figure 23 shows paśćimatānāsana practiced in this way. On the first exhale we bend only half the way forward. Staying there, we inhale and stretch the back. On the second exhalation we bend forward completely. Practicing in this way not only makes a difference in our quality of attention; it also changes the way we arrive in the final position and hold it.

Varying the Preparation

Variations are possible not just in the āsanas themselves but also in the preparations we make for them. The exercises we practice before a particular āsana can make a difference as to what we experience and where we feel the effects of the āsana. Oftentimes people will say that they did not feel anything after doing a particular āsana. If they do not feel any sensation in their muscles then they think nothing has happened. In situations like this it is helpful to change the preparation for that āsana, choosing one that moves the body in the exact opposite direction. Paying attention to the effects of both āsanas will give you a new certainty that something is really happening.

Varying the Sphere of Attention

While we are practicing an āsana we have the opportunity to direct our attention to different parts of the body. This can improve the quality of our āsana practice considerably.

Figure 24 shows two possibilities for where to place our attention in the practice of bhujaṅgāsana. We can direct our attention to the upper part of the back which is opening up as we breathe in (1), or we might direct our attention toward keeping the legs and knees on the floor (2). When beginners practice this āsana they often raise the legs off the floor as they raise the upper body. By attempting to keep the legs on the floor, the quality of work in the back is intensified.

We introduce the art of variation to bring something new and beneficial into our āsana practice. In a class I would recommend to some people that they stretch their legs fully and to others that they do the same āsana with bent knees. I would advise some to hold the breath after inhalation and others to hold their breath after exhalation. It is important to tailor your variations to match your particular needs.

Variations should never be introduced in a random way; they should only be introduced when they are warranted. We do them when we need help developing or sustaining attention, or as an aid to a particular physical need.

Respecting Classic Āsanas

It is important to understand that behind every yoga posture lies a principle; if we do not know or understand this principle we will not be able to perform the āsana or variations of it in the proper way. A teacher who respects the classic postures can help us recognize the principles they embody. What does this āsana mean? What is its purpose? What does it demand of us? Only when we have come to understand the underlying principles can we do variations of an āsana.

For example, paścimatānāsana, the seated forward bend, is a pose in which

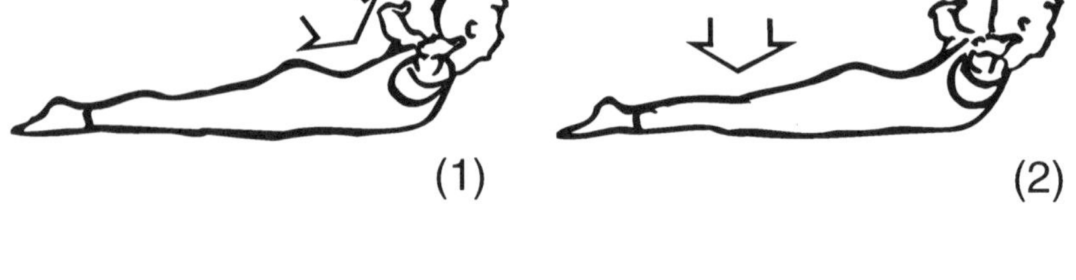

Figure 24: Shifting the sphere of attention in bhujaṅgāsana.

we sit with the legs stretched out in front of us and grasp the feet with the hands, bringing the head down toward the shins. *Paścimatānāsana* translates as "the stretching of the west," because in India we traditionally face the east when we pray or practice āsanas; in that position our back is facing west. So the real purpose of the āsana is to facilitate the movement of the breath in the back. A person practicing paścimatānāsana should be aware of the *paścimatāna* effect felt in the back of the body—not at the level of skin or muscles but *within*, at the level of the breath. Practicing paścimatānāsana means allowing the breath to flow along the back of the body.[1] It is not simply a matter of stretching the tissues, but rather of experiencing the feeling of the breath flowing through the spine.

Uṣṭrāsana, the camel pose, is a back bend performed from a kneeling position. With hands resting on the feet, the thighs are raised to vertical, as in kneeling, while the chest expands and opens on each inhalation. The principle of this pose is to facilitate the movement of breath into the chest. Space is created in the chest by stretching the intercostal muscles in the pose, and the whole front of the body is opened up. The pose allows the feeling of the breath to be experienced down the entire frontal line of the body.

"The feeling of the breath" refers to the feeling of energy or prāṇa moving in the body. The principle underlying each classic āsana has a particular implication to the movement of prāṇa in the body. A teacher who understands āsana from the point of view of whole-body feeling and the movement of prāṇa can adopt classic āsanas to the needs of each student. The student thus enjoys and benefits from the principle that is inherent to each particular posture.

The key to right practice and the appropriate variations of an āsana is to maintain the link between breath and body. Via the breath we can be with the whole body and observe the unfolding of an āsana. Rather than struggling with the body in an āsana, we monitor the āsana with the number of breaths and the breath ratio (inhale, pause, exhale, pause) that is appropriate for us. If the breath is smooth and has continuity, the āsana will be beneficial.

The breath is one of the means by which we vary āsanas. There is a natural elasticity in the body that is enhanced as we breathe in āsana practice. As the body moves the breath moves, and as the breath is stationary the body is stationary. Thus the breath and body become one movement, one process, and that is a very powerful yoga. Maintaining this link between breath and body, particularly in lengthening the exhale and pausing after the exhale, has more significance to the purpose of yoga than achieving a classic āsana for its own sake. The breath has a very important role in āsana practice. We should not compromise the easy flow of the breath to achieve the āsana.

The breath is one of the best means for observing yourself in your yoga practice. How does the body respond to the breath, and how does the breath respond to the movement of the body? The breath should be your teacher.

1. *Haṭha Yoga Pradīpikā* 1.29.

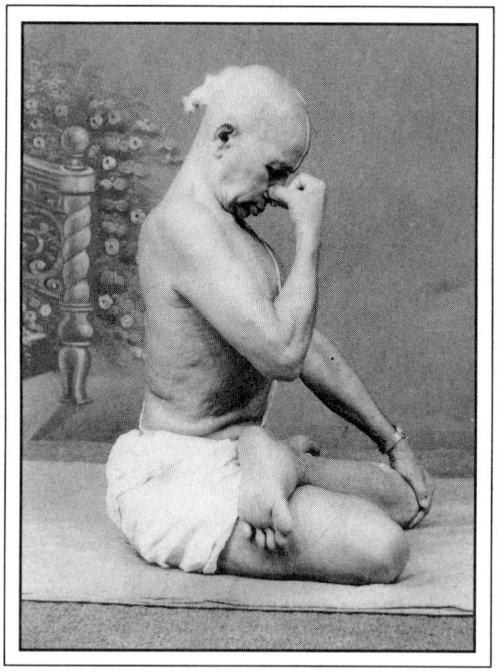

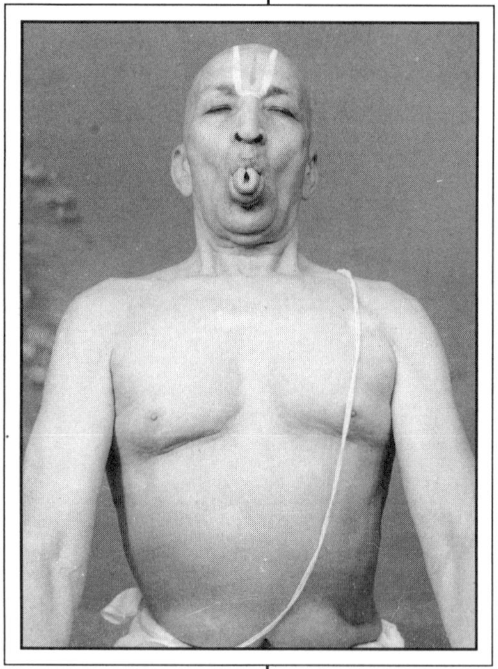

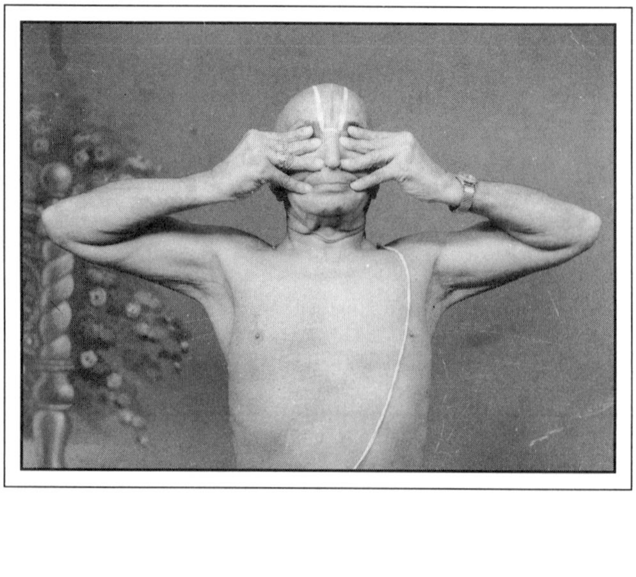

Krishnamacharya demonstrating nāḍī śodhana prāṇāyāma (top), śītalī prāṇāyāma (middle), and ṣaṇmukhi mudrā.

6

Prāṇāyāma

Yoga recommends two possible ways for achieving the qualities of sukha, comfort and lightness, and sthira, steady alertness. The first is to locate knots and resistances in the body and release them. This happens only gradually (krama) as we employ the concept of viṅyāsa krama—giving due consideration to correct preparation and appropriate counterposes as we practice. The means we use to release blocks and resistances must not adversely affect the body. We must proceed carefully. If we force the body we will experience pain or other unpleasant feelings and the problems will, in the long run, get worse instead of better. The body can only gradually accept an āsana. It is by proceeding gently that we will feel light and be able to breathe easily in the position and therefore really benefit from it.

The second possible means for realizing the concept of sthirasukha consists of visualizing the perfect posture. For this we use the image of the cobra Ananta, the king of the serpents, carrying the whole universe on his head while providing a bed for the Lord Viṣṇu on his coiled body. Ananta must be completely relaxed in order to make a soft bed for the lord. This is the idea of sukha. Yet the snake cannot be feeble and weak; it must be strong and steady in order to support the universe. That is the idea of sthira. Together these qualities give us the image and the feeling of a perfect āsana.

There is a common misconception that āsanas are only positions for meditation. If we look at Vyasa's commentary on the *Yoga Sūtra* though, we see that most of the āsanas he lists there are so complicated that with the best will in the world we could not attain a state of dhyāna in them. We can work with these postures and experience what they feel like, but we cannot remain in them for long. It is clear that not all of the āsanas given there are intended for meditation. Many of the āsanas that we work with and those that are described in the various books on yoga are of quite a different sort. They are valuable because they enable us to sit upright and stand for long periods of time and to meet with greater ease the many demands made on us by our daily lives.

In the *Yoga Sūtra* there is another very interesting claim made about the effects of āsanas. It says that when we master āsanas we are able to handle opposites. To be able to handle opposites does not mean going around half-naked in cold weather or dressing in warm woolen clothing when it is hot. Rather, it means becoming more sensitive and learning to adapt because we know the body better; we can listen to it and know how it reacts in different situations.

Practically speaking, we should be able to stand for a few minutes with ease; we should be able to sit for a while easily as well. One advantage of āsana practice is that it helps us get used to different situations and be able to cope with different demands. If we want to practice prāṇāyāma, for example, we have to be able to sit comfortably erect for a period of time. Āsanas help us focus on the breath rather than the body during prāṇāyāma practice, for if we can sit comfortably and effortlessly erect there is nothing to distract us from our concentration on the breath.

Prāṇāyāma: The Breathing Exercises of Yoga

The word *prāṇāyāma* consists of two parts: *prāṇa* and *āyāma*. *Āyāma* means "stretch" or "extend," and describes the action of prāṇāyāma. Prāṇa refers to "that which is infinitely everywhere." With reference to us humans prāṇa can be described as something that flows continuously from somewhere inside us, filling us and keeping us alive: it is vitality. In this image, the prāṇa streams out from the center through the whole body.

Ancient texts such as the *Yoga Yājñavalkya* (see appendix 1) tell us that someone who is troubled, restless, or confused has more prāṇa outside the body than within. The amount of prāṇa outside the body is greater when we feel unwell; at those times the quality of prāṇa and its density within the body is reduced. Too little prāṇa in the body can be expressed as a feeling of being stuck or restricted. It can also show as a lack of drive or motivation to do anything; we are listless or even depressed. We may suffer from physical ailments when prāṇa is lacking in the body. And finally the *Yoga Sūtra* mentions disturbances in the breath, which can take very different forms.[1] On the other hand, the more peaceful and well-balanced we are, the less our prāṇa is dispersed outside the body. And if all the prāṇa is within the body, we are free of these symptoms.

If prāṇa does not find sufficient room in the body there can be only one reason: it is being forced out by something that really does not belong there—let's call it rubbish. What we are trying to do when we practice prāṇāyāma is nothing more than reduce this rubbish and so concentrate more and more prāṇa within the body.

Our state of mind is closely linked to the quality of prāṇa within. Because we can influence the flow of prāṇa through the flow of our breath, the quality of

1. In the *Yoga Sūtra* 1.31, Patañjali calls these symptoms of a disturbed mind *duḥkha* (the experience of suffering), *daurmanasya* (negative attitude), *aṅgamejayatva* (physical ailments), and *śvāsapraśvāsa* (breathing disturbances).

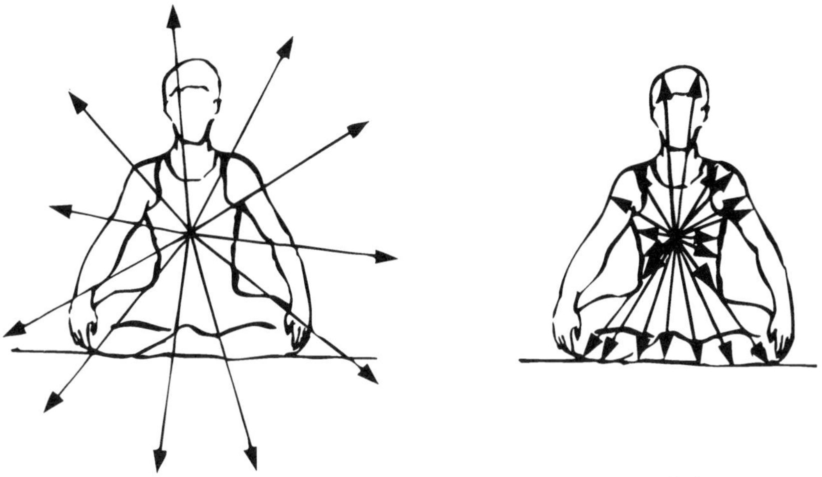

Figure 25: A sick or restless person disperses prāṇa beyond the body (1) because there are blocks hindering the flow of prāṇa within. A peaceful, healthy person keeps more prāṇa within the body (2).

our breath influences our state of mind and vice versa. In yoga we are trying to make use of these connections so that prāṇa concentrates and can freely flow within us.

Various sources call prāṇa the friend of the puruṣa (consciousness) and see in the flow of prāṇa nothing but the working of the puruṣa. If we remember how the degree of clarity created by the power of the puruṣa within us is directly linked to our state of mind, then a close connection between our mind and prāṇa is obvious.

Prāṇa can be understood as the expression of puruṣa, but it is to be found both inside and outside the body. See figure 25. The more content a person is and the better he or she feels, the more prāṇa is inside. The more disturbed a person is, the more prāṇa is dissipated and lost. One definition of the word *yogi* is "one whose prāṇa is all within his body." In prāṇāyāma we want to reduce the amount of prāṇa outside the body until there is none leaking out.

Whatever happens in the mind influences the breath; the breath becomes quicker when we are excited and deeper and quieter when we relax. In order to influence our prāṇa we must be able to influence the mind. Our actions often disturb the mind, causing prāṇa to exude from the body. Through daily prāṇāyāma practice we reverse this process, as a change in the breathing pattern influences the mind.

The idea of prāṇa existing within or beyond the body can be understood as a symbol for our state of mind. When the mind is as clear as transparent glass there is nothing that could disturb the body; there is no rubbish lying about. On the other hand, if we notice hesitancy, discontent, fear of doing something because it might be innapropriate, and so forth, we can assume that there are blockages in the system. These blockages do not just occur in the physical body; they exist even more in the mind, in consciousness. Every kind of rubbish we find in ourselves was originally produced by avidyā, that is, incorrect knowledge. The idea that yogis are people who carry all their prāṇa within their body therefore means that they are their own masters.

The link between mind and breath is most significant. The *Yoga Sūtra* says that when we practice prāṇāyāma the veil is gradually drawn away from the mind and there is growing clarity. The mind becomes ready for deep meditation.[2] Following the *Yoga Sūtra,* we can say that prāṇāyāma is first and foremost awareness of the breath: I am more aware that I breathe; I am conscious of my inhalation and my exhalation and perhaps of the pauses that naturally occur between breaths. The next step is then to answer this question: How do I remain conscious of my breath?

In prāṇāyāma we focus our attention on the breath. In the practice of prāṇāyāma it is therefore very important to keep an alert mind, for the processes that are being observed are very subtle. There is no visible movement of the body as in āsana practice; we must acutely sense and feel the movement of the breath within. The only dynamic process is breathing. Patañjali makes a few practical suggestions for keeping our attention on the breath. For example, we can focus on a place in the body where we can feel or hear the breath. Or we can try to follow the movement of the breath in the body, feeling the inhalation from the center of the collarbone, down through the rib cage to the diaphragm, and following the exhale upward from the abdomen. Another means for paying attention to the breath is to feel where it enters and leaves the body at the nostrils. It is also possible to listen to the breath, especially if you make a slight noise by gently contracting the vocal chords, a prāṇāyāma technique known as *ujjāyī.*

Suggestions like these help us keep our attention on the breath and prevent our practice from becoming merely mechanical. The goal of prāṇāyāma is not to bring the inhalation and exhalation into a certain relationship with each other, or to establish a particular length of breath. If exercises such as these help us concentrate on our prāṇāyāma, that is wonderful. But the true aim of the various techniques and breath ratios of breathing in prāṇāyāma is first and foremost to give us many different possibilities for following the breath. When we follow the breath, the mind will be drawn into the activities of the breath. In this way prāṇāyāma prepares us for the stillness of meditation.

The breath relates directly to the mind and to our prāṇa, but we should not therefore imagine that as we inhale, prāṇa simply flows into us. This is not the case. Prāṇa enters the body in the moment when there is a positive change in the mind. Of course, our state of mind does not alter with every in-breath or out-breath; change occurs over a long period of time. If we are practicing prāṇāyāma and notice a change of mind, then prāṇa has long before entered the body. Changes of mind can be observed primarily in our relationships with other people. Relationships are the real test of whether we actually understand ourselves better.

2. *Yoga Sūtra* 2.52.

Without prāṇa there is no life. We can imagine that prāṇa flows into us as we inhale, but prāṇa is also the power behind breathing out. As well, prāṇa is transformed in the body into various powers, and is involved in processes that ensure that we rid ourselves of what we no longer need. This does not just relate to physical elimination processes—it is the power of prāṇa that can free the mind from blocks and thereby lead us to greater clarity. The out-breath fulfills this function: it releases what is superfluous and removes what would otherwise become blocks to the free flow of prāṇa within.

The Forms of Prāṇa

There are five forms of prāṇa, all having different names according to the bodily functions with which they correspond. These forms of prāṇa are:

- *udāna-vāyu,* corresponding to the throat region and the function of speech
- *prāṇa-vāyu,* corresponding to the chest region
- *samāna-vāyu,* corresponding to the central region of the body and the function of digestion
- *apāna-vāyu,* corresponding to the region of the lower abdomen and the function of elimination
- *vyāna-vāyu,* corresponding to the distribution of energy into all areas of the body

We will concern ourselves with two forms: prāṇa-vāyu and apāna-vāyu.

That which enters the body is called prāṇa and that which leaves it is called apāna. The term *apāna* also refers to the region of the lower abdomen and all the activities that take place there. Apāna describes that part of prāṇa that has the function of elimination and provides the energy for it, and it also refers to the lower belly and the rubbish that collects there when the power of prāṇa is not in a state of equilibrium. When a person is slow and heavy we sometimes say that he has too much apāna. Apāna as prāṇic energy is something we need, but apāna as refuse left from activating this energy actually prevents prāṇa from developing within. All forms of prāṇa are necessary, but to be effective they must be in a state of balance with each other. If someone has a lot of rubbish in the region of the lower abdomen then he or she consumes too much energy there, and this imbalance should be addressed. The goal is to reduce apāna to an efficient minimum.

Apāna as waste matter accumulates because of many factors, some of which lie within our control. The practice of yoga aims to reduce these impurities. People who are short of breath, cannot hold their breath, or cannot exhale slowly are seen as having more apāna, whereas those who have good breath control are considered to have less apāna. An overabundance of apāna leads to problems in all areas of the body. We have to reduce the apāna so that we can bring more prāṇa into the body.

When we inhale, prāṇa from outside the body is brought within. During inhalation, prāṇa meets apāna. During exhalation, the apāna within the body moves toward the prāṇa. Prāṇāyāma is the movement of the prāṇa toward the apāna and the movement of the apāna toward the prāṇa. Similarly, holding the breath after inhalation moves the prāṇa toward the apāna and holds it there. Holding the breath after exhalation moves the apāna toward the prāṇa.

Agni, the Fire of Life

What happens within this movement of prāṇa and apāna? According to yoga we have a fire, *agni*, in the body, situated in the vicinity of the navel, between the prāṇa-vāyu and the apāna-vāyu. The flame itself is constantly changing direction: on inhalation the breath moves toward the belly, causing a draft that directs the flame downward, just like in a fireplace; during exhalation the draft moves the flame in the opposite direction, bringing with it the just-burned waste matter. It is not enough to burn the rubbish; we must also rid the body of it. A breathing pattern where the exhalation is twice as long as the inhalation is aimed at providing more time during exhalation for freeing the body of its blockages. Everything we do to reduce the rubbish in the body is a step in the direction of releasing our blockages. With the next inhalation we bring the flame back to the apāna. If all the previously burned waste has not left the body, the flame will lose some of its power.

Certain physical positions are beneficial for the meeting of fire and rubbish. In all inverted postures, the agni is directed toward the apāna. This is the reason yoga attributes so much significance to the cleansing effects of inverted postures. Cleansing is intensified when we combine inverted postures with prāṇāyāma techniques.

All aspects of prāṇāyāma work together to rid the body of apāna so that prāṇa can find more room within. In the moment when waste is released, prāṇa fills the space in the body where it really belongs. Prāṇa has its own movement; it cannot be controlled. What we can do is create the conditions in which prāṇa may enter the body and permeate it.

The *Yoga Sūtra* describes the flow of prāṇa with this lovely image: If a farmer wants to water his terraced fields, he does not have to carry the water in buckets to the various parts of his fields; he has only to open the retaining wall at the top. If he has laid out his terraces well and nothing blocks the flow of the water, it will be able to reach the last field and the furthest blade of grass without help from the farmer.[3] In prāṇāyāma we work with the breath to remove blockages in the body. The prāṇa, following the breath, flows by itself into the cleared spaces. In this way we use the breath to make possible the flow of prāṇa.

Understanding prāṇa as an expression of puruṣa, we have as little possibility for working directly on prāṇa as we have of influencing our puruṣa directly. The way to influence prāṇa is via the breath and mind. By working with these

[3] *Yoga Sūtra* 4.3.

through prāṇāyāma, we create optimal conditions for the prāṇa to flow freely within.

Practical Aspects of Prāṇāyāma

Just as the activities of the mind influence the breath, so does the breath influence our state of mind. Our intention as we work with the breath is to regulate it so as to calm and focus the mind for meditation. Often people ask if prāṇāyāma is dangerous—I assure you that we can practice prāṇāyāma as safely as we practice āsanas or anything else. Prāṇāyāma is conscious breathing. As long as we pay close attention to the reaction of the body during prāṇāyāma, we have nothing to fear.

Problems can arise when we alter the breath and do not recognize or attend to a negative bodily reaction. If someone is laboring to breathe deeply and evenly, it will immediately become apparent; he or she will feel the need to take a quick breath in between the long, slow breaths. One important precept of Āyurvedic medicine is never to supress the body's natural urges. Even during prāṇāyāma practice we should let ourselves take a short breath if we feel the need to do that. Prāṇāyāma should only be practiced by people who can really regulate the breath. Those who suffer from chronic shortness of breath or other breathing disorders should not attempt prāṇāyāma until they are ready for it. Āsanas that increase the volume of the lungs and free the muscles of the ribs, back, and diaphragm can help prepare one for prāṇāyāma. For example, a back bend and a forward bend counterpose are helpful in preparing for prāṇāyāma. An appropriate āsana practice will encourage development of prāṇāyāma. Prāṇāyāma can and should be practiced in the early days of a person's discovery of yoga, and should absolutely be undertaken only with the guidance of a good teacher.

The object of prāṇāyāma practice is to emphasize the inhalation, the exhalation, or retention of the breath. Emphasis on the inhalation is called *pūraka prāṇāyāma*. *Recaka prāṇāyāma* refers to a form of prāṇāyāma in which the exhalation is lengthened while the inhalation remains free. *Kumbhaka prāṇāyāma* focuses on breath retention. In kumbhaka prāṇāyāma we hold the breath after inhalation, after exhalation, or after both.

Whichever technique we choose, the most important part of prāṇāyāma is the exhalation. If the quality of the exhalation is not good, the quality of the whole prāṇāyāma practice is adversely affected. When someone is not able to breathe out slowly and quietly it means that he or she is not ready for prāṇāyāma, either mentally or otherwise. Indeed, some texts give this warning: if the inhalation is rough we do not have to worry, but if the exhalation is uneven it is a sign of illness, either present or impending.

Why this emphasis on exhalation? Yoga's essential aim is to eliminate impurities and reduce avidyā. Through this elimination alone, positive results come about. When the blockage is cleared from a sewer pipe, the water *has* to flow. If something in us is preventing a change from occurring, then we need only to remove the obstacle and the change can take place. The exhalation is vitally important because it transports impurities from the body, making more room for prāṇa to enter.

Often when prāṇāyāma is discussed it is the holding of the breath that is emphasized. Yet the ancient texts talk about the total breath, not simply kumbhaka, breath retention. The *Yoga Sūtra* discusses the breath in this order of importance: *bāhya vṛtti* or exhalation as the most important, then *abhyantara vṛtti* or inhalation as secondary, and finally *stambha vṛtti* or breath retention.[4] All three of these are aspects of prāṇāyāma. Do not become interested only in holding the breath; many people think they can progress quickly along the yoga path by practicing breath-retention techniques, but in fact problems often arise with this emphasis.

The most important tenet of prāṇāyāma is this: Only when we have emptied ourselves can we take in a new breath, and only when we can draw the breath into us can we hold it. If we cannot breathe out and in fully, how are we going to hold our breath? Breath-retention exercises must be done in such a way that they never disturb the in- and out-breaths. When we reach the stage where we have improved our ability to breathe in and out and to hold the breath, then breath-retention may become important because as it is held the breath is at rest, and with it so hopefully is the mind.

Prāṇāyāma Techniques

Ujjāyī

In one prāṇāyāma practice called *ujjāyī*, or throat breathing, we deliberately contracting the larynx slightly, narrowing the air passage. This produces a slight noise in the throat as we breathe. *Ujjāyī* translates as "what clears the throat and masters the chest area." You should ask for the help of a teacher in deciding whether this breathing technique is suitable for you, and if not, which one would be better.

Ujjāyī breathing has many variations. For example, we can breathe in through the throat, then completely close one nostril and breathe out through the other nostril, which is only partly closed. This technique is called *anuloma ujjāyī*.[5] In a prāṇāyāma technique called *viloma ujjāyī*, we breathe in through the nostril and breathe out through the throat. This technique is used to lengthen the inhalation. In ujjāyī prāṇāyāma it is important to follow this rule: when we regulate the breath through the nostril, we *never* breathe through the throat at the same time.

Nāḍī Śodhana

In the technique for lengthening both the exhalation and the inhalation, we breathe alternately through the nostrils and do not use the throat at all. We

4. *Yoga Sūtra* 2.50.

5. *Anuloma* refers to something that follows the normal way. For example, the Vedas describe a ritual carried out in a prescribed sequence as *anuloma*. Because ujjāyī is described in the *Haṭha Yoga Pradīpikā* as the technique of making the sound in the throat only on the inhalation and then exhaling through the nose, this way of breathing is called anuloma ujjāyī.

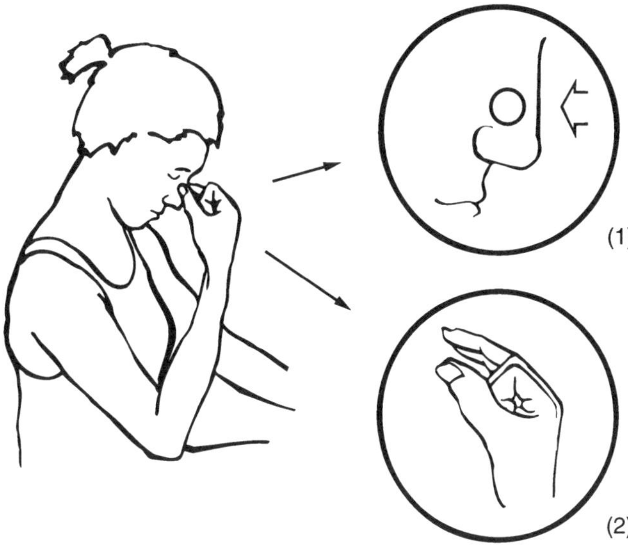

Figure 26: The hand position for nāḍī śodhana. The place where the cartilage begins (1) is the narrowest part of the nasal passage. We place the thumb and ring finger there in the position called mṛgi mudrā (deer mudrā) (2) to regulate the breathing by gentle pressure. Seen from the side, the shadow in this hand position looks like the head of a deer. Many hand mudrās are traditionally described with animal names.

breathe in through the partially closed left nostril, breathe out through the partially closed right nostril, breathe in again through the partially closed right nostril, and then breathe out through the partially closed left nostril, and so forth. We control the opening of the nostril by means of a hand mudrā. The name of this breathing technique is *nāḍī śodhana*—*nāḍī* is the passage or vein through which the breath and energy flow; *śodhana* means "cleansing." Figure 26 shows the hand position for nāḍī śodhana. Normally we work with ujjāyī for a long while before we introduce nāḍī śodhana to our practice.

Alternate nostril breathing should not be practiced if you have a cold or if your nasal passages are blocked in any way. Forced breathing through the nose may lead to complications. In prāṇāyāma it is important to follow this rule: under no circumstances should anything be forced. If you use the nostrils for breath control they must be unobstructed. If they are not, you must practice throat breathing.

Śītalī

Another very useful breathing technique includes using the tongue. During inhalation we curl up both edges of the tongue so that it forms a kind of tube, then we breathe in through this tube. During inhalation the air passes over the moist tongue, cooling down and refreshing the throat. In order to be sure that the tongue remains moist, we roll it back as far as possible against the palate during the entire exhalation so that the next breath is just as refreshing as the first. We can breathe out either through the throat or alternately through the nostrils. This technique is called *śītalī prāṇāyāma. Śīta* means "cool."

Those people who find it impossible to roll the tongue in this way can achieve the same cooling effect by means of another technique in which they open the lips and teeth a little as they breathe in and place the tongue carefully in the space between the upper and lower teeth, a position in which the air can still flow over the tongue. They again breathe out through the throat or through alternate nostrils. This type of breathing is called *śītkarī prāṇāyāma*.

The techniques of ujjāyī, nāḍī śodhana, and śītalī help us to direct our attention to where the breath is in the body. This focus helps us collect the mind, an essential contribution to the physical effects of whichever prāṇāyāma technique we are practicing.

Kapālabhātī

Kapālabhātī is a breathing technique used specifically for cleansing. If we have a lot of mucus in the air passages or feel tension and blockages in the chest it is often helpful to breathe quickly. In this practice we deliberately breathe faster, and at the same time use only abdominal (that is, diaphragmatic) breathing, not chest breathing. In kapālabhātī the breath is short, rapid, and strong. We use the lungs as a pump, creating so much pressure as they expel the air that all the rubbish is cleared from the air passages, from the lungs up through the nostrils. *Kapāla* means "skull," and *bhāti* means "that which brings lightness." Kapālabhātī is a good thing to do when we feel heavy or foggy in the head. If we have problems with the sinuses or feel numb around the eyes, kapālabhātī can help to clear this area as well.

Bhastrika

The word *bhastrika* means "bellows." In bhastrika breathing the abdomen moves like a pair of bellows. If one nostril is blocked, then we draw the air in quickly through the open nostril and breath out strongly through the blocked one.

The kapālabhātī and bhastrika breathing techniques share the same general principle, namely that we clear the nasal passages with the force of the breath. Certainly we must be very careful with these techniques because there is a danger of creating tension in the breath. We may also become dizzy when we breathe rapidly; for this reason we always conclude the practice of kapālabhātī with some slow breaths. It is important not to breathe rapidly too many times, but after a few rapid breaths take several slow ones in which we emphasize the long exhalation.

The Gradual Process of Prāṇāyāma

When we take up the practice of prāṇāyāma, we should proceed gradually, step by step. Because we are starting something new, directing our attention toward the breath—not the body—it is important to rest for several minutes after we finish our āsana practice and before we begin prāṇāyāma. The time between āsana practice and prāṇāyāma practice is not just to rest the body; it also helps the mind to make the transition from one practice to the other.

Without a rest between the two we might easily develop tensions, because the body cannot make an immediate transition. We must always rest between āsana and prāṇāyāma practice.

In practicing prāṇāyāma it is important to find a sitting position in which we can remain for a lengthy period and then get up without feeling stiff. The important aspect of our prāṇāyāma posture is that the spine remains upright. Many people find kneeling comfortable; others can easily sit cross-legged in the lotus pose; it is even acceptable to sit on a chair. (People recovering from such problems as heart disease can lie back in an armchair for their breathing exercises.) Because in prāṇāyāma we are dealing primarily with the breath, in sitting for prāṇāyāma the body must not disturb the breath. In āsana practice we are concerned first and foremost with the body. While we use the breath in our practice of āsanas, we must for prāṇāyāma adopt a posture in which we can pay as little attention as possible to the body. The only demand on the body during prāṇāyāma is that we feel comfortable and keep our spine erect.

Figure 27 shows some possible positions for prāṇāyāma practice. Padmāsana or the lotus pose (1) is a good position in which to practice prāṇāyāma and bandha, provided we can maintain it comfortably. The other cross-legged poses, siddhāsana (2) and sukhāsana (3), are a little less strenuous and just as effective. A few people can sit for long periods in vīrāsana (4), but most of us

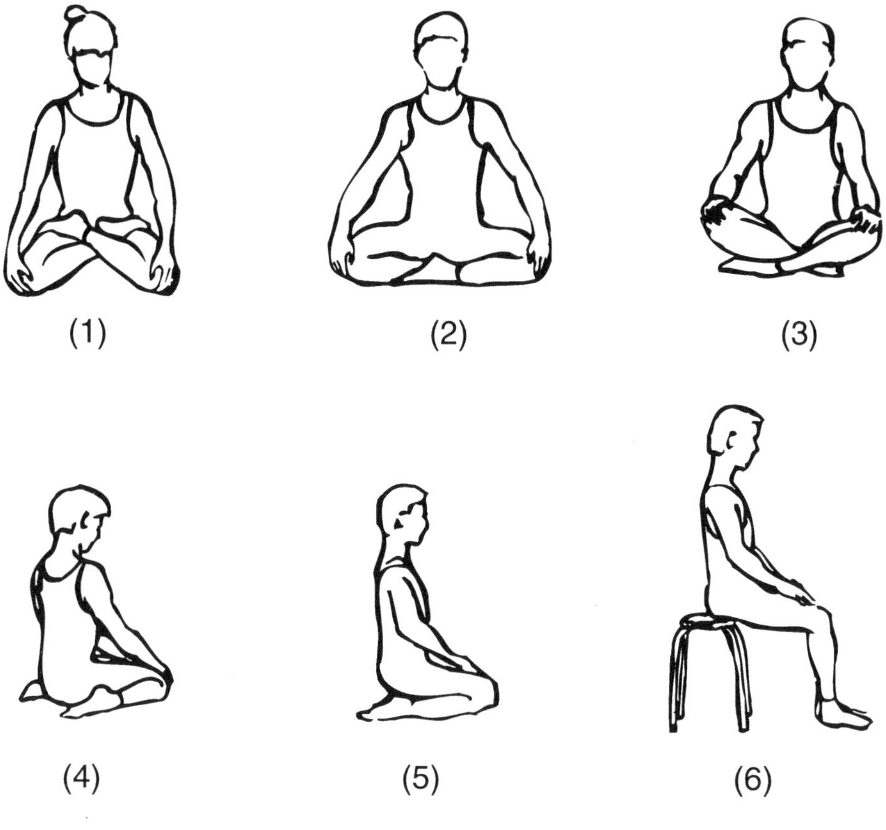

Figure 27:
Positions for prāṇāyāma.

tend to round the lower back in this position. In vajrāsana (5) there is a tendency to hollow the back. Another good position for prāṇāyāma is sitting upright on a stool (6).

The seated position we choose should be determined by the intended duration of our prāṇāyāma practice. Let's say we want to take twelve breaths, each one five seconds in and five seconds out. That would only take about three minutes. There are a number of positions in which we could sit comfortably for three minutes. But let's say we plan our practice to include inhalations and exhalations longer than five seconds, that we plan to practice breath retention, and that we want to do twenty-four breaths. The seated position that was comfortable for three minutes may not be suitable for this longer practice. We must then choose an easier position. The longer the prāṇāyāma practice, the easier seated position we need.

Breath Ratios

In addition to the various breathing techniques, the ratio of the different phases of the breath to each other in prāṇāyāma is very significant. I have already described how the different phases of breath can be emphasized in various ways. It is also possible in prāṇāyāma to fix the ratio between the inhalation, the retention afterward, the exhalation, and the retention after that. The many possibilities for these ratios can be divided roughly into two categories:

1. The inhalation, the exhalation, and the breath retention are all the same length—we call this *samavṛtti prāṇāyāma* (*sama* means "the same" and *vṛtti* means "to move"). This type of prāṇāyāma practice is good for people who use a mantra in their breathing exercises; they can make the inhalation, the exhalation, and the retention of each breath last for the same number of mantra repetitions.

2. The different phases of the breath are of different lengths—we call this *viṣamavṛtti praṇayama*. The general rule in this practice is to let the exhalation be twice as long as the inhalation.

In prāṇāyāma practice a very important issue is how to find an appropriate breath ratio for our individual needs. We cannot always breathe in the same breath ratio—it may be that we need a new ratio in order to maintain our attention on the practice, or because we have to take into account another immediate need. If the breath ratio is too easy, our prāṇāyāma practice will become mechanical. If it is too complicated, there can be resistance which will itself cause problems.

The choice of a suitable breath ratio must take into account two factors: what is possible and what our goals are. What is presently possible depends on how well we can inhale, hold the breath, exhale, and again hold the breath. We can easily discover this by observing our breathing during āsana practice. We can get a good idea of the limits of our breath by seeing if the breath wavers as the body makes demands on it in certain postures.

Here is an example of how we observe our breath in different āsanas in order to find out which breath ratio is suitable for our needs. Let's choose three different postures: a forward bend such as paśćimatānāsana, a backward bend such as bhujaṅgāsana, and sarvāngāsana or the shoulderstand, a posture in which the throat area is restricted and the abdominal organs press on the diaphragm. In these āsanas, let's make the inhalation and the exhalation the same length, say, six seconds each. Now imagine the result is this: the breath is comfortable and free in the forward bend; in the backward bend both the inhalation and the exhalation are shorter; and in the shoulderstand the exhalation is fine but the inhalation is too short. From this experiment we can see that we have difficulties lengthening the inhalation.

I shall explain further. We can likely make the exhalation as long as desired in the forward bend because the contraction of the diaphragm and abdomen is not restricted, so the exhalation is easy. In the same way we are able to breathe out for as long as desired in the inverted posture. Normally it is harder to breathe out slowly in this position precisely because the weight of the abdominal organs on the diaphragm pushes out the air easily and so speeds up the exhalation. If someone can control the exhalation despite this, then it will be easy for them to lengthen the breath in prāṇāyāma. The short inhalation in bhujaṅgāsana, a posture that encourages the inhale as the natural breath rhythm, and the short inhalation in the shoulderstand show that the inhalation phase of our breath cycle is somewhat restricted. Āsanas can tell us a lot not just about the body; if we set a breath ratio in which the inhalation and exhalation are the same length and observe the breath over a certain period in various āsanas, we can also learn a lot about the breath.

From this example we can design a prāṇāyāma practice in which the exhalation is longer than the inhalation. We might choose to breathe in a 1:2 ratio, that is, making the exhalation twice as long as the inhalation. In doing this we encourage the complete emptying of the lungs, which in turn encourages a more voluminous inhale. To strengthen the inhale we must work with the exhale.

Before we pose questions like this in our own practice we should always first consider the more obvious things. If we are beginners in yoga who have just done a few exercises and now want to practice prāṇāyāma, we should not set ourselves on ambitious goals such as being able to hold the breath following inhalation after one months' practice, and following exhalation after two months. Our goals in the beginning should focus much more on finding out what we need in order to develop a deeper interest in our practice. We should increase the length of the breath retention after inhalation and exhalation only gradually. At every stage it is important that we feel well, both in body and breath, after each correctly chosen prāṇāyāma session. If we pay attention to this we can finally practice in such a way that every kind of prāṇāyāma becomes possible for us.

Our goals determine what should soon be possible; they have to do with our needs and the direction our yoga practice is taking. We must accept where we are and move in the direction we want to go. The notion of moving from the point we are currently at to the point we want to reach is always present in yoga. Indeed this is one of the definitions of yoga.

Focus in Prāṇāyāma

There are certain techniques that will help us maintain concentration in prāṇāyāma. In concentrating on the breath, we can focus on the flow of the breath, the sound of the breath, or the place where the most work is occurring. The latter will be determined by the phase of breathing we are in. For example, during exhalation and in holding the breath following exhalation, our concentration is directed toward the abdomen. Conversely, it is directed toward the chest region when inhaling and holding the breath following inhalation.

Even though it seems like such an easy thing, it is actually very difficult simply to follow the movement of the breath. In the moment when we concentrate on the breath it has a tendency to change; we are inclined to control the natural breathing ratio, to disturb it. When we follow the breath we tend to go in one of two directions—either we occupy ourselves with the feel of the breath or we simply observe it. If we just observe it we do not have to do anything with the activity of the breath itself. It is like watching the flow of a river. When we are able to do this we find ourselves almost in a state of meditation. This is the reason why we are sometimes advised simply to observe the breath: as we do this our mind quiets down. It is not easy, but it is marvelous.

There are other techniques that help us maintain concentration in prāṇāyāma. One of these is called internal gazing, a practice in which we hold the eyes in a steady position, eyelids closed. We use our eyes so much that it is not easy to keep them still. Whether we are looking or listening, smelling or tasting, our eyes are always involved somehow or other; consequently they are often strained. Closing the eyes is a very important moment in prāṇāyāma. In internal gazing we direct the eyes as if we were looking at the belly, the navel, the tip of the nose, or the point between the eyebrows. Or we hold an image before our eyes, such as the full moon, the rising sun, or the sign of a mantra.

Gazing is an exercise. When we first begin practicing this kind of gazing we run the risk of getting headaches if we do it during inhalation and exhalation. It is advisable to begin gazing in your chosen manner only while holding the breath. That is easier as everything is still while the breath is held.

Internal gazing is not natural. Normally the eyes are moving constantly, even when they are closed. In this technique of internal gazing we try to keep our eyes on a fixed point. In a certain way it is like ignoring the other senses. The effect is to rest the senses.

Another technique for helping us maintain our concentration during prāṇāyāma uses the hands and fingers. We often see hand positions like this in pictures and statues of the Buddha. Hand positions are called *hasta mudrā*. The word *hasta* means "hand"; *mudrā* has many meanings, but here we can understand it simply as a symbol.

Many different hand positions are possible. The position of one hand resting in the other is called *dhyāna mudrā,* the mudrā of contemplation. In the *cin mudrā,* the thumb and index finger of the left hand are formed into a circle. (The right hand is used to regulate the breath at the nostrils.) When our mind wanders during prāṇāyāma the fingers move apart, and we can notice that we have become inattentive. In this way the mudrā can also be a way of making sure we concentrate on the breath.

In order to use these focusing techniques to full advantage, it is best to stay with one technique through the course of one days' practice. It is much simpler to discover something when you focus your attention on one technique than if you spread your awareness over many experiences. If you go from one focus to another during the course of twelve breaths you might easily lose your concentration altogether.

Finally, a word on counting. It is said we should take at least twelve breaths in any one session of prāṇāyāma. The number twelve relates to an old Indian ritual in which we count on the fingers by placing the thumb in the various positions on the hand each time we breathe in, starting at the base of the index finger. Figure 28 shows the order in which the breaths are counted.

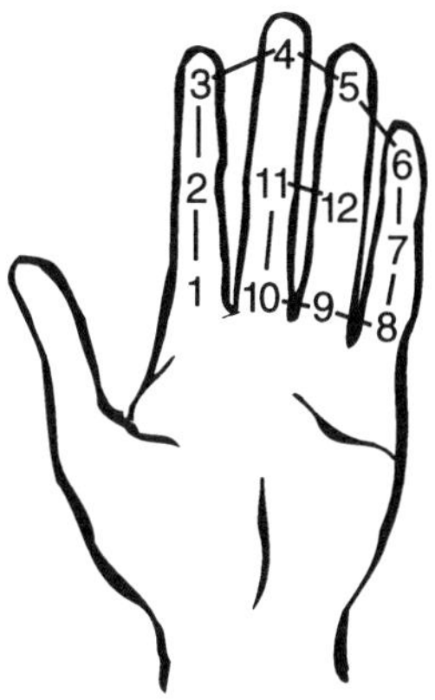

Figure 28: The traditional method for counting breaths in prāṇāyāma.

Further Thoughts on Prāṇāyāma

Q: I find it difficult to count while I am holding my breath.

A: That is interesting. Holding the breath actually gives us a moment in which nothing happens, a moment in which it should therefore be possible to do something like count. It is even said that the best moment for introducing a mantra is not the inhalation or the exhalation, but while you are holding the breath. Some mantras are very long. And we can even recite these exactly as we hold the breath because we do not have to concentrate on breathing. It is said that a moment of breath retention is a moment of meditation, a moment of dhyāna.

So your observation surprises me. Perhaps you should use the finger counting method: Simply place the thumb on a finger joint as you breathe in, then move the thumb rhythmically on the joint, one beat per second, in order to count the length of the retention. That can sometimes help. The ultimate goal is not to have to use any techniques.

Q: Should we really be able to practice prāṇāyāma without counting the breaths or the ratios between the phases of the breath?

A: Yes. What else is prāṇāyāma than being with the breath? But that is very difficult and it's why we have so many techniques. Normally our body has its own rhythm and we are not conscious of our breath. As we count we are occupied with our breath. Lots of people say that prāṇāyāma is boring; they say that just sitting there and doing breathing exercises is quite ridiculous. There seems to be more challenge in āsanas—they produce a visible result.

But when we are totally occupied with prāṇāyāma, who is bothered about numbers then? Counting and types of breathing, ratios and techniques—these are just the means, not the goal. The goal is not to use any technique at all. When we can simply be with the breath, actively observing the breath, then we are practicing the highest form of prāṇāyāma. But that is easier said than done.

Q: Can you say something more about holding the breath after the exhalation?

A: We use this kind of breathing when we want to focus our work in the abdominal area. Holding the breath after exhalation is in general more difficult than holding it after inhalation.

Q: Can you relax the diaphragm during breath retention after inhalation or exhalation?

A: If you breathe in correctly there is no particular reason to relax the diaphragm deliberately. But if you raise the chest too much on inhalation, the lungs will be extended beyond their natural limit and the diaphragm will be sucked in and upward. You will know this has happened if you feel a slight restriction in the throat after inhalation. This is when you must consciously relax the diaphragm. On the other hand, when you contract the abdomen too strongly as you exhale, the air flows out too quickly and you cannot control it well. Similarly, the air flow on inhalation can no longer be controlled if the abdomen is still contracted after exhaling, no matter how complete the exhalation may have been. If you hear or feel a choking sound as you begin to breathe in, it is a sure sign that you have contracted the abdomen too strongly. You can feel all that in the throat.

Every time we do too much we cause tensions in the diaphragm. If we have contracted the abdomen too strongly on exhalation, we must deliberately relax the diaphragm then as well.

Q: Do you have to prepare in the same way every day for a difficult prāṇāyāma practice?

A: We can prepare in various ways; certainly it is always necessary to do some preparation. If we are aiming at a particular breath ratio and choose the āsanas well for our preparation, then the preparation can be relatively short. If we want to practice holding the breath after inhaling and exhaling, for instance, we will not do a lot of strenuous postures beforehand.

Q: Do you always do prāṇāyāma after āsanas?

A: It is better to do prāṇāyāma after āsanas, provided they are not too strenuous and help us to breathe well. There are exceptions, but as a rule we do āsanas before prāṇāyāma.

Q: Can we develop the ability to gaze?

A: Yes, of course. To begin, you gaze internally at the center of the breath's movement, that is, at the area of the diaphragm. During inhalation you direct your gaze there and as you hold the breath you hold your gaze there too. When you breathe out, let the eyeballs roll downward toward the navel. The next step would be to hold your gaze on the same point during your whole prāṇāyāma practice irrespective of whether you are breathing in or out. So begin by gazing only while you hold the breath and then try it as you breathe in and hold the breath. After a few months you will probably be able to gaze without any problems for your whole prāṇāyāma practice.

Q: Do we really use the eye muscles during gazing or do we just imagine that?

A: The eye muscles cannot be relaxed during gazing; we are using them. But the various gazing techniques have different effects. Many people are so tense that their eyebrows are always furrowed. I recommend that these people look down as they breathe both in and out. When the eyeballs are turned downward the area between the eyebrows simply cannot be so tense. Gazing at the point between the eyebrows may create muscle tension. If there is too much tension in this place the technique is not appropriate. Gazing must be practiced gradually, otherwise it will lead to headaches.

Q: Do you use the yoga technique of candle gazing for meditation purposes?

A: Gazing at a candle is a form of external gazing. In India we have a custom whereby we gaze at the sun through a certain hand position every morning. The idea behind this is to make ourselves familiar with the shape of the sun so that we can visualize it with our inner eye during prāṇāyāma. Gazing at a candle, which we call *trāṭaka*, is something similar, but it is not necessarily linked to prāṇāyāma. Sometimes it is used as an eye exercise. Gazing in prāṇāyāma is directed to the inside rather than to the outside, because in prāṇāyāma we are orienting ourselves to what is within.

Q: Can't we be distracted in holding a mudrā during prāṇāyāma if we are concerned about our hand position?

A: Of course. Precisely for this reason we practice all these techniques gradually. If you were to learn prāṇāyāma with me I would not even mention these techniques for a long time, and would only introduce them gradually and carefully. Whatever we try in order to gather our energies must be done gradually. If we do anything too quickly, it blows us apart.

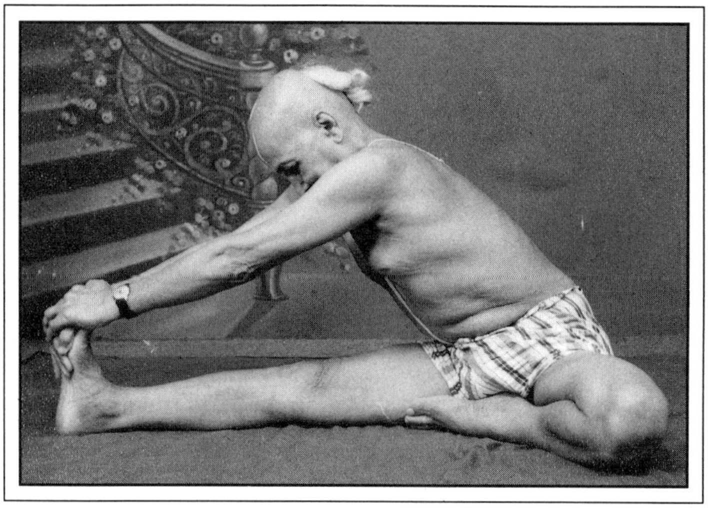

Krishnamacharya demonstrating mahāmudrā.

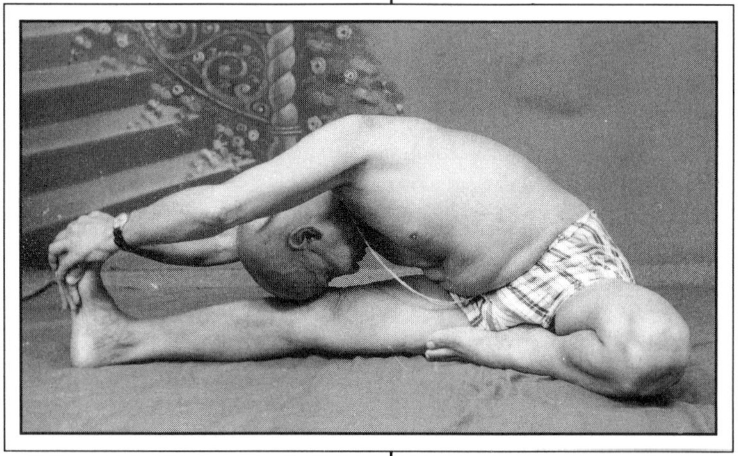

Krishnamacharya in jānu śīrṣāsana.

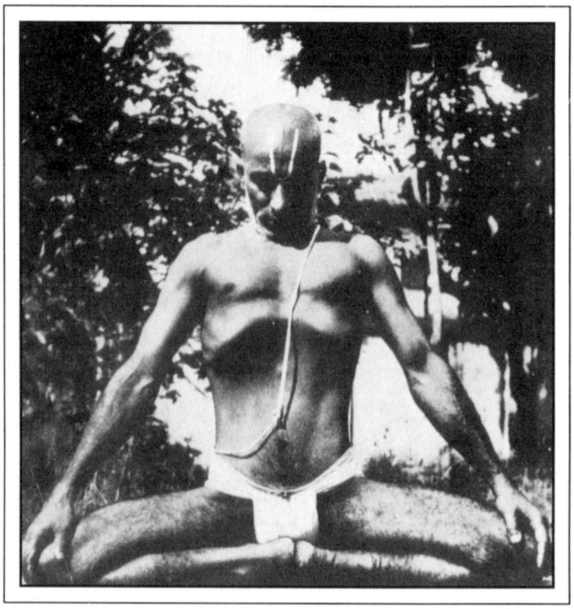

Krishnamacharya in mulabandhāsana demonstrating all three bandhas.

7

The Bandhas

The bandhas play an important role in the cleansing processes of yoga. I have already explained how prāṇāyāma helps to reduce waste matter in the body by directing the agni, the fire of life. Bandhas are the means by which this process can be intensified. The old texts tell us that by using the bandhas, the agni can be directed to the exact place where the rubbish has settled and is blocking the flow of energy in the body. The bandhas intensify the effect of the fire. The word *bandha* means "to bind or tie together, to close." In the way it is used in yoga, *bandha* also means "to lock." When we execute a bandha we lock certain areas of the torso in a particular way.

The three most important bandhas are the *jālandhara bandha*, the *uddīyāna bandha*, and the *mūla bandha*. Jālandhara bandha involves the neck and upper spine and makes the whole spine erect. Uddīyāna bandha focuses on the area between the diaphragm and the floor of the pelvis. Mūla bandha involves the area between the navel and the floor of the pelvis.

Bandha Techniques

To learn the bandhas you must work with a teacher—that is the only way to learn these techniques safely. In learning the bandha techniques you always begin with jālandhara bandha; you should practice this bandha for a while after mastering it, before attempting to learn the other two.

Jālandhara Bandha

Figure 29 shows the positions of the three bandhas discussed here. To begin jālandhara bandha, we lift the spine so that it is very straight. The head is then pulled back a little, the neck is stretched, and the chin is lowered. As long as the chin is down and the back is straight we are in jālandhara bandha. This bandha is possible to perform with many, though not all, āsanas.

Uddīyanā Bandha

Only when you are certain of and well practiced in jālandhara bandha should uddīyanā bandha be attempted. In this technique the diaphragm and the lower abdomen are raised. As you begin to exhale you contract the abdomen. By the end of the exhalation the abdomen should be fully contracted, drawn up and back toward the spine. With this contraction the diaphragm rises. When this bandha is mastered, the navel moves toward the spine and the rectal and back muscles contract. At the completion of uddīyāna bandha the whole abdominal area is hollow.

In this practice it is very important that both the contraction and the relaxation of the abdomen occur slowly. If the breath is held for ten seconds after the exhalation, for example, then you should take at least two seconds to release the abdomen. If the abdomen is not fully relaxed after uddīyāna bandha, the following inhalation will be restricted and you will experience a choking feeling. It is easy to get the right feeling for uddīyāna bandha in some of the easier āsanas such as taḍāka mudrā and adhomukha śvānāsana (see figure 30).

Mūla Bandha

Mūla bandha develops out of uddīyāna bandha: we release the upper abdomen and diaphragm but maintain the contraction in the lower abdomen. In other words, the area below the navel remains contracted while the area above it is released. We move from uddīyāna bandha into mūla bandha, holding the breath after the exhalation for both. We can maintain mūla bandha during the following breaths, even while inhaling.

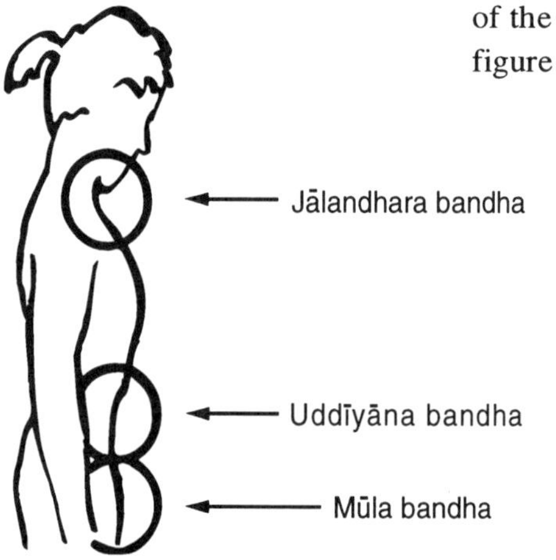

Figure 29: The position of the jālandhara, uddīyāna, and mūla bandhas.

Bandhas and Āsanas

We should begin practicing the bandhas in simple āsanas so that the body can get used to them. Figure 30 illustrates some of these āsanas. The easiest position is lying flat on the back with the arms resting on the floor over the head (1). We can practice uddīyāna bandha in this position, which is called *taḍaka mudrā*. Taḍāka refers to the big pools on the temple grounds in India. Hollowing the abdomen in this position reminds us of one of these pools. Another simple position for practicing the bandhas is adhomukha śvanāsana, the downward-facing dog pose (2). Anyone who can easily practice the bandhas in these positions is ready to try them in a sitting position such as mahāmudrā (3). Mahāmudrā, the great mudrā, is essentially only called this when all three bandhas are involved. The position of the heel in the perineum supports the mūla bandha.

With the exception of jālandhara bandha, the bandhas can also be carried out in inverted positions such as the headstand. The bandhas are easy in this āsana

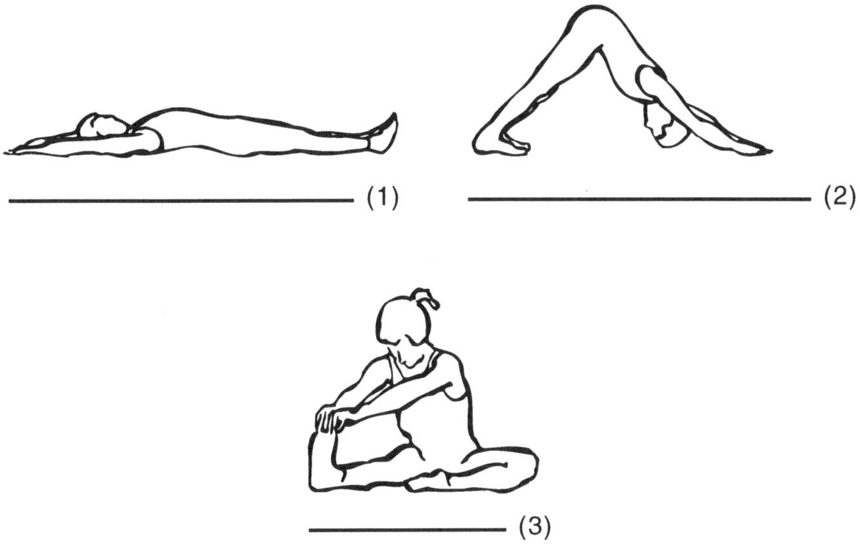

Figure 30:
Easy āsanas in which to practice the bandhas are taḍāka mudrā (1) and adhomukha śvanāsana (2). Only when the bandhas have been mastered in these positions should you think of practicing them in mahāmudrā (3).

because raising the rubbish to the flame (with uddīyāna bandha) and holding it there (with mūla bandha) is greatly assisted by the body mechanics of the posture. In all inverted postures, the rubbish is raised to sit above the flame. The flame burns up toward the rubbish and the rubbish moves down toward the flame.

If we master the breath in the shoulderstand, then this is also a good posture in which to practice the bandhas. The best āsanas therefore for practicing bandhas are a few of the inverted postures and all postures in which we are lying flat on the back or sitting with a straight spine. The practice of bandhas is very difficult or impossible in āsanas such as backbends and twists, and are therefore best avoided.

A word of caution: Do not use bandhas throughout the entire āsana practice. Like all other yoga techniques, bandhas should be practiced artfully and not obsessively. The help of a good teacher is essential.

Bandhas and Prāṇāyāma

Only when we can comfortably execute the three bandhas in the āsanas discussed above are we advanced enough to introduce them in our prāṇāyāma practice. Let's consider how the bandhas intensify the cleansing effect of prāṇāyāma. Jālandhara bandha positions the torso in such a way that the spine is held erect. This makes it easier for the prana to move the flame toward the rubbish that needs burning. Uddīyāna bandha then raises the rubbish up toward the flame, and mūla bandha helps us leave it there long enough for the rubbish to be burned.

These three bandhas can be used during both āsana and prāṇāyāma practice. Jālandhara bandha can eventually be maintained during the whole process of inhalation, exhalation, and holding the breath. Uddīyāna bandha can only be done during breath retention following exhalation. Mūla bandha, like jālandhara bandha, can be maintained during the whole prāṇāyāma practice.

Because uddīyāna bandha is only done as you hold the breath after exhalation, one of the most important prerequisites for anyone who wants to practice it is that you must be capable of holding the breath for a long time after exhalation without sacrificing the quality of either inhalation or exhalation. If this is not possible then you must not consider doing this bandha. If you want to do jālandhara bandha, you must make sure you are not tense in the neck or back so that you can hold your spine erect without any trouble while you keep the chin down. If you try to draw the chin down when your neck is stiff, greater tensions and pains will develop. Only jālandhara bandha can be practiced with kapālabhātī and bhastrika prāṇāyāma. You should not do the bandha in śītalī prāṇāyāma, because in that exercise you are moving the head up and down.

If the bandhas are to be practiced during prāṇāyāma, we must first establish a ratio of breathing—that is, inhalation, exhalation, and holding the breath—that we can maintain comfortably during twelve breaths without bandhas. We can then gradually introduce the bandhas. As in our daily āsana practice, we follow the principle of vinyāsa krama, building up to the strenuous practice of bandhas step by step. We then taper off gradually and finish our prāṇāyāma practice with simple breathing. We intensify our practice until we make progress in the preceding step, practicing patiently without forcing the body or the breath.

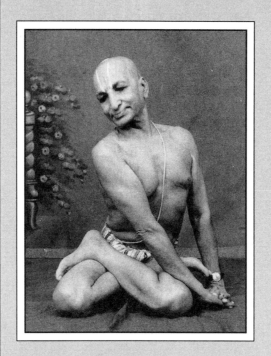

Top: Krishnamacharya demonstrating padmāsana paravṛtti.

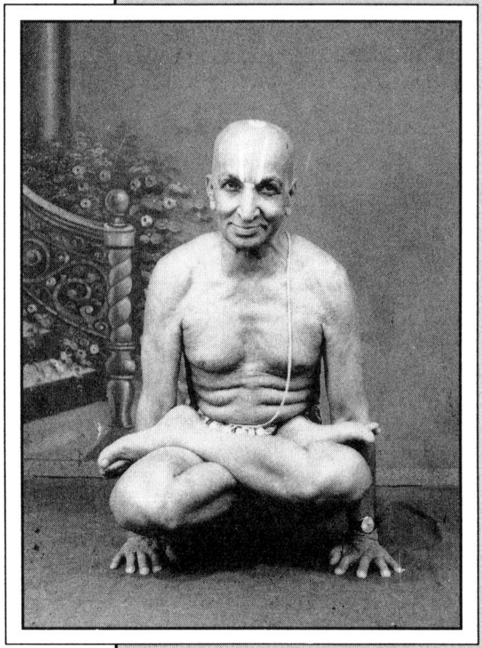

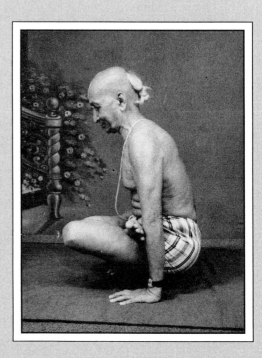

Middle and bottom: Two views of Krishnamacharya in tolāsana.

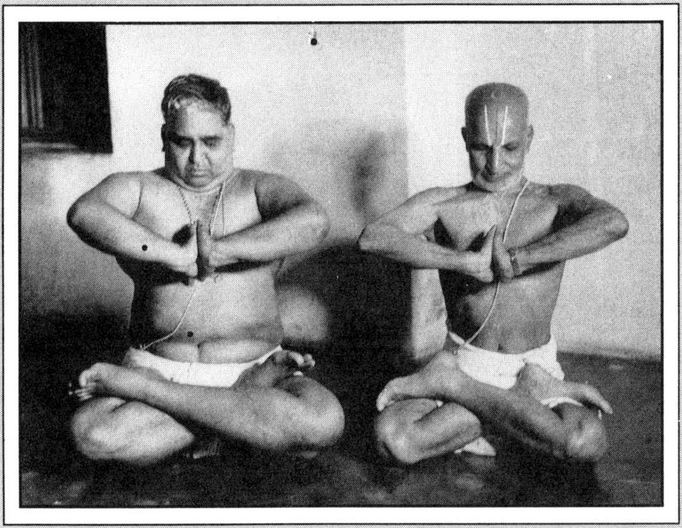

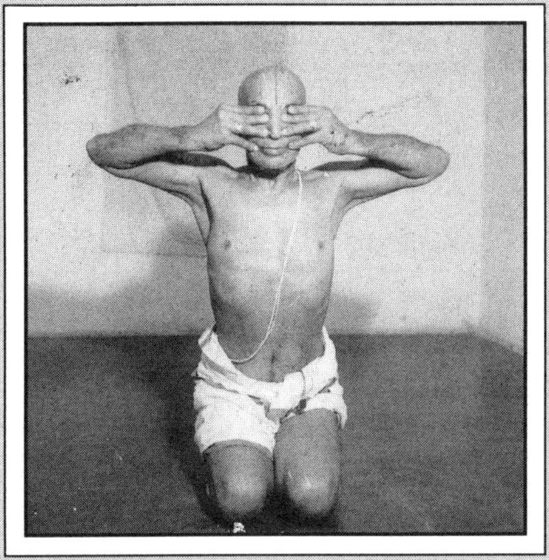

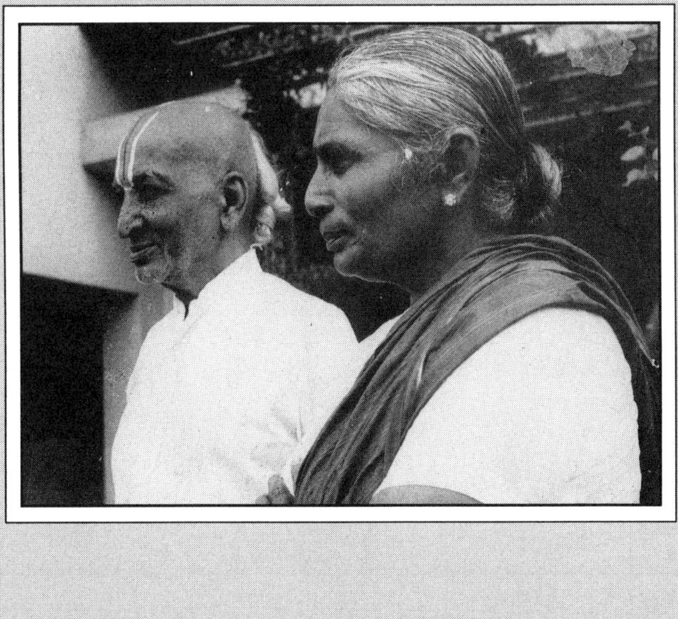

Part II
The Understanding of Yoga

Top: Krishnamacharya teaching padmāsana.

Center: Krishnamacharya demonstrating sanmukhī mudrā.

Bottom: Krishnamacharya and his wife, Namagiriamma.

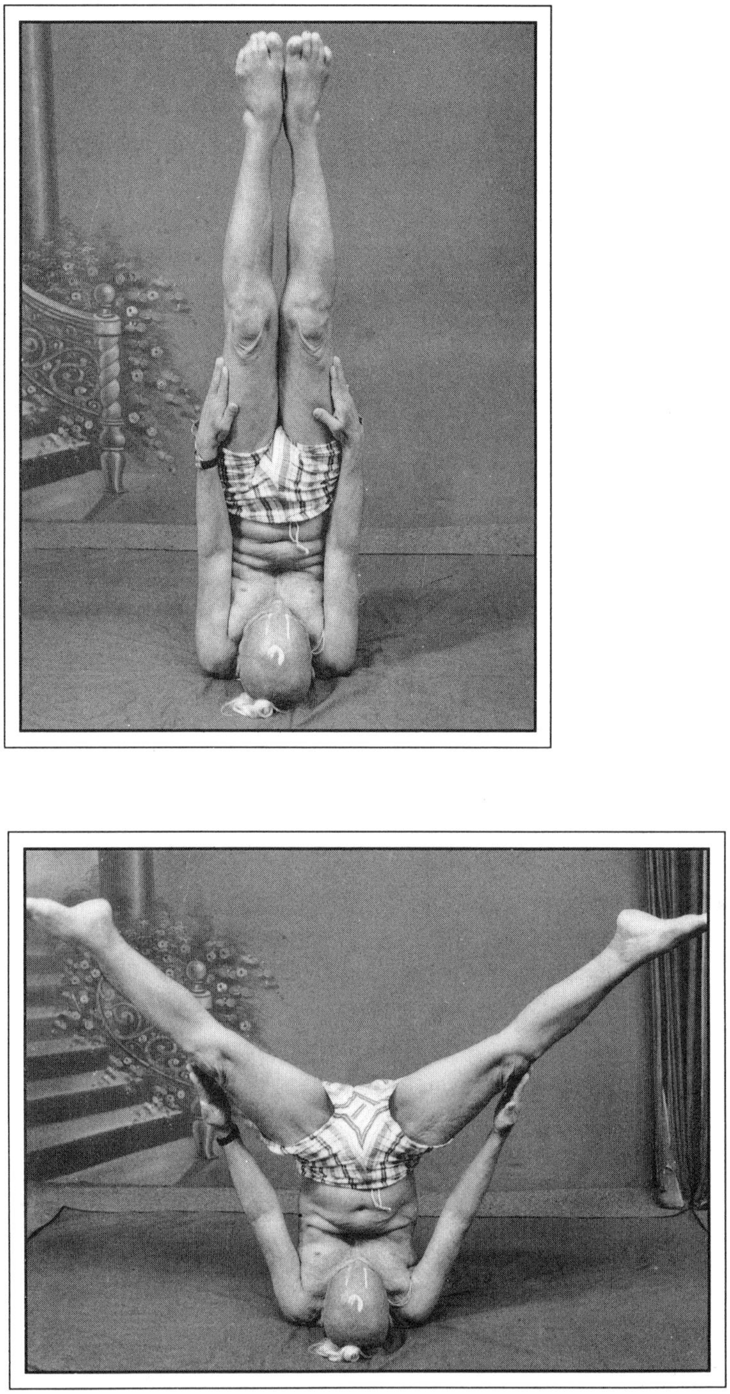

Krishnamacharya in two variations of niralamba sarvāngāsana.

8

The Things That Darken the Heart

There are many definitions of yoga, and I have already mentioned some of them:

- yoga as the movement from one point to another, higher one
- yoga as the bringing together, the unifying of two things
- yoga as action with undivided, uninterrupted attention

These definitions of yoga have one thing in common: the idea that something changes. This change must bring us to a point where we have never been before. That is to say, that which was impossible becomes possible; that which was unattainable becomes attainable; that which was invisible can be seen. One of the basic reasons many people take up yoga is to change something about themselves: to be able to think more clearly, to feel better, and to be able to act better today than they did yesterday in all areas of life. In these endeavors yoga can be of great help, and it requires no prerequisites that must be fulfilled before we set out on this path. Just because yoga originated in India does not mean that we must become a Hindu in order to practice it. On the contrary, it is not even expected of a Hindu that he or she practice yoga. Yoga does not require a particular belief system and, if we already have one, it is not challenged by yoga. Everyone can begin, and the point at which we start is very personal and individual, depending on where we are at the time.

Why do we set out on this journey at all? Because we sense that we do not always do what might be best for ourselves or others. Because we notice that we often do not recognize the things around us and in us clearly enough. And why does this happen? Because the veil of avidyā clouds our perceptions. We can, in any given moment, be right or wrong in our assessment of a situation, but this is something we cannot tell at the time. If our view of a situation is false, then avidyā is present and the ensuing action will be clouded by it. In this way avidyā influences both our action and the results of our action, which we will sooner or later have to confront. We have already talked about the fact that from the yogic point of view everything is real and there is no illusion. Even avidyā, the source of so many problems, has a value and is real. Everything we see and experience is accepted. This concept is called satvāda. Yoga also claims that everything is in a state of change and flux. We will not see things tomorrow in the same way that we saw them today. This concept is called *pariṇāmavāda*.

If we follow yogic thinking further, we find that there is something that can perceive this constant change in things because it is itself not subject to change. This is puruṣa, something deep within us that is really able to see and recognize the true nature of all things, including the fact that they are in a state of constant change. But puruṣa is also cloaked with the same veil of avidyā that covers the mind.

I have already described how avidyā is expressed and experienced in four different ways. One way is asmitā, the ego: "I am right"; "I am sad"; "I am a yoga teacher." These are statements of asmitā. We identify completely with something that might possibly change, and may no longer belong to us tomorrow. Another form of avidyā is rāga, the desire to have something whether we need it or not. A third form is dveṣa, which manifests as refusing things and having feelings of hatred. And finally there is abhiniveśa or fear—afraid of death, we cling to life with all our might. These are the four possible ways in which avidyā is expressed.

The essential purpose of yoga practice is to reduce avidyā so that understanding can gradually come to the surface. But how can we know whether we have seen and understood things clearly? When we see the truth, when we reach a level that is higher than our normal everyday understanding, something deep within us is very quiet and peaceful. Then there is a contentment that nothing can take from us. It is not the kind of satisfaction derived from gazing at a beautiful object. It is much more than this. It is a satisfaction deep within us that is free from feeling and judgment. The center of this contentment is the puruṣa.

Yoga is both the movement toward and the arrival at a point. The yoga that we are practicing and in which, through practice, we can make progress is called kriyā yoga. The *Yoga Sūtra* defines kriyā yoga as being made up of three components: tapas, svādhyāya, and īśvarapraṇidhānā. Tapas does not mean penance or castigation, but is something we do in order to keep us physically and mentally healthy. It is a process of inner cleansing: we remove things that we do not need. Svādhyāya is the process of gradually finding out where we are, who we are, what we are, and so forth. Our āsana practice begins with precisely these questions. We take the first step by observing the breath and body. We do this over and over again, hoping that we will with time develop a deeper understanding of ourselves and our current state. In this way we also learn to recognize what our next steps will be. If we follow the *Yoga Sūtra*, this close connection with svādhyāya holds true for every kind of yoga practice. The literal meaning of īśvarapraṇidhānā is "to yield humbly to God." In kriyā yoga there exists the free choice of accepting God or not. The meaning of īśvarapraṇidhānā in the context of kriyā yoga relates much more to a special kind of attention to action: we place value on the quality of the action, not on the fruits that can develop out of it.

Our normal course of action is first to decide on a goal and then, bearing it in mind, start working toward it. But it can easily happen that our goal changes or even disappears. For instance, someone thinks it necessary to make a million dollars and spends two or three years working toward this end. Suddenly this person discovers that this goal is really of no use; the goal loses its meaning and is replaced by another quite different goal that is much more important. We should remain flexible so that we are still able to react to changes in our expectations and old ideas. The more distanced we are from the fruits of our labors, the better we are able to do this. And if we concentrate more on the quality of our steps along the way than on the goal itself, then we also avoid being disappointed if we perhaps cannot attain the exact goal that we had set for ourselves. Paying more attention to the spirit in which we act and looking less to the results our actions may bring us—this is the meaning of īśvarapraṇidhānā in kriyā yoga.[1]

Avidyā changes according to whether it is manifested as asmitā, rāga, dveṣa, or abhiniveśa. Sometimes it will manifest itself as anxiety; other times it will appear as attachment, rejection, avarice, and so forth. The four aspects of avidyā are not always present in the same proportion. Although they are normally all there, generally one or two are dominant and the others are lurking in the background.

If we feel modest for a while it does not mean that we have overcome our self-seeking tendencies. We never know when a particular form of avidyā will appear even more clearly. It is like sowing seeds; as soon as they receive water, fertilizer, and air, they begin to grow. Every seed grows best under different conditions and at different times. So it can happen that a desire (rāga) drives us to do something that our pride, our ego (asmitā), had forbidden. Or our desire to be noticed (asmitā) may become so great that it overcomes our anxiety (abhiniveśa) because we have to prove what great heroes we are.

We should never sit back smugly when it seems as though we are free of avidyā. Because the four faces of avidyā do not always appear on the surface, we must remain aware of the fact that their power and intensity can go on changing. Sometimes avidyā is scarcely visible in any of its forms and sometimes it overwhelms us. Because there are so many levels of avidyā we must remain watchful and alert in our actions, and maintain our efforts to lessen its influence on us. If somebody enjoys a clear mind and spirit for years on end, that certainly shows great progress. But suddenly avidyā can hit him or her

1. The question of the attitude we adopt toward our action is central to the definition of īśvarapraṇidhānā given in the *Yoga Bhāṣya*, the oldest commentary on the *Yoga Sūtra*. There it is written: "Īśvarapraṇidhānā is the yielding of all action to God, the renunciation of the desire for the fruits of all action."

again like an earthquake. That is why we emphasize that our practice of yoga, the striving for a deeper understanding, must go on until avidyā is reduced to a minimum.

A few days' yoga practice and contemplation may help for a short time, but the benefits will not last forever. We have to place one stone on another; it is a gradual process. We have to engage in these practices constantly because, although we may be further on today than yesterday, tomorrow we may slip back a step. We are required to be constantly active until the seeds of avidyā are burned and cannot germinate any more. As long as the seed is there we can never know if it will sprout or not. The practice of yoga helps to prevent these seeds from germinating and growing again. Avidyā is as closely related to nonaction—even nonaction has consequences. The *Yoga Sūtra* claims that whether our actions have positive or negative effects is determined by the degree of influence avidyā has over them.[2]

The *Yoga Sūtra* makes a distinction between two kinds of action: action that reduces avidyā and brings true understanding, and action that increases avidyā. We increase avidyā by feeding it and reduce avidyā by starving it; our actions encourage or discourage the growth of avidyā. Everything we do in yoga—whether it is āsana practice, prāṇāyāma, or meditation, whether it is attentive observation, self-searching, or the examination of a particular question—all have as their goal the reduction of avidyā.

Nothing We Do Is Without Consequence

Each of our actions shows its effects either immediately or after a period of time. Every action has a consequence. This can take the form of a residue left behind by an action, which in its turn influences the following action. For example, someone toward whom we have behaved in a friendly manner will take something of our friendliness into his or her next encounter. It is a continuous process: the first action influences the next and so on, ad infinitum. That is the reason why it is best for us to remain alert in all our actions.

What possibilities are there for preventing actions with negative consequences, actions that we may later regret? One possibility is *dhyāna,* which in this context means "reflection."[3] Reflection can take many forms. For example, when faced with an important decision, you could imagine what would happen if you did the exact opposite of what your instincts suggest.[4] Try to make the consequence of your decision as real as possible in your imagination. No matter what it is or what you feel, before you make an important decision and take action you should give yourself the opportunity to consider the matter with an open mind and a certain degree of objectivity. Dhyāna in this respect is a quiet, alert consideration, a meditation. The aim is to free yourself of preconceptions and avoid actions that you may later regret and that may create new troubles (duḥkha) for you.

2. *Yoga Sūtra* 2.12 ff.

3. *Yoga Sūtra* 2.11.

4. *Yoga Sūtra* 2.33 and 34 present this idea as *pratipakṣabhāvana.*

Dhyāna strengthens self-sufficiency. Yoga makes us independent. We all want to be free, although many of us are dependent on psychologists, gurus, teachers, drugs, or whatever. Even if advice and guidance are helpful, in the end we ourselves are the best judge of our own actions. No one is more interested in me than me. With the help of dhyāna we find our own methods and systems for making decisions and better understand our behavior.

There are other ways of distancing ourselves from our actions than reflecting on how it would be if we were to act differently from what we intend. We might go to a concert or go for a walk or do something else that calms the thoughts. All the while the mind goes on working unconsciously, without any external pressure. In the pursuit of other activities we gain a certain distance. However short it may be, time becomes available to cast the mind over everything surrounding the decision that has to be made. Perhaps with ease and distance we will make a better decision. Stepping out of a situation in order to get a better look at it from another standpoint is called *pratipakṣa.* The same word describes the process of considering other possible courses of action.[5] The time spent in dhyāna is extremely important. Through self-reflection our actions gain in quality.

Another notion closely linked to avidyā is that of duḥkha. Sometimes terms such as "suffering," "troubles," or "sickness" are used to explain the meaning of duḥkha, but it is best described as a feeling of being restricted. Duḥkha is a quality of mind that gives us the feeling of being squeezed. It is not to be compared with physical pain. There does not need to be any physical pain to experience a feeling of great duḥkha. The level on which duḥkha works is the mind. Duḥkha is nothing but a certain state of mind in which we experience a limitation of our possibilities to act and understand. Even if we do not have a need to express our feelings in tears, somehow we feel disturbed deep within ourselves, painfully bound and restricted.

When we feel a sense of lightness and openness within, then we are experiencing the opposite of duḥkha, a state that is called sukha.[6] The concept of duḥkha plays an important part not only in yoga but in every significant philosophy of India. There is duḥkha at different times in the life of every human being. We all have the goal of eliminating duḥkha. That is what the Buddha taught. That is what Vedānta strives for. That is what yoga tries to achieve.

Duḥkha Arises from Avidyā

What is the relationship between duḥkha and avidyā? Every action that stems from avidyā always leads to one or another form of duḥkha. It very often happens that we do not see our avidyā as selfishness, desire, hate, or fear, but can only perceive the result, the duḥkha. Duḥkha can be expressed in many different forms; we never know how before it besets us. Sometimes we might

5. *Yoga Sūtra* 2.33.

6. A literal translation can help us understand these terms, which are used again and again in the *Yoga Sūtra*; *kha* means something like "space," and *su* translates as "happy," "fortunate," or "good." A graphic metaphor for duḥkha as the opposite of sukha is a dark room.

literally feel as if we are choking; other times we only notice duḥkha in our thoughts and feelings. Irrespective of what form it takes, however, duḥkha will certainly occur whenever our actions have arisen out of avidyā. An action that is supported by a clear mind cannot conceal any duḥkha within it. Consequently, there are actions that somehow never have any negative aspects, and there are others that we thought would be good but later on we recognize that they brought us duḥkha.

Duḥkha can even arise out of our efforts to progress along the path of yoga. When we see something that we would like to have, there is no duḥkha initially present. Duḥkha begins to take hold when we cannot get what we want. People often feel that they suffer from this kind of duḥkha precisely when they are in the process of improving their lives. They become so thirsty for real insight that they cannot reach this new quality of understanding and action as quickly as they would like.

In the great spiritual literature of India there are many stories of people who strive to become better but are in such a hurry, and therefore achieve so little, that they develop duḥkha and are unhappy. And this happens despite the fact that they have tried to change something for the better.

We also talk of duḥkha when we cannot make ourselves comfortable in a new situation. Duḥkha can arise from being used to certain things and insisting on nothing else. When our habits are disturbed we feel unwell. If we cannot continue life in our habitual way, we experience it as a disturbance. This form of duḥkha arises from our own actions, which have brought to us a feeling of satisfaction.

Duḥkha can also be generated from the other direction. Sometimes the process of leaving an old track that we realize is not good for us is painful and can cause duḥkha. That is the reason why it is sometimes difficult to lay aside a certain behavior that we recognize as unproductive. The separation from a pattern we are used to can be very painful. It is up to us to find out why so that we can overcome the situation.[7]

Duḥkha Arises out of the Guṇa

To understand duḥkha we must understand the three qualities of mind described by yoga. These three qualitites—tamas, rajas, and sattva—are collectively known as the *guṇa*. [8]

Tamas describes the state of heaviness and slowness in feeling and decision. Let's say that a feeling of great lethargy comes upon you when you are supposed to give a speech. You would suddenly have great difficulty in remaining alert, your audience (and you yourself) would be discontented, and finally you would experience duḥkha. This kind of lethargy is what is meant by tamas. A different situation exists when it is really time to go to sleep but the mind says, "Come on, let's go! Let's go to the movies! You must go to the movies! How can you want to go to bed now?" This quality of mind would like action, would like to dance. This quality is called rajas, and also produces

7. The different aspects of duḥkha discussed here are thus distiguished: from the inability to perceive or accept a change arises *pariṇāma-duḥkha*; from the situation where a need cannot be fulfilled arises *tāpa-duḥkha*; from the difficulty in giving up habits arises *saṃskāra-duḥkha*. A discussion of the various causes of duḥkha can be found in the *Yoga Sūtra* 2.15.

8. The concept of the three guṇa is not presented in detail in the *Yoga Sūtra*, but is referred to in 2.18, and presupposed in the *Yoga Sūtra* constantly. It is explained in the texts of the Sāṃkhya, where the guṇa are comprised of those three qualities that are peculiar to everything material (to which also belong our thoughts, our feelings, and the whole range of our mental activity), but not puruṣa. Even the movement of the three guṇa can be reason for duḥkha. See the *Yoga Sūtra* 2.15.

duḥkha. The third quality of mind describes the absence of the other two. There is neither heaviness and lethargy nor raciness and restlessness, but only clarity. This is called sattva, and from this quality of mind alone can arise no duḥkha.

These three qualities are subject to their own cycles—sometimes one prevails, sometimes another. Only sattva, clarity, is totally positive in the sense of leading to a reduction of duḥkha. Rajas and tamas can both lead to duḥkha. For instance, if I really need sleep and want to go to sleep, then my mind is tamas, and that is good. But if I am to give a lecture or would like to listen to one, a state of mind that is predominantly tamas causes considerable difficulties.

All the factors that lead to the occurrence of duḥkha work in us as forces that reduce our space and freedom and ultimately limit us. If we are alert enough we can be aware of the play of these forces within us all the time. Through our yoga practice we are attempting to become more aware of these movements within, to reduce the limitations that result from them and to avoid the occurrence of duḥkha in the future. When we become aware of duḥkha and see it as something to face, we are also able to find a way to get rid of it. That is why becoming aware of duḥkha is the first step toward freeing ourselves from it.

Finally, yoga claims that there is a state called *kaivalya* in which someone is free of the external concerns that cause such disturbances and generate duḥkha.[9] Let's say I have a radio that means a lot to me. One day my son breaks it. I am furious and become angry with him even though he did not do it deliberately. Actually I should not have become angry—it is only a radio after all. While I should not actually encourage my son to be careless, I must also be flexible enough to see what really happened. A little flexibility always reduces duḥkha.

9. *Yoga Sūtra* 2.25. The concept of kaivalya represents a central concern of yoga. The last chapter of the *Yoga Sūtra* bears the title "Kaivalya" or "Freedom."

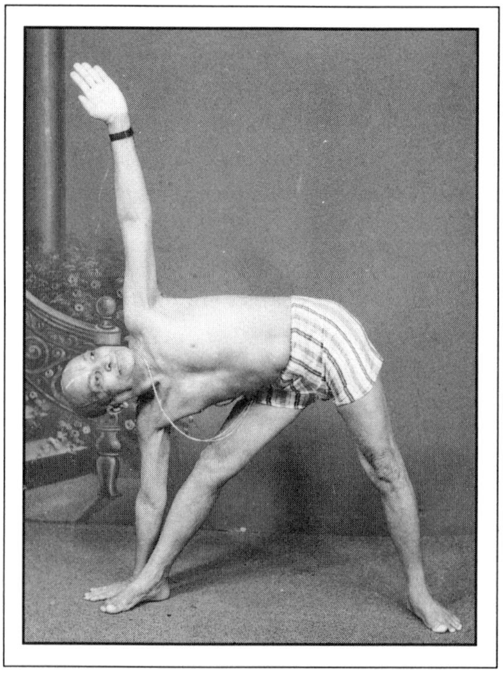

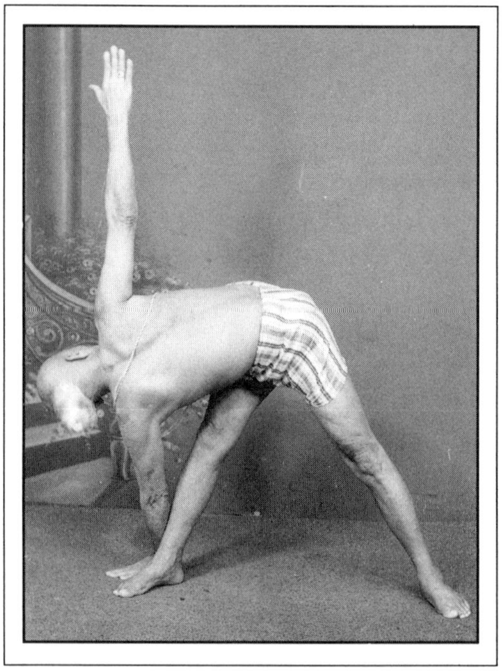

Krishnamacharya in trikonāsana variations: utthita (above) and parivṛtti.

9

Actions Leave Traces

I have already discussed how the incorrect knowledge of avidyā affects our actions. Sometimes we do not see things as they are and act out of misunderstanding. Often that action does not have an immediately negative outcome, but sooner or later we begin to suffer from its effects. One action arising from a faulty perception can influence the next, and thus we become gradually less free. We simply walk the same old track, and the result is duḥkha, a feeling of being restricted, of not being free. Duḥkha arises when we do not get what we want; it arises from desire. Duḥkha also results from wanting to repeat a pleasant experience that actually cannot ever be repeated because the situation has changed. Another form of duḥkha is experienced when we become habituated to having something and suddenly do not have it any more. In this case duḥkha arises because we have to give up something we are used to.

Duḥkha: The Lot of Those Who Seek

The *Yoga Sūtra* states that although duḥkha can be found everywhere, we do not always perceive it, and indeed there are some people who never become aware of it at all. But it is precisely those who are searching for clarity who often experience duḥkha particularly strongly. Vyasa's commentary on the *Yoga Sūtra* gives a wonderful example of this. (The commentaries on the *Yoga Sūtra* are discussed in appendix 1.) It says that dust that lands on the skin is harmless, but if only a tiny particle gets into the eye, it is very painful. In other words, someone who is searching for clarity becomes sensitive because the eyes must be open, even if what they see is sometimes very unpleasant. Someone who is searching feels or sees things long before other people do. He or she develops a special insight, a particular kind of sensitivity. We should see this positively—this insight or sensitivity can be as useful as a warning light in a car. It tells us that there is something wrong and we would be wise to find out what it is. Someone who is searching for clarity always sees more suffering than someone who is not. This awareness of suffering results from greater sensitivity. The person who is not searching for clarity does not even know what brings him or her happiness or sorrow.

We have already talked about how the movement of the three parts of the mind, the guṇa—rajas, tamas, and sattva—causes duḥkha to arise. Rajas is active, fiery, the one that induces us to act. Sometimes it pushes our mind into a state of constant activity and we cannot be still: that state is characterized by restlessness and agitation. Tamas is the opposite of rajas; it is a fixed, immobile, heavy state of mind. Sattva is the quality of insight that is white, clear, and transparent. It is a state in which neither of the other two guṇa predominate. According to the relationship between rajas and tamas, duḥkha will take different forms. Our goal is to reduce these two guṇa until our mind achieves a state of sattva.

Recognition of duḥkha is a process that can be broken down into seven stages. The first is to understand that something is not right. For example, we might feel that something habitual in our life needs to be avoided, or we might feel compelled to do something that veers from our normal course. Perhaps we do not know exactly what action to take, but we have at least become aware of a problem. This is the first of the seven steps, and anyone seeking understanding is more prone than other people to this feeling that something is not right. The other steps are too complex for our discussion. Vyasa's commentary on sūtra 2.27 of the *Yoga Sūtra* addresses the seven steps toward true recognition of duḥkha.

According to the *Yoga Sūtra*, our mind possesses five faculties which we call *vṛtti*, "movements" or "activities."[1] The first activity of the mind is *pramāṇa*, direct perception through our senses. *Viparyaya*, incorrect understanding, is the next possible activity of the mind. The third faculty, *vikalpa*, is the power of the imagination. It describes knowledge or understanding based on ideas that have nothing to do with the present moment or material reality. The fourth faculty is *nidrā*, dreamless sleep. The fifth is *smṛti*, memory, that activity of the mind that can store an experience or observation.

These faculties work together; with the exception of nidrā, we experience a mixture of them every second of the day. These mental activities, alone or in any combination, do not necessarily conceal a form of duḥkha but can have an influence on how much duḥkha is present. Dreams, for instance, arise from a combination of the various activities. Whether a dream causes us duḥkha or not depends on its effects. The effects of a dream can be good or bad, depending on what we do with it or what it does to us.

Puruṣa Sees by Means of the Mind

What is the relationship between *citta*, the mind, and puruṣa, the part of us that sees? The *Yoga Sūtra* says that the puruṣa can only see by means of the mind.

[1] *Yoga Sūtra* 1.6–11.

If the mind is colored, then the perception will also be colored, which will in turn affect the puruṣa. If, however, the mind is clear, then its powers of observation are at their best. As the puruṣa observes through and with the help of the mind, the quality of its observation depends totally on the quality of the mind. The mind is the instrument through which the puruṣa perceives, yet the energy and power that the mind needs in order to see comes from the puruṣa.[2] Since we cannot work directly with the puruṣa, we focus on the mind. Through yoga, the mind steadily becomes more transparent, so the puruṣa is able to see more clearly and make this seeing accessible to us.

Very often it is the mind that decides where our attention is directed. It does this because it has been conditioned to do so. The conditioning of the mind that lets it continually take the same direction is called saṃskāra. Saṃskāra is the sum total of all our actions that conditions us to behave in a certain way. Saṃskāra may be positive or negative. Through yoga we attempt to create new and positive saṃskāra rather than reinforcing the old saṃskāra that has been limiting us. When this new saṃskāra is strong and powerful enough, then the old, distressing saṃskāra will no longer be able to affect us. You could say we then begin a completely new life. When the new behavior patterns become stronger, the old ones become ineffectual.

When we practice āsanas we carry out actions that are not determined so much by our habits, and yet still lie within the range of our abilities. So we plan a sequence of exercises and as we execute them, the mind clears a little. We are no longer so bound by our habits. When that happens we might find out that we should change our practice plan a bit, recognizing with greater clarity what is good for us. This kind of reorientation is called *parivṛtti. Vṛtti* means "movement" and *pari* translates as "around."

Imagine you are driving a car and suddenly a tree appears right in front of you. In your mind's eye you see what would happen if you kept driving in the same direction: you would crash into the tree. To avoid that outcome you immediately turn toward another direction. *Parivṛtti* describes this ability to foresee what is going to happen and to redirect oneself accordingly. Instead of letting the mind travel further in the same direction, we practice āsanas or do something else that will help us to see more clearly. This activity may perhaps enable us to see that we were not on the right path. If the reorientation does not help, then it is likely that our mind, rather than our puruṣa, will decide what we do next. Some philosophers have described this well by saying that the mind is a loyal servant but a terrible master. The mind is not the master, but it often behaves as if it is. That is why it is beneficial to do something that gives the puruṣa a chance to do what it is meant to do, namely, to see clearly. If we only glide through familiar waters, then the mind takes over the rudder and the puruṣa cannot really do anything at all.

Ideally, when we take up the practice of yoga we begin a process that offers us a way of stopping what is harmful to us. We do not have to stop doing something deliberately. We do not have to do anything ourselves, but rather

2. Patañjali uses the word *draṣṭṛ* for puruṣa, "the seer," and *dṛśya* for "what is seen." According to Patañjali, avidyā arises when you confuse the two. This confusion is called *saṃyoga*, a word that means that two things have become so entangled with each other we can no longer tell them apart. In the moment of saṃyoga the seeds of suffering are sown.

Asmitā is an expression of saṃyoga. We talk of asmitā when the puruṣa and the citta are mixed up in an inseparable notion of I-ness. The mind is essentially an instrument of perception, and puruṣa is the perceiver. The mind has the quality of being able to change, whereas the puruṣa does not. The association of these two distinct entities often causes problems. See the *Yoga Sūtra* 2.6 and 2.17–24.

whatever it is simply fades out because we have redirected ourselves toward something positive.

The expression of puruṣa allows us to see how the mind functions and how to work with it. Puruṣa does not destroy the mind but gives us control over the mind: we know our strengths and weaknesses, and know what causes us more or less suffering. We use the word *viveka* to describe this clarity of puruṣa. *Viveka* means to see both sides, to be able to see what we are and what we are not, to discriminate. When we used the word *asmitā* we defined it as ego; asmitā can also be described as a state in which puruṣa and citta are mixed together, so that the two function as a unit even though they cannot really become one. When the difference between puruṣa and citta is clear, then viveka is present.

Sometimes it can be helpful to understand the reasons for our old, negative saṃskāra, for there are many kinds of saṃskāra. It is only the powerful saṃskāra that cause us problems, while the weaker ones perhaps reinforce those that are more influential. In a given situation it may well be that we were acting in good faith and were doing everything right, and yet our actions plunged us into trouble. At these times a quiet mind can help us sort out why this happened. Consideration of the situation helps us to be more alert the next time.

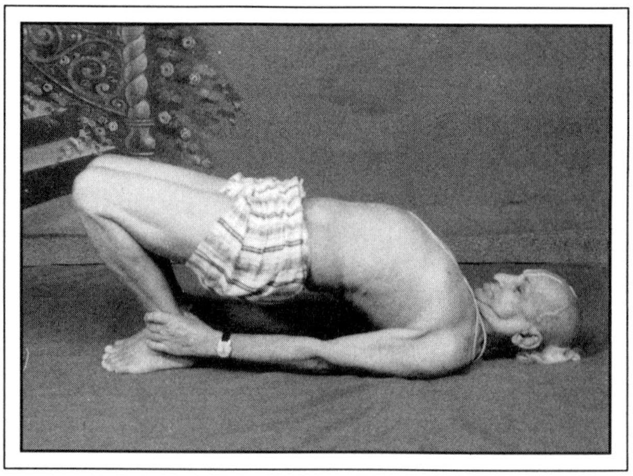

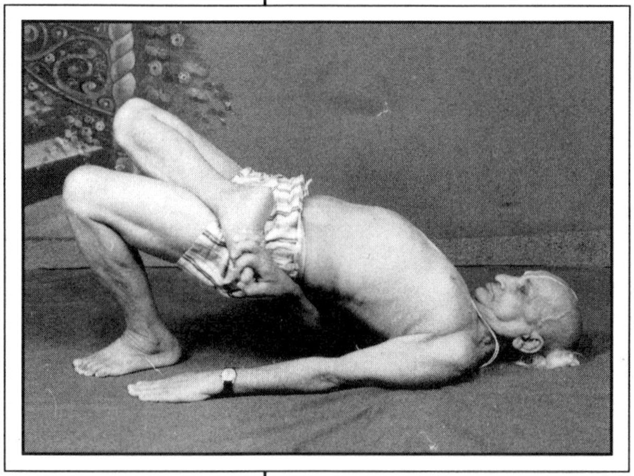

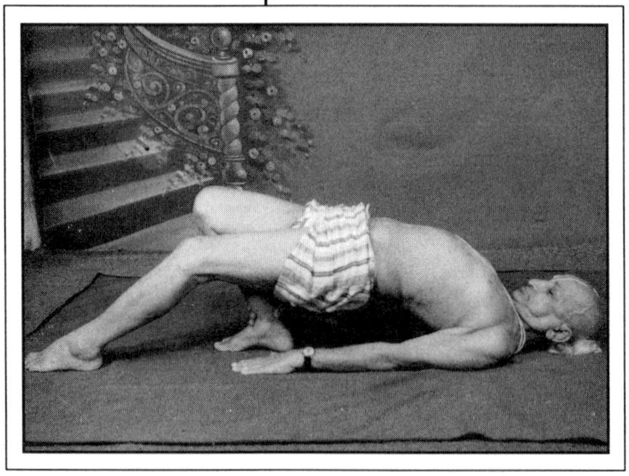

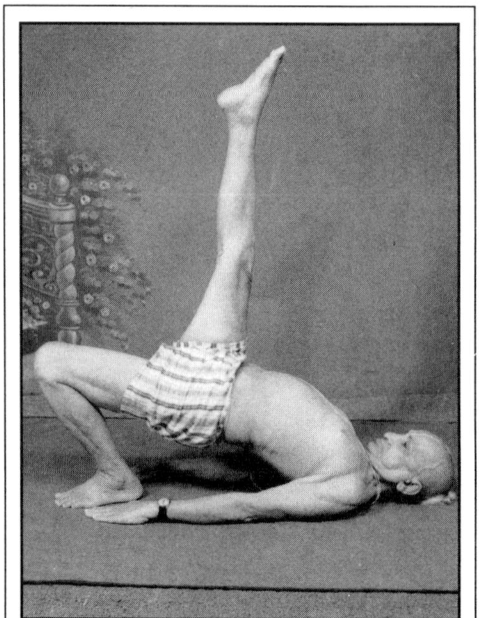

Krishnamacharya in dvipāda pītham sequence.

10

The World Exists to Be Seen and Discovered

Yoga follows the teachings of the Sāṃkhya, which divides the universe into two categories: puruṣa and prakṛti. Puruṣa is that part of us capable of real seeing and perception. It is not subject to change. Conversely, prakṛti is subject to constant change and embraces all matter, even our mind, thoughts, feelings, and memories. All prakṛti can be seen and perceived by puruṣa. (The *Yoga Sūtra* uses the terms *draṣṭṛ* for puruṣa and *dṛśya* for that which is seen.)

Everything that falls into the realm of prakṛti has a common source called *pradhāna*, a word that refers to the original matter from which all things are formed, the spring from which all life flows. In the beginning there was no connection between pradhāna and puruṣa. But then they came together and germinated, like a seed. This seed is prakṛti. The whole material world grew from this seed. First came *mahat*, the great principle. Out of mahat came the *ahamkāra*, the sense of I. Out of ahamkāra came *manas*, the power behind the senses, and from there the so-called *tanmātras* and the *indriyas*. Tanmātra refers to the sound, touch, form, taste, and smell of material objects. The indriyas, the eleven senses, include all our mental activities; our passive perceptive senses such as hearing, feeling, seeing, tasting, and smelling; our active faculties of speech; manual dexterity; locomotion; evacuation; and procreation. From the tanmātras came the *bhūtas*, the five elements: space, air, light, water, and earth.

What I have just described is an all too brief summary of the yogic theory of evolution. The world as we see it is a combination of these aspects constantly interacting with one another. Everything that happens in the external world influences us, and what happens within us in its turn has an influence on our relationship with the external world.

We can most easily understand what the puruṣa is if we think of what is absent from a corpse. In death the puruṣa vanishes. (Where it goes is not revealed in the *Yoga Sūtra*.) The body, the brain, and the sense organs are still present, but they are lifeless because the puruṣa is gone. Yet for the puruṣa there is no death. For the puruṣa change does not exist—and what is death but change? Our mind cannot see the puruṣa. Only because we sometimes experience moments of clarity do we know that there is a puruṣa. It is the constant witness to all our actions. This witness is active, but it is not influenced by what it sees. Because the puruṣa works through the mind, it can only see when the mind is clear.[1]

It is hard to imagine that puruṣa and prakṛti can exist independent of each other. In humans the two are always interrelated. Why do we confuse puruṣa and prakṛti? According to the teachings of yoga, this confusion, saṃyoga, permeates human existence. At the same time, those who search for clarity can learn the difference between right and wrong understanding. In this respect yoga is optimistic: through the insightful perception of problems and confusions we move toward clarity.

Just because some of us look for solutions to problems, and in the process attain a certain degree of clarity, does not mean that the puruṣa of others will see more clearly. Other philosophical systems believe that there is only one puruṣa; however, in yoga it is believed that even though one person solves his or her problems, it does not mean some part of the burden has been lifted from all of humanity.[2] While there are different puruṣa, there is only one prakṛti, one common universe for us all. It is the relationship between the individual puruṣa and the one praktri that is special. For this reason alone, our way of looking at things such as our bodies, our senses, and our habits are all different. Observation can only occur when the puruṣa has the energy and inclination to go out from within and come back with impressions of the outer world. Herein lies a great difference with modern physics, according to which you need light for the image of an object to come to the eye. Even when light is present, as well as an object that can be viewed, still there must be something that calls us out to see, to think, to listen. This impulse comes from the puruṣa within, not from outside. Often there are external objects to attract our attention, yet we do not react to them. All action must come from the puruṣa. Humans cannot live without our puruṣa.

There are various opinions about how the relationship between puruṣa and prakṛti came about. Some say it is *līlā*, a divine game. Others believe there was in the beginning one entity that said to itself, "I should like to become many." A third body of opinion calls it chance. Each standpoint we take on this must remain speculative.

1. *Yoga Sūtra* 2.20.

2. *Yoga Sūtra* 2.22.

There are also many theories about what happens to our puruṣa when we die. People who believe in an energy higher than human beings, in God, say that the various puruṣa are like rivers that all flow toward the sea. Each has its own bed, its own direction, its own quality, but they all flow together into the sea.

Change is not a direct or even an indirect consequence of yoga or any other practice. We cannot depend on it. What we can count on gaining from our yoga practice is a quieter mind—somehow the heaviness and the jumpiness vanish. Yet something very personal and essential has to happen for us at the right time, and it has to touch us so deeply that we suddenly really want to pause, consider, and change the course of our actions. After that happens we simply go forward step by step. The quality of our action begins to change. The new positive saṃskāra becomes stronger and our mind remains clear.

The mind cannot observe its own changes. Something else observes these changes.[3] For this very reason we describe our puruṣa as the witness as well as the source of our action. As the source of action, our puruṣa works like the transmitter for an electric door. But what actually moves is the door. Our puruṣa is the source of our action. But we also need our puruṣa as a witness and constant observer of the functioning of the mind. In the end, clarity can prevail in the mind, but experiential understanding occurs only through the puruṣa.

If real clarity is present, we experience quietness and peace within us. If there is only intellectual clarity, we may be happy for a moment or two, but this feeling will not last. Our goal is freedom from duḥkha, from distress and suffering. To this end we must recognize duḥkha, we must know that it arises out of the incorrect understanding of avidyā, and we must know that we can avoid it.

Our aim in practicing yoga is to bring about a change in the quality of the mind so that we can perceive more from the puruṣa. Yoga attempts to influence the mind in such a way that it is possible for our puruṣa to operate without hindrances.

3. *Yoga Sūtra* 4.18–21.

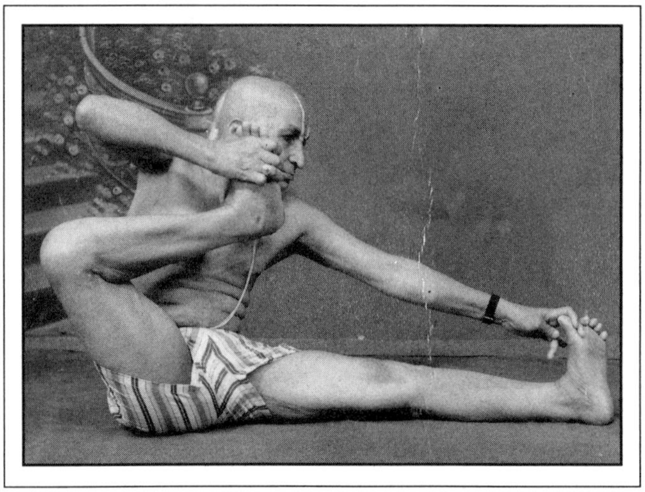

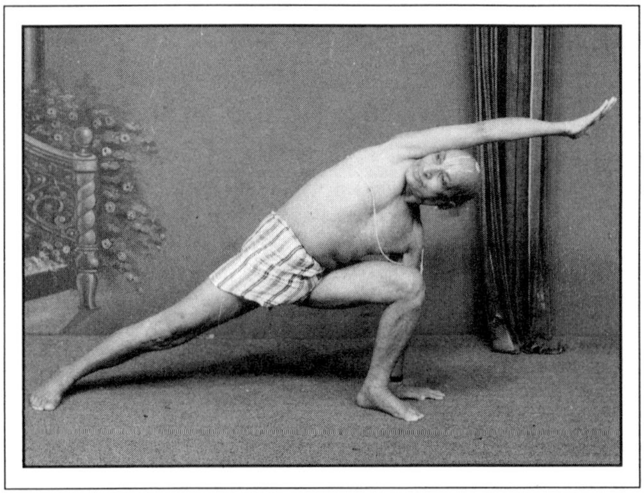

Krishnamacharya demonstrating ākarṇa dhanurāsana and utthita pārśva koṇāsana.

11

Living in the World

Yoga cannot guarantee us this or that particular benefit if we practice diligently. Yoga is not a recipe for less suffering, though it can offer us help in changing our attitude so that we have less avidyā and therefore greater freedom from duḥkha. We can understand the whole practice of yoga as a process of examining our habitual attitudes and behaviors and their consequences.

Yama and Niyama: Behavior Toward Ourselves and Others

What suggestions does yoga make about our interaction with others—our behavior toward those around us—and about our attitude toward ourselves? The attitude we have toward things and people outside ourselves is called *yama* in yoga, and how we relate to ourselves inwardly is called *niyama*.

Yama and niyama deal with our social attitude and life style, how we interact with other people and the environment, and how we deal with our problems. These all form a part of yoga, but they cannot be practiced. What we can practice are āsanas and prāṇāyāma, which make us aware of where we are, where we stand, and how we look at things. Recognizing our mistakes is the first sign of clarity. Then gradually we try to bring about some changes in the way we show our respect to nature or relate to a friend. No one can change in a day, but yoga practices help change attitudes, our yama and niyama. It is not the other way around.

Let me tell you a story about a man named Daniel and his wife, Mary. At work Daniel was always friendly to everyone, but he was often very short tempered at home. Mary was never sure when he would lose his temper. None of his friends and colleagues believed her when she told them of his actions at home, and Daniel would not admit to his short temper. Daniel suffered from back pain and, on the suggestion of a colleague, started going to a yoga class regularly. Gradually his back pain disappeared. At the end of his yoga practice his teacher used to say: "As you lie down to relax, feel your body, feel your breath, and become aware of your emotions." One day he realized in a flash that his bad temper built up on his way home from work. He recognized that he was doing to his wife what he could not do to his boss or subordinates. He went home that day and told Mary: "You are right. I am indeed a short-tempered fellow. But bear with me. I am working on it." This recognition made Mary very happy.

Yama and niyama are the first two of the eight limbs of the body of yoga.[1] Both words have many meanings. Yama can mean "discipline" or "restraints"; I prefer to think of yama as "attitude" or "behavior." Certainly a particular attitude can be expressed as discipline, which then influences our behavior. Patañjali's *Yoga Sūtra* mentions five different yama, that is, behavior patterns or relationships between the individual and the outside world.[2]

The Yamas

Ahiṁsā

The first of these behavior patterns is called *ahiṁsā*. The word *hiṁsā* means "injustice" or "cruelty," but *ahiṁsā* is more than simply the absence of hiṁsā, which the prefix *a-* suggests. Ahiṁsā is more than just lack of violence. It means kindness, friendliness, and thoughtful consideration of other people and things. We must exercise judgment when thinking about ahiṁsā. It does not necessarily imply that we should not eat meat or fish or that we should not defend ourselves. It simply means that we must always behave with consideration and attention to others. Ahiṁsā also means acting in kindness toward ourselves. Should we as vegetarians find ourselves in a situation where there is only meat to eat, is it better to starve to death than to eat what is there? If we still have something to do in this life, such as family responsibilities, then we should avoid doing anything that may cause us harm or prevent us from carrying out our duties. The answer in this situation is clear—it would show a lack of consideration and arrogance to become stuck on our principles. So ahiṁsā has to do with our duties and responsibilities too. It could even mean that we must fight if our life is in danger.

In every situation we should adopt a considered attitude. That is the meaning of ahiṁsā.

Satya

The next yama mentioned by Patañjali is *satya*, truthfulness. *Satya* means "to speak the truth," yet it is not always desirable to speak the truth come what may, for it could harm someone unnecessarily. We have to consider what we say, how we say it, and in what way it could affect others. If speaking the truth has negative consequences for another, then it is better to say nothing. Satya

1. *Yoga Sūtra* 2.29. The eight limbs or *aṅgas* are: yama, niyama, āsana, prāṇāyāma, pratyāhāra, dhāraṇā, dhyāna, and samādhi.

2. The yama and niyama are described in the *Yoga Sūtra* 2.29–45.

should never come into conflict with our efforts to behave with ahiṁsā. The *Mahābhārata*, the great Indian epic, says: "Speak the truth which is pleasant. Do not speak unpleasant truths. Do not lie, even if the lies are pleasing to the ear. That is the eternal law, the dharma."

Asteya

Asteya is the third yama. *Steya* means "to steal"; asteya is the opposite—to take nothing that does not belong to us. This also means that if we are in a situation where someone entrusts something to us or confides in us, we do not take advantage of him or her.

Brahmacarya

The next yama is *brahmacarya*. This word is composed of the root *car*, which means "to move," and the word *brahma*, which means "truth" in terms of the one essential truth. We can understand brahmacarya as a movement toward the essential. It is used mostly in the sense of abstinence, particularly in relationship to sexual activity. More specifically, brahmacarya suggests that we should form relationships that foster our understanding of the highest truths. If sensual pleasures are part of those relationships, we must take care that we keep our direction and do not get lost. On the path of serious, constant searching for truth, there are certain ways of controlling the perceptual senses and sexual desires. This control, however, is not identical with total abstinence.

India has the greatest respect for family life. According to Indian tradition, everything in life has its place and time, and we divide the life cycle into four stages: the first is the stage of the growing child, the second is that of the student striving for greater understanding and searching for truth. The third stage is centered around starting and raising a family, and the fourth is the stage where the individual, after fulfilling all family responsibilities, can devote him- or herself to becoming free from all bondages and finding ultimate truth.

In this fourth stage of life everyone can become a *sannyāsin*, a monk or nun. But a sannyāsin must then beg for food from people who are still involved in family life. The Upaniṣads advise the student to marry and raise a family immediately upon finishing his or her studies. That is why brahmacarya does not necessarily imply celibacy. Rather, it means responsible behavior with respect to our goal of moving toward the truth.

Aparigraha

The last yama is *aparigraha*, a word that means something like "hands off" or "not seizing opportunity." *Parigraha* means "to take" or "to seize." *Aparigraha* means to take only what is necessary, and not to take advantage of a situation. I once had a student who paid me tuition every month for our work together. But at the end of the course he also offered me a gift. Why should I accept this when I had already been paid sufficiently for my work? We should only take what we have earned; if we take more, we are exploiting someone else. In addition, unearned rewards can bring with them obligations that might later cause problems.

Developing the Yamas

The *Yoga Sūtra* describes what happens when these five behaviors outlined above become part of a person's daily life. For example, the more ahiṁsā—kindness and consideration—we develop, the more pleasant and friendly feelings our very presence engenders in others. And if we remain true to the idea of satya, everything we say will be truthful.

There is a wonderful story on the theme of satya in the Rāmāyana. The monkey Hanuman, Prince Rama's servant, sets out to look for Sita, his master's wife. He travels to Sri Lanka where she is being held prisoner. Toward the end of his time there he is caught by Sita's captors and his tail is set on fire. When Sita sees what pain he is suffering she calls out: "Let the fire cool!" Hanuman's pain is immediately alleviated and he shouts: "What happened? Why doesn't the fire burn me anymore?" Because Sita always spoke the truth, her words had great power and could extinguish the flames.

For those who are always truthful, there is no difference between speech and action—what they say is true. The *Yoga Sūtra* also states that a person who is firmly anchored in asteya will receive all the jewels of this world. Such a person may not in fact be interested in material wealth, but he or she will have access to the most valuable things in life.

The more we recognize the meaning of the search for truth, for what is essential, the less we will be distracted by other things. Certainly it requires great strength to take this path. The word used in the *Yoga Sūtra* to describe this strength is *vīrya*, which is closely linked to another concept, that of *śraddhā*, deep trust and loving faith.[3] The *Yoga Sūtra* says that the more faith we have, the more energy we have. At the same time we also have more strength to pursue our goals. So the more we seek the truth in the sense of brahmacarya, the more vitality we will have to do so. Parigraha is the increasing orientation toward material things. If we reduce parigraha and develop aparigraha, we are orienting ourselves more inwardly. The less time we spend on our material possessions, the more we have to spend on investigating all that we call yoga.

The Niyamas

Like the five yamas, the niyamas are not exercises or actions to be simply studied. They represent far more than an attitude. Compared with the yamas, the niyamas are more intimate and personal. They refer to the attitude we adopt toward ourselves.

3. In the *Yoga Sūtra* 1.20, Patañjali lists what people need in order to recognize the truth: faith and trust, strength and energy, and the ability never to lose sight of the goal.

Śauca

The first niyama is *śauca*, cleanliness. Śauca has both an inner and an outer aspect. Outer cleanliness simply means keeping ourselves clean. Inner cleanliness has as much to do with the healthy, free functioning of our bodily organs as with the clarity of our mind. Practicing āsanas or prāṇāyāma are essential means for attending to this inner śauca.

Saṃtoṣa

Another niyama is *saṃtoṣa*, modesty and the feeling of being content with what we have. Often we hope for a particular result to ensue from our actions, and we are just as often disappointed. But there is no need to despair—rather, we should accept what has happened. That is the real meaning of saṃtoṣa—to accept what happens. A commentary on the *Yoga Sūtra* says: "Contentment counts for more than all sixteen heavens together." Instead of complaining about things that go wrong, we can accept what has happened and learn from them. Saṃtoṣa encompasses our mental activities such as study, our physical efforts, and even how we earn our living. It is about ourselves—what we have and how we feel about what God has given us.

Tapas

The next niyama is tapas, a term that we discussed earlier. In relationship to the niyamas, tapas refers to the activity of keeping the body fit. Literally it means to heat the body and, by so doing, to cleanse it. Behind the notion of tapas lies the idea that we can get rid of the rubbish in our body. Earlier I discussed āsanas and prāṇāyāma as means by which we can keep ourselves healthy. Another form of tapas is paying attention to what we eat. Eating when we are not hungry is the opposite of tapas. Attention to body posture, attention to eating habits, attention to breathing patterns—these are all tapas that help to prevent the buildup of rubbish in the body, including excess weight and shortness of breath. Tapas makes the whole body fit and well functioning.

Svādhyāya

The fourth niyama is *svādhyāya*. *Sva* means "self" or "belonging to me." *Adhyāya* means "inquiry" or "examination"; literally, "to get close to something." *Svādhyāya* therefore means to get close to yourself, that is, to study yourself. All learning, all reflection, all contact that helps you to learn more about yourself is svādhyāya. In the context of the niyama we find the term often translated as "the study of ancient texts." Yes, yoga does instruct us to read the ancient texts. Why? Because we cannot always just sit down and contemplate things. We need reference points. For many this may be the Bible or a book that is of personal significance; for others it may be the *Yoga Sūtra*. The *Yoga Sūtra* says, for instance, that as we progress in our self-examination, we will gradually find a link with the divine laws and with the prophets who revealed them. And since mantra are often recited for this purpose, we sometimes find *svādhyāya* translated as "the repetition of mantras."[4]

Īśvarapraṇidhānā

The last niyama was discussed in Part 1. *Īśvarapraṇidhānā* means "to lay all your actions at the feet of God." Because avidyā often underlies our actions, things frequently go wrong. This is the reason why saṃtoṣa (modesty) is so important: let it suffice that we know we have done our best. We can leave the rest to a higher power. In the context of the niyamas we can define īśvarapraṇidhānā as the attitude of a person who usually offers the fruits of his or her action to God in daily prayer.

Further Thoughts on the Yamas and Niyamas

Q: What is the relationship between kriyā exercises and śauca?

A: The *Yoga Sūtra* does not mention the concept of kriyā when discussing the various niyama. The word *kriyā* means "action." In the context of your question it refers to cleansing. Something from the outside is used to clean the inside. For example, we can cleanse a blocked nostril with a light salt solution, or use a prāṇāyāma technique to reduce a breathing difficulty that might have developed from inhaling stale air. In this sense, kriyās are a vital aspect of śauca.

Q: I've often heard *tapas* translated as "self-denial" or "self-deprivation." How do you interpret tapas?

A: If by "self-denial" you mean fasting for the sake of fasting or adhering to a strict and unusual lifestyle simply for its own sake, you are talking about activities that have nothing to do with tapas. Just as when you are dealing with satya (truth), everything about tapas must help you move forward. You can incur serious physical difficulties if you do something like fast for twenty days just for the sake of it. On the other hand, if by "self-denial" you mean a sensible, well-founded discipline that helps you move forward in life, then you are talking about real tapas. Tapas must not cause suffering. That is very important.

Q: Can the yamas and niyamas help us to differentiate between a moment of true clarity and a moment of self-deception?

A: The relationships we have with the outer world—with other people and things around us—can help us to recognize a moment of self-deception. This is where the yamas and niyamas become important. If we deal uprightly and respectfully with other people we can easily tell whether we are deceiving ourselves or not. I can think I am the greatest yogi, but from what others think of me, how they relate to me and how I interact with them, I can experience very directly whether my image of myself is right or not. For this reason it is important to live in the world and observe what sort of communication we have with other people. It is very easy to deceive ourselves otherwise.

4. A mantra is a word or a syllable, traditionally given by a teacher to the student. The repetition of a mantra is known as *japa*. Japa is one of the many yoga techniques for meditation.

Q: Can the yamas and niyamas, which help to reduce avidyā and its effects, be developed through conscious willing effort?

A: We must always distinguish between cause and effect. Very often we confuse them. Mostly we follow certain behavior patterns in our lives because we have definite expectations and goals. But often we do not achieve our goals. During the course of our lives, through personal development and external events, it often happens that something totally unexpected arises. Yamas and niyamas can be both cause and effect. Today I might tell you a hundred blatant lies and feel perfectly happy about it; tomorrow I may recoil from telling even one small untruth. That is how yamas grow. There are no definite rules, and we can never predict with certainty what is going to occur. But in what has happened in the past we can find gentle hints about what may arise in the future.

Q: So we can always only observe how, for example, hate or greed appear, and then try to prevent them from reappearing?

A: First we must simply observe—the first thing we do is watch and see what is happening. Then we see what we need to be wary of. We do not simply drive onto a motorway and take off. We must be constantly looking around as we go forward.

Q: Isn't it easier to abide by yogic principles if you live in a quiet place like a monastery rather than living in the family home?

A: Both settings can be helpful. A friend of mine came to India thinking it would do him good to live alone for two or three years in the Himalayas. He found a nice place and spent three years there. He had a few books with him and practiced sādhana—indeed, he practiced intensely. One day he came to me to work on a few āsanas and to study the *Yoga Sūtra*. When he arrived in Madras he said he had the feeling that a lot had been going on for him. He seemed very happy. He used very complicated expressions such as *sabīja samādhi* when he was talking about his development in the Himalayas. Then he found a simple room to rent on the grounds of the Theosophical Society in Madras, a quiet and peaceful place where he would not be disturbed. After two days he told me he had changed his mind and wanted to look for a larger place to live. I was a bit surprised and asked him why he was all of a sudden looking for a big house. "I have gotten to know a woman. My whole life has suddenly changed." I do not judge this change of heart; I simply want to point out that my friend was not really who he thought he was.

A place like a retreat or monastery can be a help, but the real test for this experience would be a city like Madras with its teeming population. The real test for someone from Madras would be to see what it is like living in a secluded monastery. I am sure that there are people who could not last more than one day in that kind of quiet. Someone who is uncertain of themselves, on the other hand, would only last a day in Madras.

Change helps. We must look at both fire and water if we want to experience how we will react to them. That is why yama is so important, for it includes our relationships with different people at different times. In this way we can experience who we are.

Q: A changing environment, then, is important for yoga?

A: Yes, a little change is very important. The mind grows so used to things that our action quickly falls into habits (saṃskāras). We can never experience our real nature if we do not expose ourselves to change. That is why we must test ourselves sometimes by doing something completely different.

Q: I understand how we should give up living out a desire that we recognize is bad for us. Where should the emphasis of our work then lie—on giving it up or on making sure that the desire does not reappear? I notice that I get angry when a desire arises, and I am disturbed that I get so angry. It is a vicious circle.

A: We must first of all determine whether that which we consider to be a problem really is one. Think about what it means when you say "That's causing me a lot of trouble." To recognize if there really is a problem, it is often helpful to change your surroundings and look at things from a different perspective. As an example, let's say you have the opportunity to lie about something. It may be a "white lie," one that would avoid a difficult interaction. It could also be a statement of untruth that prevents your having to spend a lot of time analyzing a situation. Or it could be a lie that has no consequence—there are many different philosophical origins for a single untruth. At the moment it seems fine—you might even want to lie. But later it bothers you. You think: "How could I have lied like that? It would have been better to speak the truth or to have remained silent."

What was right in this situation? You can sort it out by discussing the whole experience with someone in an abstract way and watching his or her reaction. Or you can change your surroundings, going into a different situation from where you can view the whole encounter from a fresh perspective. Then you have the chance to look at everything again. The *Yoga Sūtra* says that if something is really causing you problems, imagine the opposite situation—this can help you sort out the right thing to do. The idea is to be open.

Encouraging a change of perspective is a matter of finding a new situation that can allow a fresh attitude to develop. This may mean reading a book, talking with a close friend, or going to the movies. Perhaps you will even discover that what you have been worrying about is not the real source of your difficulties.

In any situation, when you do not know exactly how you should behave then you should not act immediately.

Q: So whenever we are in doubt we shouldn't act?

A: If there is time to consider the situation, don't act. If there is no time, then at least give yourself a little breathing space. Whenever you are in doubt, it is best to pause. Few things are so pressing that they cannot wait for a moment of breath.

Q: It seems to me, though, that it is precisely when I am in a situation in which I am in doubt that I find it impossible to pause, especially if I am responsible for someone else in that moment. Times when doubt and uncertainty are the greatest stand out in my experience because of the fact that I cannot give myself breathing space. If it were otherwise, the stress under which I live would not seem so great. What should I do when doubts arise? Should I turn to another thought or circumstance? Should I confront my doubts? Or should I perhaps ignore them?

A: Somehow you must arrange things so that you can look at the problem from another, higher vantage point. If you succeed in doing this, that is already a sign of progress. Perhaps, if you practice yoga, things are going better for you today than yesterday, and already it is easier to look at the same problem differently. But often one makes no progress toward solving problems simply by viewing them from a different angle or discussing them with someone else. Something more may be necessary.

In yoga it is important to grow. We must develop. What was doubt does not have to remain doubt forever. My personal experience of changing my life from that of an engineer to a devoted yoga teacher—that was in 1964—was a major decision that brought with it many problems. I talked about it with many people, but the problems remained. And then suddenly one day there were no longer any problems. Somehow I was able to view the whole situation from a different vantage point and suddenly the problems were gone. When things become a little easier, the doubts disappear more easily.

The goal of yoga is to encourage us to be a little better than we were before. We become better by making an effort and by practicing patience. When we do this we will not see ourselves as beset by so many problems. Our efforts may change in intensity, but over a period of time we will gradually experience progress. We must actively seize every opportunity that helps us to progress.

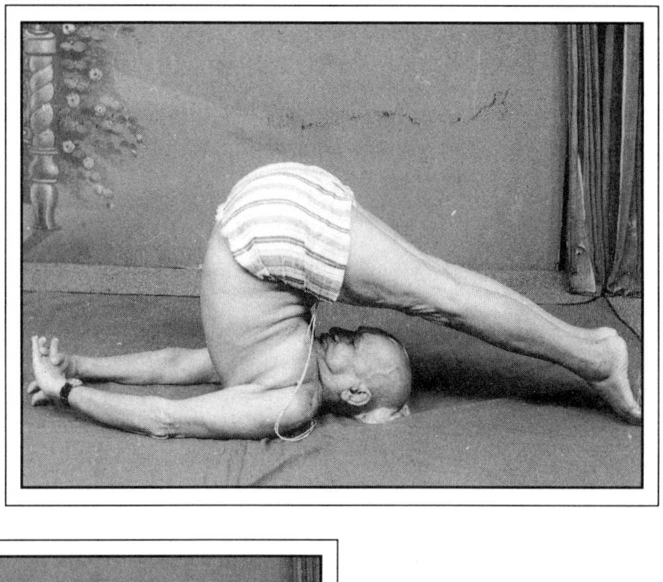

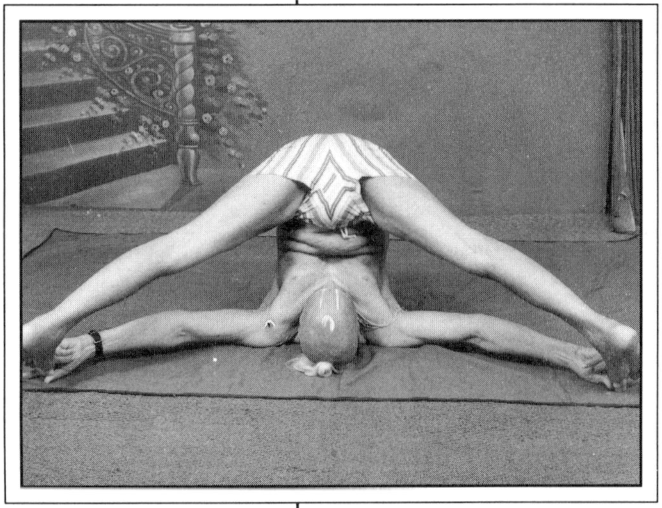

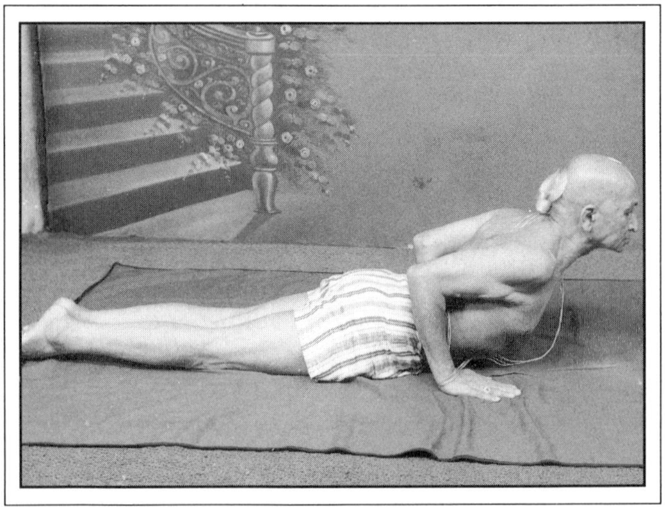

Krishnamacharya in (top to bottom) halāsana, supta koṇāsana, bhujaṅgāsana.

12

The World Exists to Set Us Free

We cannot simply start adhering to the five yamas by practicing ahiṁsā first and, when we have mastered that, proceeding to satya, and so on. Our behavior changes gradually as we progress along the yoga path, a path that is determined by the desire to better ourselves by any means. In this connection, the word *aṅga* or "limb" has a very important meaning. From conception through a child's full development, all the limbs of the fetus grow simultaneously; the body does not sprout an arm first, then a leg, and so on. Similarly, on the path of yoga all eight aspects develop concurrently and in an interrelated way. That is why the *Yoga Sūtra* uses the term *aṅga* for the eight limbs of yoga. Patañjali refers to them collectively as *aṣṭāṅga*.

Pratyāhāra

We have already discussed the first four limbs of yoga: āsana, prāṇāyāma, yama, and niyama. The fifth limb of yoga, *pratyāhāra,* has to do with our senses.[1] The word *āhāra* means "nourishment"; *pratyāhāra* translates as "to withdraw oneself from that which nourishes the senses." What does this mean? It means our senses stop living off the things that stimulate; the senses no longer depend on these stimulants and are not fed by them any more. Our eyes are drawn to a beautiful sunset as bees are drawn to honey—this is the way our senses function normally. But there is also the possibility that the most beautiful sunset on earth will not attract our attention, will not engage our senses, because we are deeply immersed in something else. Normally the senses say to the mind: "Look at this! Smell this! Touch that!" The senses register an object and the mind is drawn to it at once.

1. *Yoga Sūtra* 2.54–55.

In pratyāhāra we sever this link between mind and senses, and the senses withdraw. Each sense perception has a particular quality to which it relates: the eyes relate to the form of something; the ears to the sound, the vibration it makes; the nose to its smell. In pratyāhāra it is as if things are spread out with all their attractions before our senses, but they are ignored; the senses remain unmoved and uninfluenced.

Let me give you an example. When we are totally absorbed in the breath during prāṇāyāma, when we are completely with it, pratyāhāra occurs quite automatically. The mind is so intensely occupied with the breath that all links between mind, senses, and external objects that have nothing to do with the breath are cut. So pratyāhāra is not a state of sleep. The senses are quite capable of responding, but they do not because they have withdrawn.

As another example, when I am asked a question, I try to clarify the subject I have been discussing as I answer. As I become more involved in my response, I grow less aware of where I am. I become increasingly more engrossed in the interaction—this is another manifestation of pratyāhāra. Although I stand in front of the audience with open eyes, I am so absorbed in the content of the discussion that my senses no longer react to other stimuli. Even if there were snow falling outside the window I would not notice; nor do I hear the sounds coming from outside the room. Pratyāhāra does not mean that I look at something and say to myself: "I'm not going to look at that!" What is meant by pratyāhāra is that I create a situation in which my mind is so absorbed in something that the senses no longer respond to other objects.

When we act we must use our senses. When we speak we must use the mouth and the ears. Vairāgya, the concept of equanimity or detachment, means that we act without thinking about the possible gains to be had as a consequence of that action. Vairāgya is being detached from the results or the fruits of my action.

Pratyāhāra, on the other hand, is related to the senses. It is only about the senses. Pratyāhāra occurs almost automatically when we meditate because we are so absorbed in the object of meditation. Precisely because the mind is so focused, the senses follow it; it is not happening the other way around. No longer functioning in their usual manner, the senses become extraordinarily sharp. Under normal circumstances the senses become our masters rather than being our servants. The senses entice us to develop cravings for all sorts of things. In pratyāhāra the opposite occurs: when we have to eat we eat, but not because we have a craving for food. In pratyāhāra we try to put the senses in their proper place, but not cut them out of our actions entirely.

Pratyāhāra can be a means for controlling physical discomfort by directing the attention elsewhere. Imagine you have been sitting in the full lotus pose, completely absorbed in God or *OM*. You have not even been aware that you have been sitting for so long in this position. When you return to your normal awareness you find you have to massage your legs; you have not been aware of what has been happening in your legs and feet because your interest was focused on something else. In this sense it is possible for pain to be masked by pratyāhāra, but it is difficult to direct the senses to a particular object with the express purpose of forgetting pain because our senses always function collectively. Pratyāhāra is rather a state that occurs spontaneously. Many people say that inner gazing is a pratyāhāra technique, and in many texts this is suggested. But pratyāhāra happens by itself—we cannot make it happen, we can only practice the means by which it might happen.

Dhāraṇā

Dhāraṇā is the sixth limb of yoga. *Dhṛ* means "to hold." The essential idea in the concept of dhāraṇā is holding the concentration or focus of attention in one direction. Let me give you the example that is traditionally used to explain dhāraṇā: imagine a large reservoir of water used by farmers for watering their fields. There are channels leading away from the reservoir in different directions. If the farmer has dug all the channels the same depth, the water runs equally in all directions. But if one channel is deeper than the others, more water flows through it. This is what happens in dhāraṇā: we create the conditions for the mind to focus its attention in one direction instead of going out in many different directions. Deep contemplation and reflection can create the right conditions, and the focus on this one point that we have chosen becomes more intense. We encourage one particular activity of the mind and, the more intense it becomes, the more the other activities of the mind fall away.

Dhāraṇā is therefore the condition in which the mind focuses and concentrates exclusively on one point. This point can be anything at all, but it is always just a single object. Dhāraṇā is only one step away from *dhyāna,* contemplation or meditation.

Dhyāna

During dhāraṇā the mind is moving in one direction like a quiet river—nothing else is happening. In dhyāna, one becomes involved with a particular thing—a link is established between self and object. In other words, you perceive a particular object and at the same time continuously communicate with it. Dhāraṇā must precede dhyāna, because the mind needs focusing on a particular object before a connection can be made. Dhāraṇā is the contact, and dhyāna is the connection.

Samādhi

When we succeed in becoming so absorbed in something that our mind becomes completely one with it, we are in a state of *samādhi.* Samādhi means "to bring together, to merge." In samādhi our personal identity—name, profession, family history, bank account, and so forth—completely disappears. In the moment of samādhi none of that exists anymore. Nothing separates us from the object of our choice; instead we blend and become one with it.

Figure 31 shows the relationship between dhāraṇā, dhyāna, and samādhi. In dhāraṇā (1), we focus the mind, making contact with that on which we are focusing—the breath, a sound, an area of the body, the mind itself, the image of the moon, the notion of humility, etc. Then the mind links with the object of attention and maintains this link. There is a communication or interation between the two. This is dhyāna (2), which then leads to samādhi (3), a state in which the mind blends and becomes one with the object of meditation.

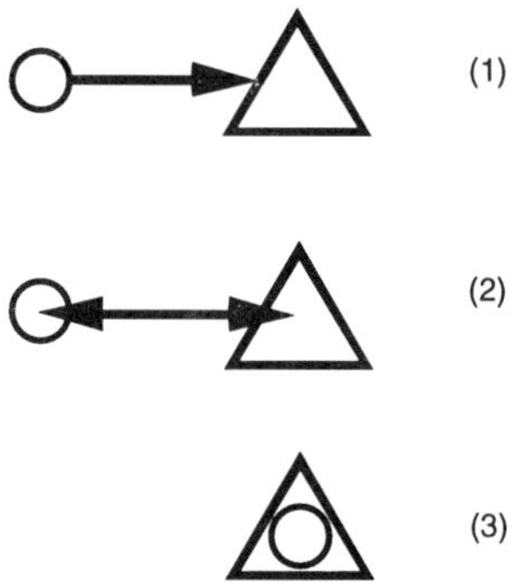

Figure 31: The progression from dhāraṇā, via dhyāna, to samādhi

Pratyāhāra, dhāraṇā, dhyāna, and samādhi cannot be practiced. I cannot simply sit down and say, "Right now I am going to do dhāraṇā." I can, though, create the right conditions to help bring about a state of dhāraṇā; I can practice āsanas and prāṇāyāma that, according to the *Yoga Sūtra*, create favorable conditions for my mind to enter the states I described above. In order to experience dhāraṇā and dhyāna, the mind must first be in a particular condition. I have to first allow the many things that are going on in my mind to settle so that my mind becomes quiet. If the workings of the mind are too powerful, I cannot enter a state of dhāraṇā. If I try to enter a state of dhāraṇā by forcing the mind while there are still many disparate things churning around in it, then I can get into great difficulties. For this reason the *Yoga Sūtra* suggests the practice of āsanas and prāṇāyāma as preparation for dhāraṇā, because these influence mental activities and create space in the crowded schedule of the mind. Once dhāraṇā has occurred, dhyāna and samādhi can follow.

So when somebody says "I am meditating," he or she actually means "I am attempting to prepare myself for dhyāna. I'd like to bring my mind into a suitable state for dhyāna to occur." To say "I am doing dhyāna" or "I am meditating" actually corrupts the concept of dhyāna because technically dhyāna is not something we can do. It is something that simply happens if the conditions are right. It is a *siddhi,* simply given. Hence all we can do is emphasize the means that help to make the conditions right for dhyāna.

Saṃyama

When dhāraṇā, dhyāna, and samādhi are concentrated on one object, the resulting state is called *saṃyama. Sam* means "together," and the word *yama* can be translated as "curbing" or "discipline." When a person is constantly focusing on one particular object, he or she will come to understand it progressively more deeply. Say for example that I want to understand how the stars move. I would have to investigate this thoroughly. I might begin by asking, "What is a star? Why does it move from east to west?" From there I would ask progressively more involved questions about the movements of the stars until my desire to know was satisfied. What happens when I do this? In a short time I learn more about this topic than any other. That is saṃyama. Instead of choosing one topic today and another tomorrow, I try to understand one particular thing well, without my interest constantly leading me elsewhere. If my interest is on āsanas, then I will find out everything about āsanas.

It is said that saṁyama releases supernatural powers, yet this is only the effect of saṃyama, not the aim. If these powers become the most important thing for me, then I lose the true meaning of saṃyama. The true goal of saṃyama is to concentrate on one object and to investigate it until we know everything about it.

Kaivalya

Kaivalya describes the effect on the personality of being in a continuous state of samādhi. This is the state of inner freedom that yoga strives for. The last thirty-four verses of the *Yoga Sūtra* are devoted to kaivalya. Derived from the word *kevala,* which translates as "to keep to oneself," we sometimes find kaivalya explained as isolation or aloofness. A person in the state of kaivalya understands the world so well that he stands apart from it in the sense that he is not influenced by it, although he may well be in a position to influence the world. It is a misunderstanding to think that someone who lives in a state of kaivalya is no longer a real person with normal human needs and functions. In reality, people in kaivalya behave like normal people, but they do not carry the burden of the world on their shoulders. They live in the world, but they are not subject to it. They are not free from sensual perception or free of the body, but they are a bit different. Wherever they happen to be, they are sure of themselves. That is kaivalya. External forces have no power over a person like this, though he knows the external world very well.

According to yoga, the purpose of the whole of creation is to give us a context for understanding what we are and what we are not. When we understand that, then there is kaivalya, and prakṛti has fulfilled its purpose.[2] A person who experiences kaivalya sees prakṛti, the material world, simply as it is, with no meaning beyond that.

By practicing āsanas we become more flexible; by practicing prāṇāyāma we gain control over our breath. It is similar with kaivalya: something gradually happens that is beyond our control. There is always a gap between our efforts and these states I am describing. There is always a spontaneity; something simply happens within us. It is similar to the moment we fall asleep: we cannot pinpoint it. Either we miss the moment or we do not sleep.

There are two forces within us: one comes from our old conditioning and habits; the other is our new conditioning that develops out of our changing behavior. As long as these two forces are operating, the mind is swinging from one to the other. But when the old force disappears, the mind no longer swings back and forth. We have reached another state, and it is felt as a continuum.

Further Thoughts on Pratyāhāra, Dhāraṇā, Dhyāna, and Samādhi

Q: What is the relationship between pratyāhāra and dhāraṇā?

A: Pratyāhāra occurs automatically in a state of dhāraṇā. The word *pratyāhāra* is often used to simply describe what happens with our senses in the state

2. *Yoga Sūtra* 2.21.

of dhāraṇā. We cannot be thinking of a thousand different things and say we are going to do pratyāhāra. Pratyāhāra is the result of a state of dhāraṇā or dhyāna or samādhi. In the *Yoga Sūtra*, pratyāhāra is mentioned first not because it occurs first but rather because it has to do with the senses and not the mind. It is therefore more external than dhāraṇā. I cannot simply decide to practice āsanas for half and hour, then pratyāhāra for twenty minutes, and then dhāraṇā for an hour. The process does not work like that.

Q: Let's look at two different situations; one in which I am totally unaware of the messages that my senses are sending to my mind, and another wherein my mind registers the messages but I decide not to react. What is the difference in these two scenarios? Say for example that I am a musician, totally absorbed in what I am playing, and I become aware that someone is waiting to speak to me. I could ignore the person, finish the piece of music, and then ask what they want. Would that be pratyāhāra? Or would it only be pratyāhāra if I had not even noticed that someone was waiting to see me?

A: We must not think that when we are in a state of dhāraṇā, dhyāna, or samādhi, our senses are dead. There are examples of wonderful poems that sages have composed while in a state of samādhi. People in samādhi can sing beautiful words. And when we sing we are using our aural senses and our voice. But how have these sages used their senses? They have used them to serve the mind and spirit, not to distract them. The senses are certainly not dead. The difference between this and our normal state is that here the senses *support* the focus of the mind on one point.

Let's say we want to describe a wonderful statue of a god that we have seen. To do this we have to look at the toes, the ankles, and so on—we must see. But in this situation our seeing only serves the purpose of describing the statue. If we start to wonder about where the stone that the statue is made of originated and what its geological make-up is, then the mind is distracted. But if we look at the feet and recognize them as the feet of the divine image sitting in the lotus position, then the senses are working in harmony with the mind. The senses are certainly not dead in this process. Pratyāhāra means that the senses *serve* the mind in the state of dhāraṇā, dhyāna, and samādhi.

Q: When someone is in a state of pratyāhāra, do they perceive things? Are the objects spontaneously and directly perceived? Is there discursive thinking or not? Do we perceive without mediating thought?

A: It all depends. For instance, thinking played a part in my example of the statue of the god. The thinking process is there, but exclusively in relation to the object. Memory is functioning only in connection with the object. In this example of pratyāhāra, there is no distraction through our senses because we are so absorbed in the object of our meditation. The senses react only to this object.

If I am expounding on something from the *Yoga Sūtra* and the smell of food from the kitchen suddenly attracts my attention, I am not in a state of pratyāhāra. But if I carry on with my explanations without being distracted by the cooking smells, then I am in a state of pratyāhāra. In dhyāna there is a medium for communication that could be thinking. But in samādhi there is not even this kind of thinking. The mind is clear. It has understood the object as it is.

Q: I'm still not clear about pratyāhāra in dhyāna.

A: The more we become absorbed in the object of our meditation, the more we can notice how our senses change their behavior. (I use the word *object* for lack of a better term. An object in this sense could be simply the image of pure white light, or it could be a sūtra. The object of meditation is anything used to help focus the mind.) In a meditative state, the senses are in accord with the state of dhyāna. Pratyāhāra occurs as a result of this state; it is not possible to achieve pratyāhāra by itself. We can certainly do things such as inner gazing and mudrā in prāṇāyāma to help us realize pratyāhāra. But those practices alone are not pratyāhāra. Pratyāhāra is rather a point at which the senses are at the service of the mind. Pratyāhāra occurs when we are in the state of dhyāna.

Various activities such as prāṇāyāma and prayers are called dhyāna, yet these are really nothing more than aids for attaining a meditative state. Some teachers recommend practice exercises for pratyāhāra. They suggest things like: "Close your eyes, breathe in deeply, and send the breath to the ankles." A technique such as this is similar to practicing prāṇāyāma—it is an exercise for focusing the mind in a certain direction so that it becomes less distracted. But it is very difficult to find a real technique for practicing pratyāhāra, for the more we think about the senses, the more active they become. We can, however, create the conditions under which the senses lose their usual significance and simply support the mind in its state of dhyāna.

Q: How does this occur? We cannot simply sit down and practice dhyāna like we can prāṇāyāma. How does dhyāna come about?

A: A certain effort is always required, and this involves two things. When we are trying to practice exercises such as prāṇāyāma, there is always something that hinders us. This is actually in the mind. There is one force in us wanting us to practice, and another, namely, our old habits, that wants to stop us. This means that when we want to practice, we must make an effort. The moment we no longer have to make any effort at all is the beginning of dhyāna. That is why Patañjali says, in the first chapter of the *Yoga Sūtra*, "Abhyāsa is necessary."[3] We have to move in a certain direction toward a particular goal. The more we do this, the less we will be distracted by the other possible choices we could have made. Then comes the day when it is no longer necessary to say: "All right—time for some practice!"

Let's say I am doing my prāṇāyāma practice and the postman brings a letter from a friend. One voice inside me whispers: "Go and read the letter!" But another voice is telling me to finish my prāṇāyāma practice first. Because of this oscillation of the mind, I have to make an effort. In the moment of dhyāna, all the effort to practice disappears.

Q: Let's say you were a student and had to write a paper. You already have an idea for it. When you sit down and begin to concentrate you are in a state

3. *Yoga Sūtra* 1.12. The state of yoga is achieved by simultaneously strivinging (abhyāsa) and letting go (vairāgya).

of dhāraṇā. When you really get involved in the effort to understand it and put it on paper, is that then dhyāna?

A: Yes.

Q: And in this example, what would be a state of samādhi?

A: Imagine you get stuck in the middle of writing the paper. You do not know how to go on, so you take a break from your work for a while and do something else. Suddenly, in the middle of whatever else you are doing, it comes to you in a flash: "I've got it!" You haven't actually got the whole paper in your head, but you've understood how to proceed. Then you sit down again at your desk and finish the paper. At this point you have completely merged with the subject—become one with the subject—and can therefore easily finish the paper. That is samādhi.

Q: Is the difference then that in dhyāna there is still a consciousness that I am thinking, while in samādhi the knowledge simply comes?

A: Yes, in samādhi the gap between the mind and the object we are focusing on is much smaller, and the understanding so immediate, that we no longer have to think. In the first chapter of the *Yoga Sūtra* there is a description of how samādhi happens: first of all we reflect. This is called *vitarka*. Once we have done this, the next step is to study the object; this is *vicāra*. As the intent study becomes more refined, we suddenly understand. In this moment we experience a feeling of profound happiness, which we call *ānanda*, and we know with certainty that we are one with the object of our meditation—this is *asmitā*.[4] Finally we feel that we understand what we wanted to understand. The term *asmitā* refers here to the merging of mind with the object of meditation. This is the process of samādhi: first there is oscillation in the mind, then the superficial logic is reduced and the process becomes an inner, deep, subtle one. Finally, reflection becomes refined to the point where I know that I understand. There is no longer any doubt.

Q: I am still not clear about the difference between dhāraṇā and dhyāna.

A: Let me give you another example. When I begin a class I have normally thought about it and planned it, but I do not know how I will actually proceed. So I start the class by asking if there are any questions arising from what we discussed in the previous class. That is the beginning of dhāraṇā: I have not yet made the connection; I am just orienting myself so that I know how to continue speaking to the students about yoga. Dhāraṇā is the preparation and orientation. The deeper I immerse myself in what we are talking about, the more I approach a state of dhyāna. In the state of dhāraṇā, I am more susceptible to distractions than when I am in dhyāna. That is the difference.

Q: Do we have to sit in a certain place for dhāraṇā, dhyāna, and samādhi, or could we experience them in different settings—as we watch a beautiful sunset, for example?

A: Yes, you can experience these states in the company of a beautiful sunset. It is actually useful to use external objects as meditation objects, especially at the beginning. This is why there are statues in our temples and crosses

4. *Yoga Sūtra* 1.17.

in a Christian church. These objects of worship are there to help beginners experience dhāraṇā, but that is only the first step. Whether you sit or stand is irrelevant. You can walk and hardly notice your action if you are absorbed in something. There are certain schools in India that teach walking meditations. If something as simple as walking disturbs our dhāraṇā, then our concentration is not strong. But at the start it is always best to begin with the easiest thing—a comfortable sitting position and, as a meditation tool, an object that is pleasing to us. Let's say you did not believe in Śiva, one of the highest gods in the Hindu pantheon, and I said to you: "Meditate on the god Śiva!" There will be conflict in you. You must instead start with something to which you can relate. In yoga it is said that you must begin where you are and with what you like. After all, the object of meditation is actually unimportant. What is important is that the chosen object does not cause you any problems or hinder you from focusing your mind. That is why I suggest you choose an object that suits your temperament and faith. A Muslim in India would have enormous difficulties meditating on the word *OM*, the holy sound of the Hindu culture.

Q: In dhyāna, does the individual and the object of meditation retain individual and separate identities?

A: Yes. In dhyāna there is a feeling that "I" am in a meditative state. The consciousness of the self is present. Many people use the word dhyāna to describe someone who is nearly in a state of samādhi, as if in dhyāna there is only the object. But we should understand these three states as three steps or stages: first, there is dhāraṇā, where we concentrate on our chosen object and close off from external distractions; then there is dhyāna, the connection or communication between self and object. Finally there is samādhi, where we have so deeply immersed ourselves in the object that the sense of self no longer seems to exist.

Q: Does the object of our attention retain its distinct identity in samādhi?

A: Of course. It is not the object that meditates—we are meditating. The object can change, as all things may change, but that is not the result of samādhi. On the other hand, what we experience in relation to the object may vary enormously from person to person. Suppose we want to think about the concept of Īśvara. We read about it widely and begin to investigate it thoroughly. The more we go into it, the more we understand. Not because Īśvara itself changes but because we understand more. We are not altering the object of our research; we have no control over that. Our understanding of the subject is what changes because the mind becomes clearer and we can see what was previously hidden from us.

As another example, to investigate the nature of anger is dhyāna, but to find ourselves in a state of anger is not dhyāna. In all the classical texts the emphasis is placed on what actually occurs in the state of samādhi. The Sanskrit word *prajñā* translates as "very clear understanding." The old texts say that in samādhi, *ṛta prajñā* prevails—that is, what is seen is the truth. This means that in samādhi we arrive at a real understanding of the object, even if the object is anger. We can see where it comes from, how it has arisen, and what effects it has. If anger has taken possession of us, however, we lose ourselves in it. In such a state the mind is completely covered with avidyā, whereas in samādhi avidyā does not cloud the mind at all. That is why in a state of samādhi we can often see things that were previously hidden from us. Whether we are experiencing samādhi or not is not shown by sitting cross-legged with closed eyes and a meaningful expression on our face. We know we are experiencing samādhi if we can see and understand things that we could not see or understand before.

Q: It is said that in yoga we should try to recognize the difference between puruṣa and prakṛti. Now you are talking about samādhi as a state in which there is no gap between subject and object. How do these two concepts relate to each other?

A: The gap does not exist anymore because there is observation. I said that we see and recognize something which was previously hidden from us. For example, when we look into a mirror we see ourselves in it. But what we really see is the mirror's reflection of us, not our real selves. Now the image in the mirror and our person seem to merge into each other, yet we can still distinguish between the two. When we look into the mirror we cannot take away the image of our face without turning away from ourselves. That is to say, what is seen merges with that which sees. This also implies that anything standing between them has vanished. As I said, our puruṣa sees an object through the mind. If the mind is colored, we cannot see clearly. If the mind is very clear, then it is almost as if it does not exist. We see the object exactly as it is. The problems we have to deal with in life arise from the way the consequences of our actions have settled in our mind; that is, they arise from our saṃskāra. We are not able to distinguish the colored image that exists in the mind from the real object. For instance, I may say "Yes, I understand," and then five minutes later say "Oh, but I'm not clear about that." The same "I" that thought it understood is now saying it does not understand. In the state of samādhi the "I" is almost nonexistent; the confusion of the mind is gone. But to understand this fully we have to experience it.

Q: Can a student of yoga who is beginning to experience these various states do this alone, or should I ask for the help of a teacher?

A: As in any situation, a little advice is always helpful. Theoretically everything seems very simple, but in practice there are many difficulties. For example, what do you choose as an object and then where do you begin—how do you focus on it? Since we all have a different starting point, it is best that you find someone you respect and relate to easily and let that person guide you. A teacher can help you if only because he or she can observe you. When the *Yoga Sūtra* was written it was taken for granted that students went to a teacher; that is why there is no specific reference to a teacher in the texts. Originally yoga was passed on by word of mouth; only much later was it written down. Students lived with their teachers until they got to know them well. I think it is best to have some personal guidance.

Q: Can the state of dhyāna occur in āsanas? Can we use the body as the object and allow the communication between the mind and the body to grow into dhyāna?

A: Yes. Actually, the third chapter of the *Yoga Sūtra* deals with this. If your meditation object is the Pole Star, you can understand the movements of all stars,[5] and if you meditate on the navel cakra, you can reach an understanding of the whole body.[6] It is certainly possible to use the body as your meditation object. In this way, you come to understand more about the body. If you choose the breath as your object of meditation, then your understanding of the breath grows.

Q: Can we then reach a state of samādhi during āsana practice? Wouldn't it interrupt the movement?

A: Haven't we got all the necessary elements in āsana practice—mind, object, and relationship between them? So what is the problem? It is only that our focus is different when we are doing āsanas. For example, if we want to feel a twist, then our mind only has to focus on it completely, and then we understand what a twist is. There are many possible objects for dhyāna when we are doing āsanas. It could be the whole concept of āsana, or it could be a detail—something particular such as a twist, the flow of the breath, or something else. What we see in dhyāna depends on what object we have chosen. We often find suggestions for what we should direct our attention toward, depending on the purpose of our meditation. That is why we have so many different gods in India. We look at smiling Viṣṇu and experience something particular. We look at the powerful goddess Durga and experience another feeling. The kind goddess Śakti awakens in us something different again. The particular meditation object we choose influences our understanding.

Q: When you were talking about samādhi you said that it contains three elements: the person who is looking, the object, and the connection between the two. And when you were talking about dhyāna, you said that the person who is looking and the object being looked at merge into each other and a connection develops. If I understood you correctly, you also said that in samādhi only the object remains; neither the person observing nor the connection between observer and observed is important. What then has happened to the connection between them?

A: With regard to dhyāna, I said that the observer and the observed meet and make a connection. What I wanted to say with regard to samādhi is that in this state there are no thoughts. Thinking is absent; there is no need for it because we are so closely linked to our object. It is irrelevent to say "This is like this and that is like that." We, the observers, are certainly still there, but we have such a profound, intense understanding of what we are observing that there is no need to think or analyze. That is what I meant to convey in saying that the connection no longer exists.

Of course, there are various stages and degrees of intensity in samādhi. What I have just described is more developed than those where thinking and communication are still present.

Q: Is it true that every time we learn something, we have a little taste of dhāraṇā, dhyāna, and samādhi?

A: Definitely! It does not have to be such a profound process as is described

5. This statement is the theme of 3.28 of the *Yoga Sūtra.*

6. *Yoga Sūtra* 3.29.

in yoga books, but it is still the same. When we understand something our mind has to be actively involved. That is dhāraṇā and dhyāna.

There is also the question about whether the states of dhāraṇā, dhyāna, and samādhi are permanent. Someone in a state of samādhi is totally in this state, that is, only samādhi prevails. It is almost as if the person in samādhi cannot remember that he or she has ever had a restless, confused mind. But when the same person is again in a state of restlessness and confusion, there is at best only a memory of samādhi.

It is usually the case that we alternate between dhāraṇā, dhyāna, and samādhi on the one hand and states of restlessness and confusion on the other. In samādhi, we are not even aware that we were ever confused. A confused person may vaguely remember his or her samādhi state, but that is all. As a person gets more involved, he or she spends more time in samādhi, and experiences less restlessness. It may get to the point where that person is always in a state of samādhi. We hope for this!

Q: Is then the ultimate goal of yoga to be always in a state of samādhi?

A: The ultimate goal of yoga is to always observe things accurately, and therefore never act in a way that will make us regret our actions later.

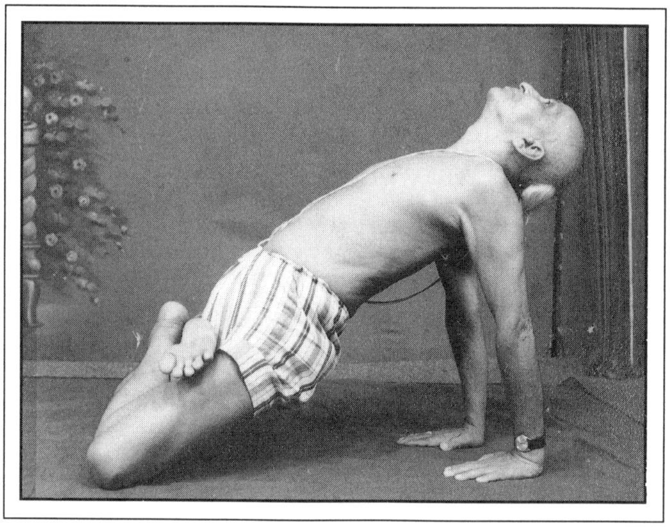

Krishnamacharya in padmāsana ūrdhvamukha (above) and padma bhujaṅgāsana.

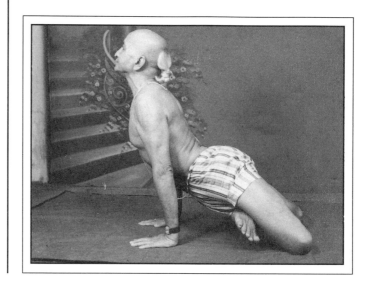

13

The Qualities of the Mind

In the first chapter of the *Yoga Sūtra*, Patañjali defines yoga as a certain state of mental activity, one that he calls *nirodha.*[1] A level of mental functioning characterized by consistent focused attention, nirodha is the fifth and highest level of the mind. We only attain nirodha by successively recognizing and conquering the lower levels of the mind's activities. The lowest level of the mind can be likened to that of a drunken monkey swinging from branch to branch: thoughts, feelings, and perceptions come and go in rapid succession. We are hardly aware of them and can find no thread linking them. This level of the mind's activity is called *kṣipta.*

The second level of the mind is called *mūdha*. Here the mind is like one of a heavy water buffalo standing for hours on end in one place. Any inclination to observe, act, or react has nearly disappeared. This sort of state of mind can arise from many causes. We might feel this heavy after eating too much or as a result of getting too little sleep. Some medications can cause this state of mind. Some people go into a state of mūdha when they lose a loved one. Mūdha can also be a reaction to a deep disappointment, when something that was deeply desired cannot be reached. And it sometimes arises in people who, after many unsuccessful attempts to make something of their lives, simply withdraw and do not want to know about anything anymore.

Vikṣipta is the word used to describe the third level of the mind. In vikṣipta, the mind is moving but the movement lacks consistent purpose and direction. The mind encounters obstacles and doubts. It alternates between knowing what it wants to do and uncertainty, between confidence and diffidence. This is the most common state of mind.

The fourth level of mind is called *ekāgrāta*. Here the mind is relatively clear; distractions have little influence. We have a direction and, most important of all, we can move forward in this direction and keep our attention on it. This state

[1]. *Yoga Sūtra* 1.2.

corresponds to dhāraṇā. By practicing yoga we can create the conditions that gradually move the mind from the kṣipta level to the ekāgrāta level.

When ekāgrāta is fully developed, it peaks at nirodha. This is the fifth and final level at which the mind can operate; at this level, the mind is linked completely and exclusively with the object of its attention. Mind and object seem to merge into one.

This is a difficult concept to understand, so I will give you another example. Before I give a lecture on the concept of nirodha, I think a lot about the five levels of the mind and find that many ideas arise relative to what I'm considering. Many related experiences and memories come to mind. But where I begin to speak to my audience and answer their questions, as I become more engrossed in explaining nirodha, I see how I should proceed. Fewer questions arise in my mind. I get to the stage when I do not get lost in side issues and I am not particularly aware of my audience. I am no longer worried about what they think of my examples. What I say comes much more from an inner closeness to the topic I am discussing. In this process my mind has focused completely on one thing: explaining nirodha. It is as if my mind is almost enveloped in this interest. Nothing else concerns me, and all my understanding of the concept of nirodha is fully with me. Nothing but the topic I am explaining exists for me.

This is the state of mind that is meant wherever the term nirodha is used in the *Yoga Sūtra*. The syllable *rodha* is derived from the root *rudh*, "to be wrapped in"; *ni-* is a prefix that indicates great internal intensity. *Nirodha* describes a state in which the mind focuses exclusively on one thing without being disturbed by other thoughts or external distractions.

The word *nirodha* also has another meaning, which is sometimes translated as "limit" or "restraint." This interpretation can indeed be justified, not in the sense that we limit or restrict the mind to one particular direction, but rather it works conversely: the mind has moved so strongly and intensely toward one area and has become so absorbed in it that nothing else can penetrate it and all other mental activities cease. So if nirodha means "limit," it is because the restraints and cessation of all other mental activities are a natural consequence. In this sense, *nirodha* means "total absorption." Patañjali thus defines yoga as *citta vṛtti nirodha*. The mind has one and only one activity (citta vṛtti), and all other activities that could distract the mind are absent.

Some people ask whether yoga isn't a matter of eliminating the activities of the mind. It shows insufficient knowledge and understanding of the *Yoga Sūtra* if you come to the conclusion that the many mental faculties we have—those of observation, inference, memory, imagination, inactivity, and hyperactivity, for example—are detrimental and need to be eliminated. Yoga understands that these faculties are indeed necessary for living. However, exposed to the influences that constantly assail it, the mind develops its own way of working if it is left to its own devices. In the end it becomes incapable of using the many faculties it possesses because it cannot find any stability and clarity. That is the reason why the *Yoga Sūtra* says that all mental faculties can be either positive or negative.[2]

In yoga we are simply trying to create the conditions in which the mind becomes as useful as possible for our actions. This can only happen gradually—every shortcut is an illusion. It is a step-by-step process, one that includes a great number of techniques from which one must choose intelligently according to the individual need. The *Yoga Sūtra* gives many suggestions, which together comprise our yoga practice, the yoga sādhana. Asana practice, breathing exercises, study of the *Yoga Sūtra*, surrender to God, detachment from one's own action, visiting a holy person, and investigating the nature of dreams are all part of the process.

Every person is different and has a unique set of life experiences. That is why there are so many suggestions for helping the student on the yoga path. In one way or another, you can bring your mind into a state in which it understands and can act with complete involvement. And who is not searching for opportunities to understand things more clearly, to make new discoveries and rectify faulty perceptions? If you can say anything about what happens in the state of nirodha, it is this: you see and you know. Whatever the mind may be preoccupied with, it sees and understands it so completely that there is little left to learn. If you go into this process further, you can catch a glimpse of what lies beyond normal observation and experience. Therein lies the basis of yogic wisdom. A yogi or yogini has not seen something others can never see; rather, he or she sees what others do not yet see.

2. *Yoga Sūtra* 1.5. This passage states that there are five activities of the mind, and they can be used for better or for worse. These five activities, discussed in the following sūtras, are correct perception, false perception, imagination, dreamless sleep, and memory.

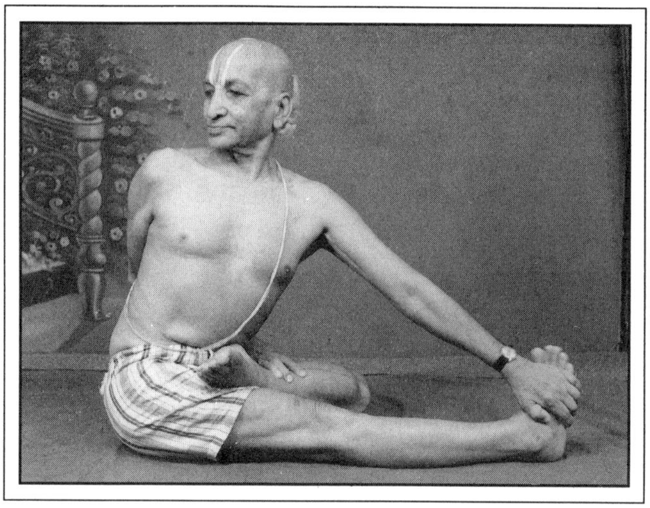

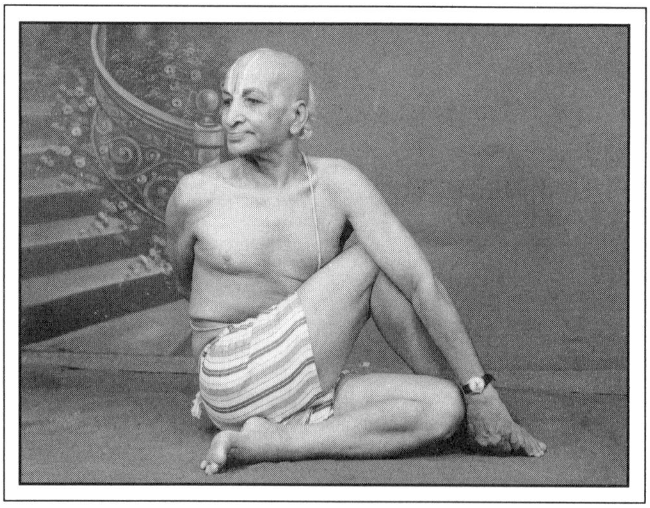

Krishnamacharya demonstrating variations of ardha matsyendrāsana.

14

Nine Obstacles on the Yoga Way

I have discussed the potential the mind has to become focused (dhāraṇā), to enter into ongoing communication with a chosen object (dhyāna), and finally to merge completely with it (samādhi). These are natural states of mind that can arise spontaneously, but there are always obstacles arising that prevent their occurrence. Recognizing these obstacles can help us prepare the mind for attaining a state of great clarity. The question is, therefore, what are the obstacles and what can help us get them out of the way? Patañjali describes the obstacles *(antārayas)* as rocks lying on the path traveled by someone who has set off on the yoga journey. The student is constantly stumbling over them, making detours, or getting stuck. Let us consider these nine obstacles, see how they come about, and learn how we can get rid of them.

The nine obstacles listed by Patañjali are illness, lethargy, doubt, haste or impatience, resignation or fatigue, distraction, ignorance or arrogance, inability to take a new step, and loss of confidence. They are manifested in symptoms like feeling sorry for oneself, a negative attitude, physical problems, and breathing difficulties.[1]

Obstacles

Obviously it is an obstacle to my yoga practice when I feel unwell or am ill. *Vyādhi,* illness, disturbs the mind so much that I must first do something to improve my health before I can go on.

Another obstacle that directly affects my state of mind is subjection to my moods. Sometimes I feel good and know I can tackle anything; at other times

1. *Yoga Sūtra* 1.30–31.

I might feel lethargic and lacking enough energy to do anything. This heaviness and lethargy, *styāna*, can be caused by eating too much, by eating the wrong kinds of food, by cold weather, or by the very nature of the mind. Of the three guṇa, tamas describes this lethargy, this heavy state of mind. If tamas takes over we can hardly do anything, even things we are accustomed to doing. We can scarcely move.

For some people, doubt is the greatest obstacle to progressing in yoga. I am not referring here to svādhyāya, the kind of self-examination that can help us progress. Svādhyāya is an intrinsic part of yoga. The doubt Patañjali speaks of is *saṃśaya*, a regular and persistent feeling of uncertainty, as for example when we are in the middle of doing something and suddenly ask: "How shall I go on? Is it worth it even for another day? Perhaps I should look for another teacher. Perhaps I should try another way altogether." This kind of doubt undermines our progress in yoga.

Sometimes we act hastily and carelessly, especially when we want to reach our goal quickly. *Pramāda*, haste, can create problems; acting in haste, we slip back rather than make progress. Because we have not spent enough time analyzing and reflecting on what we are doing, we grind to a halt in our practice.

Another obstacle is the kind of resignation or exhaustion which we call *ālasya*. It manifests in such thoughts as: "Perhaps I am not the right person to be doing this." There is a lack of enthusiasm and very little energy. When this happens, we must do something to regain our motivation and enthusiasm. Lack of enthusiasm is a serious obstacle on the yoga path.

The next obstacle can crop up when our senses gain the upper hand and begin to see themselves as masters rather than servants of the mind. Sometimes this happens without our even noticing it, which is hardly surprising since from birth we are trained to look here, see this, listen to that, taste this, touch that. It can easily happen that the senses take over out of habit and little by little steer us imperceptibly in the wrong direction. *Avirati*, distraction, is a great obstacle.

The most dangerous of all obstacles occurs when we think we know everything. We imagine we have seen the truth and have reached the zenith, when in reality we have simply experienced a period of calm that makes us say: "This is what I have been looking for! I've found it at last! I've made it!" But the feeling of having reached the top rung on the ladder is only illusion. Illusions like this are very common. They are nothing but ignorance and arrogance—*bhrāntidarśana*.

Another stumbling block can arise when, just as we've been thinking we have made some progress, we suddenly notice how much there still is for us to do. We can grow very disappointed at this point and become fickle in mood. We suddenly have no interest in trying again, in finding another way to begin, in taking the next step. We start saying: "No more for me. I thought that was it, but now I feel like a fool, even more stupid than before. I just don't want to go on." We are incapable of taking another step. This is called *alabdhabhūmikatva.*

As you see, the obstacles can consist of ordinary reality such as a physical illness, or they can be as subtle as an illusion of being better than you really are. When you become aware of the illusion you have been harboring and look reality squarely in the face, it is unfortunately all too easy to then view yourself as smaller and less important then you really are. This leads to loss of confidence, the last obstacle described by Patañjali. You may have reached a point you have never reached before, but you lack the power to stay there and fall back, losing what you have gained. Patañjali calls this *anavasthitatvani.*

These are the obstacles that may be encountered on the yoga path. We do not necessarily meet them in the order I have described, and not every student has to deal with all of them.

At no stage on the yoga path should we think we have become masters. Rather, we should know that the feeling of being a little better today than yesterday exists just as much as the hope that we will be a little better in the future. These feelings will come and go until we reach the point where there is no better and no worse.

Overcoming Obstacles

Just as yoga identifies the obstacles you may encounter along the way, so too does it suggest ways to help you overcome them. It is a great help to work with someone who can show you how to stick with the discipline you have chosen. Say you have a certain teacher with whom you are studying. It may happen that in the course of your work with that teacher you come across something new, only to discover later that it leads nowhere. The consequence of this may be that you begin to desire a different, "better" teacher. When the same thing happens with the new teacher you look for another—and the cycle continues in this way. The *Yoga Sūtra* tells us not to do this, but to instead maintain the relationship with your teacher, for if you do you will reach a deeper understanding and a greater degree of trust in him or her. It is also likely that the teacher, when he or she senses your trust, will be better able to discover what it is you need to be taught. Following one teacher and one direction helps you discover the ways and means of avoiding and overcoming the various obstacles discussed earlier.[2]

Prāṇāyāma is another technique often recommended as an aid to overcoming obstacles. For this purpose, the exhalation is of particular importance; Patañjali suggests practicing prāṇāyāma with a long quiet exhalation, and holding the breath afterward.[3] Simple techniques like this can be of tremendous help in overcoming obstacles.

Another method for dealing with blocks on the yoga path is to investigate the senses in order to quiet the mind.[4] We can explore such questions as: How does the tongue function? How does this taste on the tip or in the middle or at the root

2. *Yoga Sūtra* 1.32.

3. *Yoga Sūtra* 1.34.

4. *Yoga Sūtra* 1.35.

of the tongue? How do I observe things? How do I hear sounds? It is not what we discover that is important, but rather that we quiet the mind and get to know ourselves better. Another possibility for stilling the mind is to begin examining the concept of puruṣa. The Upaniṣads locate the puruṣa somewhere in the region of the heart, describing it as a small "muscle" in the heart area, in the depths of which can be found a tiny opening shaped like a lotus bud. If we concentrate our attention on this and look into our puruṣa, the mind becomes quiet and peaceful.[5]

One more effective technique recommended in the *Yoga Sūtra* is to find out about people who have experienced much suffering (duḥkha) throughout their lives, and have overcome it.[6] By talking to or reading books written by such people, we can also find out how they solved their problems, which may in turn help us find solutions to our problems. In India there are many temples, each with its unique story of why it was built and what tradition it follows. Standing in front of a temple, we contemplate and investigate the meaning of the sculptures, the symbols used, and the people who made them, and as we do this we can discover some very moving stories. We gradually understand what a particular symbol signifies and what real meaning it can have for us. The more we allow ourselves to discover such things, the freer the mind becomes.

When we are in a state of confusion and agitation, it is helpful to look for the cause within ourselves. It may be that something that arises continually and may therefore be very familiar to us is really something we know very little about. We can also ask ourselves where our dreams come from and what the underlying meaning of the dreams are, or what it is that sleeps and what happens when we wake up. Many people say that in deep, dreamless sleep we the children, the puruṣas, are sleeping in the lap of the father, Īśvara. An investigation into deep sleep can therefore not only help us to learn more about this state, but can also contribute to a feeling of well-being and peacefulness. We might even ponder what makes it possible for life itself to continue. Quietly investigating all these things can help the mind to become more still.[7]

But suppose none of the suggestions mentioned so far appeal to you. What do you do? You could try a form of meditation that makes use of a visual object. For example, you can visualize something and then reflect on what it means to you. In India we often meditate like this on the images of gods. As we visualize a particular god in the mind's eye, we recite his or her name 108 or 1008 times, if we are following the tradition. We immerse ourselves in the ideas and concepts associated with that particular god. We read poems about the god written by our great poets; we call the god over and over again by name. This kind of meditation helps the mind to become quieter and more clear and prepares us for dhyāna, the merging of the ego with the object of meditation. We do nothing except focus our attention on the god.

If you try this technique you should be sure that you use objects that will actually bring peace to your mind and spirit, not ones that will cause more distraction. There is a verse in the *Yoga Sūtra* that says that we can meditate

5. *Yoga Sūtra* 1.36.

6. *Yoga Sūtra* 1.37.

7. *Yoga Sūtra* 1.38.

on anything we like.[8] But we should never lose sight of the fact that in choosing our meditation object, we must find one that is pleasing and calming to us.

Īśvarapraṇidhānā

The most important method for removing obstacles on the way to greater clarity is īśvarapraṇidhānā, submission to Īśvara.[9] The concept of īśvarapraṇidhānā stems from the belief that there is a spiritual being higher than we are; we give ourselves to this higher being, believing it can help us. We devote all the fruits of our labors to this being.

What is Īśvara? First of all it is a name, a concept that, as I have said, describes the highest divine being. Īśvara does not belong to the material world (prakṛti), or to the seer in us (puruṣa). Īśvara is distinguished by these qualities: Īśvara sees all things as they are; his action is perfect; he is omniscient, the first teacher, a source of help and support. Unlike us, Īśvara is not subject to the influence of avidyā. Although he is acquainted with avidyā, he remains untouched by it, which is why he never acts wrongly, never has acted wrongly, and never will act wrongly. Unlike us, he has never been covered with the veil of avidyā, and for this reason he can see things that we cannot see. This is why he can lead and direct us.

Īśvara does nothing that could have a negative outcome or regrettable consequence. He is beyond the vicious cycle in which actions produce bad effects that cause new conditioning that in turn leads to action with negative effects. Like our puruṣa, Īśvara sees—that is one of his greatest qualities. For this reason, the *Yoga Sūtra* calls him a puruṣa, but a very special one: *viśeṣa puruṣa*. The word *viśeṣa* means "extraordinary." Īśvara is extraordinary in that he is not subject to avidyā, knows no negative action that could cause regret, and is not susceptible to duḥkha, suffering. For this reason he possesses the extraordinary ability of knowing and understanding everything. Yoga uses the word *sarvajña* to describe this special quality. *Sarva* means "everything," and *jña* translates as "to know." Īśvara is all-knowing—he knows everything always, and at every level. This quality he alone possesses; we as human beings do not. That is why he is the great teacher, the master who is honored as guru. Patañjali calls Īśvara the First Guru. He is the teacher who surpasses all others. The honor accorded him rests on the fact that he knows everything. Anyone who calls on him says: "You who know, share your knowledge with me!"

Yoga does not describe Īśvara in a particular form. If you want to have a relationship with this being, you use a special symbol that represents him. This symbol is the sound *OM*. You will not find any mention of *OM* in Patañjali's *Yoga Sūtra*. Instead you will find the term *prāṇava*, which has the same meaning.

It is possible to enter into relationship with Īśvara, to contact him, by reciting the sound *OM*. The more we recite *OM*, and at the same time bearing in mind that *OM* means Īśvara, the more we will come to know Īśvara. In the process

8. *Yoga Sūtra* 1.39.
9. *Yoga Sūtra* 1.23.

of reciting *OM*, the mind merges into this sound symbol and the concept of Īśvara. There will then come a moment when we grow quiet and take another step on the yoga path.

What is our relationship to Īśvara? We accept him as the great teacher; we call upon him to help us because we know that he can. Turning to Īśvara for help is called īśvarapraṇidhānā. Yielding to Īśvara is one of the ways Patañjali suggests for overcoming the obstacles we may encounter on our journey.[10]

Unfortunately I cannot find an English word for Īśvara; perhaps it is God or the Divine Power. What is important is that yielding to this higher being is an expression of a belief that something exists that is higher than ourselves, something in which we can place our trust. With faith in this being, we devote all our efforts to him and so make progress along the way. For many people, īśvarapraṇidhānā has no meaning. For them it is more important to find other ways of overcoming obstacles. What is always important is that we never try to force anything in situations where there seems at first to be no way to move. We must just create space for ourselves, for the mind. Whether it is through īśvarapraṇidhānā, or with the aid of breathing techniques, whether it is by approaching a teacher or investigating our senses—whenever there is confusion in our minds we must try to create space. There are many possibilties for getting out of a difficult situation. Ways and means can always be found for overcoming the obstacles we meet. Yoga is open to a wide variety of approaches.

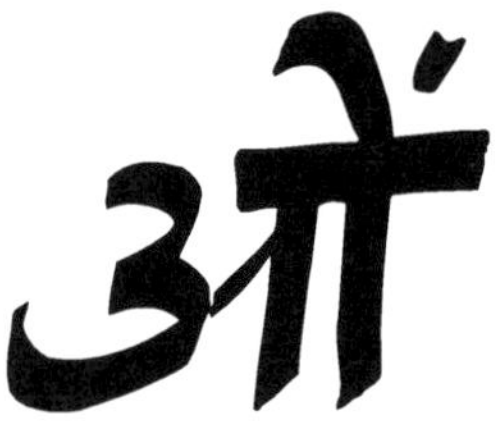

Figure 32: The Sanskrit Symbol for OM.

Īśvara and the Sound of *OM*

The reasons why the audible symbol *OM* has been chosen to call on Īśvara are interesting indeed. With the sound *OM* we say everything.

If we analyze *OM* as it is written in Sanskrit, we see that it is made up of *A*, *U*, *M*, and a symbol representing resonance. So *OM* has four aspects. The first is the *A*, a sound that comes from the belly, is formed in the open throat, and is voiced with the mouth open. As with many alphabets, *A* is the first letter of the Sanskrit alphabet. The second aspect is the *U*, a sound that is formed in the middle of the mouth. The mouth is not as wide open as it is for sounding the *A*. With the third sound, *M*, the mouth closes. The sound rises to the nasal passages, from where the resonance, the fourth aspect of *OM*, issues forth.

U stands for continuity and connection, and *M* is the final consonant in the Sanskrit alphabet. So getting from *A* to *M* through *U* represents everything that can be expressed in letters and words. And everything which can be expressed in words is Īśvara. When I sound *A*, I must open my mouth, which stands for the process of creation. *U* symbolizes the continuance of creation, which is constantly renewing itself. *M* symbolizes the end and dissolution. Following *M*, the sound carries on a while. This sound has no alphabetical symbol to represent it. We can therefore say that Īśvara is not only that which can be expressed in words, but also that which cannot be expressed in words. This is the full meaning of *OM*.

10. *Yoga Sūtra* 1.23–29.

The Upaniṣads say that *A* represents the waking state, *U* the dream state, and *M* the state of deep dreamless sleep. The fourth state, sounded in the resonance following *M,* is samādhi. This parallel points to the one who stands behind all four states, the only one who is truly awake: Īśvara. There is One who is present in all these states, One who never sleeps and never dreams, One who is always awake, always watchful, One who knows about everything and yet is beyond everything. If I repeat *OM* with these ideas in the back of my mind, I will gradually become immersed in Īśvara and my mind will become so saturated with Īśvara that I will become very still. Then I can go on my way again. For this reason, īśvarapraṇidhānā is one of the strongest ways for dispelling the obstacles we meet as we move forward in life.

Further Thoughts on Īśvara

Q: If I try chanting *OM,* must I have an idea of what Īśvara is?

A: Whenever we say *OM,* we mean Īśvara. Īśvara is beyond avidyā; Īśvara is the One who has known, does know, and always will know everything. So if Īśvara can guide us, we assume we can become better. Saying *OM* is actually a form of meditation in which the meditation object is a concept with the name Īśvara. As Īśvara is beyond all naturally occurring forms that we are able to imagine, we need a symbol for it, and that symbol is *OM.* When we say *OM* we think of it as the aural representation of Īśvara. Whenever we chant this sound we must give ourselves time for our mind to consider what it really means.

Both the repetition of the sound (japa) and the meaning must be present in the *OM.* Otherwise there is a danger that the repetition will become mechanical. If we repeat a mantra like parrots we will not gain anything. The meaning of the *OM* is important, for the deeper we look into it, the more we will see in it. And each new discovery will lead to another.

Q: Isn't *OM* a Hindu symbol?

A: Yes, but the Hindu *OM* is not written the same way as the yoga *OM.* We must not confuse the two. Let me tell you a story. A few years ago I was invited to a big international conference on yoga. On the first day, a Muslim yoga teacher showed me the conference brochure. On the cover was the Hindu symbol for *OM.* I turned it over and on the back was the same symbol. I opened it and found the same *OM* on every page used as a logo to separate the announcements of the various activities and events. A number of people were wearing T-shirts with a huge Hindu *OM* printed on the front or the back. I don't know how many people were wearing pendants with the same symbol on them, and there was even a dog there named OM!

I must admit I was most embarrassed by this teacher who knew India well and was asking me the meaning of this ubiquitous display of the Hindu *OM.* For us *OM* is not a gadget or a decoration. We regard it with the utmost seriousness and respect.

I suggested to the conference director that I give a lecture on the abuse of the symbol. I explained the value of the symbol for us and talked about the great respect and care with which we have been taught to regard it.

I also tried to help people understand that this symbol does not belong just to yoga, saying there had been some mistakes made in the way it was being used at this very conference. I naively believed that my audience would appreciate these things, but in fact some of them were so attached to their pendants and T-shirts that they became very angry at my intervention.

I think this story exemplifies the confusion that exists between Hinduism and yoga, even among teachers of yoga. The symbol *OM* also belongs to the Buddhist and Jain traditions; it is not exclusive to Hinduism. To misuse it wittingly is to act with disrespect toward all these groups.

Q: If I give myself over to the protective guidance of Īśvara, what does my puruṣa do? How am I to understand what you have said in the past about puruṣa being the master?

A: You have problems and are unable to overcome certain obstacles—puruṣa is certainly not in charge at this time! For this reason, you entrust yourself to another master. Just think for a moment of a situation in which you are having difficulties with your practice. You need help. But what kind? Whatever form of help you get, it has only one goal—to restore your equanimity and bring clarity to your mind. When your mind is a little quieter, you begin to move again. You do not need anyone to push you. The moment you get stuck you can try a little prāṇāyāma or do a few āsanas; that may be enough. Yoga offers you many possibilities; foremost among them are devotion, faith, and complete trust in Īśvara.

When I discuss how the Sāṃkhya philosophy and yoga see the relationship between puruṣa, body, and mind, the highest entity is puruṣa, then the mind, then the senses, and lastly the body. In the course of our lives this relationship gradually becomes inverted and puruṣa is pushed to the bottom. Puruṣa is ruled by the mind, the mind by the senses, the senses by the body. That is our everyday situation. The aim of yoga is to turn this process around and restore puruṣa to the place it really should occupy. The real quality of the human being is that it can be guided by that something that has the ability to perceive. That something is our puruṣa. The problem is always only that we lose sight of our puruṣa, even forgetting that it exists.

Machines and the outside world control us completely. Yoga attempts to restore us to our true nature, wherein puruṣa is the master that mind, senses, and body obey. These three rank lower than puruṣa and are meant to serve it.

Q: If this is so—if all these things are meant to serve the puruṣa—is the puruṣa then meant to serve Īśvara?

A: The question you pose does not arise in yoga. There is no master-servant relationship between puruṣa and Īśvara. What I am trying to say is this: someone who is attempting to improve him- or herself and suddenly cannot make any more progress can turn to various sources and techniques for help. Of these, one of the most important is to turn to Īśvara for guidance. By so doing there is more room, more space created in the mind, and the clearer the mind becomes, the more chances there are for our puruṣa to play its true role and enable us to understand our situation. Īśvarapraṇidhānā can therefore be helpful to us because only Īśvara is, was, and always will be beyond avidyā. That is how it is. Whether our puruṣa is there to serve Īśvara is irrelevant.

Q: Can you say that devotion to Īśvara is the best way to overcome obstacles?

A: That varies from one person to another. If someone comes to me with difficulties and I immediately say: "Why don't you just pray?" it is very likely that I am not responding at all appropriately to that person. Many people would turn down a suggestion like that at once. "Don't tell me to pray!" they would say. "I have no time for God." I used to be like this myself. When I went through the *Yoga Sūtra* with my father the first time, I said to him: "Please don't preach Īśvara to me. I want to know about yoga. I don't want to learn how to pray." Nowadays I would not say that, but I have not always been the way I am now.

I repeat what I have said before: we must teach a person what he or she can accept at the time, not what we think would finally be best for them. We do well to respect the fact that, to some people, the concept of Īśvara means nothing at all. Over the years I have had a lot to do with people who, when they first took up yoga, had the same attitude I used to have. I don't know how it happens, but in the course of time their attitude toward the concept of Īśvara almost always changes. A kind of respect develops, and gradually they begin to accept the existence of something that is higher than we are. They would never have been able to accept this at the beginning of their practice. This happens with people of very different backgrounds, and this change almost always occurs. We cannot make devotion to Īśvara a prerequisite for starting yoga studies. To be open is essential in yoga. Everything is real, but everything changes. So only when someone is ready to talk about Īśvara do I ever mention the concept.

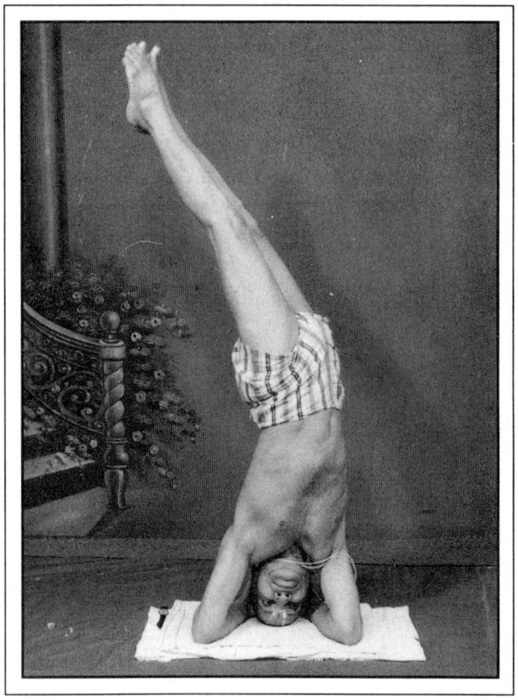

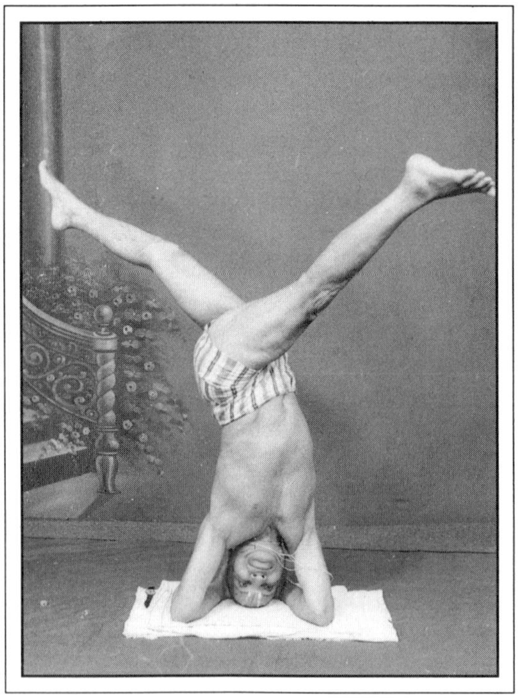

Krishnamacharya, age 79, in śīrṣāsana parivṛtti (above) and viparīta koṇāsana parivṛtti.

15

The Many Paths of Yoga

Yoga offers several methods for attaining clarity of mind, each with its own emphasis. In the *Bhagavad Gītā* alone, eighteen different forms of yoga are named. I shall discuss the following nine: jñana yoga, bhakti yoga, mantra yoga, rāja yoga, karma yoga, kriyā yoga, tantra yoga, kuṇḍalinī yoga, and haṭha yoga.

Jñāna yoga

Jñāna means "knowledge." Jñāna yoga describes the search for real knowledge. Traditionally this search begins by listening to the words of a teacher who explains the old yoga texts to his or her students. This is followed by reflection, discussion with others, and clarification of doubtful points, which leads to the gradual recognition of the truth and a merging with it.

The underlying assumption of jñāna yoga is that all knowledge lies hidden within us—we only have to discover it. The *Yoga Sūtra* says that the moment the mind is freed from the bonds of avidyā, jñāna occurs spontaneously. Previously it was locked in and therefore unavailable to us. The state in which this true understanding occurs is none other than samādhi. Dhyāna is the way to samādhi.

Bhakti yoga

The term *bhakti* comes from the root *bhaj,* which means "to serve." It does not mean to serve a person, however, but rather to serve a power greater than ourselves. This is the idea discussed in connection with the practice of īśvarapraṇidhānā.

By whatever means, in bhakti yoga we serve the divine being, which is the ultimate source of help and guidance. Following bhakti yoga, we offer all our thoughts and actions to this higher power. In everything we see, and in every other human being, we recognize God—truth. We act out of a conviction that we are serving God. We always carry his name within us. We meditate on him. We go into his temples. We are completely devoted to him. That is bhakti yoga.

Mantra yoga

A mantra can be a single syllable such as "ram," a number of syllables, or a whole verse. One of the most often used definitions of a mantra is something that protects the person who has received it. It is not something we can find in a book or buy somewhere.

Traditionally a mantra is given to a student by a teacher, at the time when the teacher knows exactly what the student needs. This process can take years. A mantra given in any other way may perhaps show some results at first, but they will not last. The mantra receives its special meaning and power through the way it is given and the way it is put together. Often there is a special image, either real or imaginary, that is linked to the mantra and visualized while the words are repeated. If we are aware of its meaning and maintain our practice over a period of time, repeating the mantra as we were taught, mantra yoga can have the same effect as jñāna yoga or bhakti yoga.

Rāja yoga

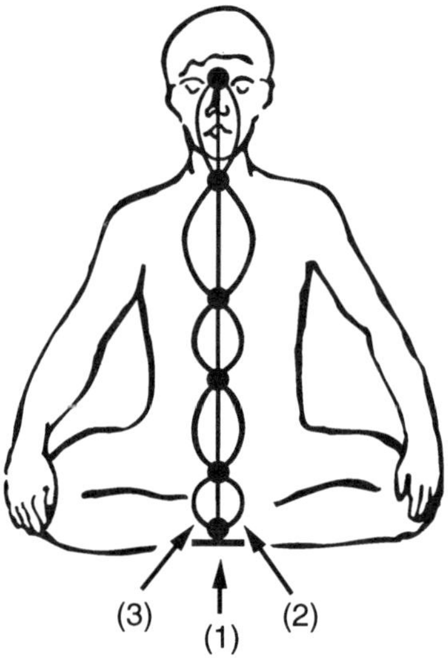

Figure 33: The position of the suṣumṇā (1), iḍā (2), and piṅgalā (3) nāḍīs, and their six points of convergence, known as the cakras.

The translation of the word *rājā* is "king." In the context of rāja yoga, it describes a king who is always in a state of enlightenment. The king stands for something in us that is more than what we usually consider ourselves to be. Rāja can also refer to the divine being or power mentioned in connection with bhakti yoga.

The way toward accepting the existence of Īśvara is often described as rāja yoga. In this respect, God or Īśvara is then the king referred to by the word *rājā*. In the Vedas we find many uses of the word *rājā* in connection with Īśvara.

There are other definitions of rāja yoga for those who do not want to link it to Īśvara. You can say that there is a king in each one of us; we understand this concept as puruṣa. This puruṣa, or the king within, normally remains hidden by our everyday actions. It is concealed by the workings of the mind, which is driven this way and that by sensual impressions, memories, and fantasies. It is avidyā, of course, which conceals our puruṣa so that many of us are unaware of its existence. When this process is reversed and the mind becomes master of the senses, we find clarity and peace, and our puruṣa can take the place it rightfully should have.

Whether the king is puruṣa or Īśvara, rāja yoga refers to the kind of yoga where the king takes his rightful place. In the *Yoga Sūtra* it says that when there is no more restlessness in the mind, puruṣa will unfold and see. That is rāja yoga.

Karma yoga

Karma is action. The *Bhagavad Gītā* ascribes a central place to karma yoga, stating that in life we can only act, but we should not be affected by the results of our action. If the fruits of our efforts do not correspond to our expectations, we should not be disappointed, for the effort itself is often imperfect. Our actions should indeed never be determined by any expectations, for we can never be sure of the results of our actions. We should also not take the credit when things turn out well, for we are not necessarily personally responsible for successes any more than we are responsible for failures. And it could well be that we see things in a different light tomorrow. We must involve ourselves through action, but leave the rest to God and expect nothing. This is the explanation of karma yoga given in the *Bhagavad Gītā,* and this definition corresponds to that of īśvarapraṇidhānā in chapter 2 of the *Yoga Sūtra.*[1]

Kriyā yoga

There are many different ideas about the definition of kriyā yoga. The *Yoga Sūtra* describes it as the whole spectrum of practices known as yoga. Everything that we can actually practice is kriyā yoga, and the *Yoga Sūtra* names three aspects that together define kriyā yoga: tapas, svādhāya, and īśvarapraṇidhānā.[2]

Tapas are practices such as āsana and prāṇayama that can help us to remove blocks and tensions, both physical and mental. Svādhyāya means searching, asking questions, looking into ourselves. And īśvarapraṇidhānā, as explained above, is action not motivated by outcome. When these three aspects are linked together in our practice, we are on the kriyā yoga path.

Haṭha, Kuṇḍalinī, and Tantra yoga

If we want to understand haṭha, kuṇḍalinī, and tantra yoga, we must look closely at a concept that is central to all three, namely, the concept of kuṇḍalinī. The fundamental idea, shared by all types of yoga that talk about kuṇḍalinī, is that there are certain channels or nāḍī in the body through which prāṇa can enter and leave. There are many nāḍī, but in the context of kuṇḍalinī we need only concern ourselves with the three most important ones: iḍā, piṅgalā, and suṣumṇā, all three of which run along the spine. Suṣumṅā runs straight up the spinal column, whereas iḍā and piṅgalā cross over the spinal column and back a number of times. The iḍā nāḍī passes the left nostril and the piṅgalā nāḍī passes the right nostril. Both have other names such as *ha* and *ṭha*, the two syllables that make up the word *haṭha. Ha* represents iḍā and the cool energy of the moon *(candra)*; *ṭha* represents piṅgalā and the hot energy of the sun *(sūrya).* The nāḍī meet at the six points in the body recognized as the cakras. Figure 33 shows the locations of the cakras along the central axis of the spine. There is one between the eyebrows, one in the throat, one in the heart region, one in the navel, one just above the base of the trunk, and one at the base of the spine.

Ideally, prāṇa flows unhindered along all these passages, but this can only happen when they are not blocked by impurities and rubbish. Normally prāṇa

1. We are reminded of Vyasa's commentary on sūtra 2.1, in which he says "Īśvarapraṇidhānā is the dedication of all actions to God or the renunciation of the desire for the fruits of all action."

2. *Yoga Sūtra* 2.1.

cannot reach suṣumṇā but only flows through the iḍā (ha) and piṅgalā (ṭha) nāḍī, and often insufficiently at that. When it is possible for the prāṇa to enter the suṣumṇā nāḍī, the prāṇa of ha and ṭha unite (yoga), which is why we call the process of getting there haṭha yoga.

The suṣumṇā or central nāḍī is regarded as the ideal path for prāṇa. If prāṇa flows through this central passage, it is concentrated in the body to such a large degree that its effects can spread throughout the body in an ideal way. None of it gets lost outside the body. When I was describing the purpose and effect of prāṇāyāma, I said that the state in which prāṇa leaks out of the body is one in which avidyā prevails. How and where prāṇa flows in the body, therefore, has direct consequences for our state of mind: if we cannot keep enough prāṇa in the nāḍī, if blocks hinder its flow and it cannot keep flowing in the right direction, it dissipates outside the body and results in the mind becoming dark and restless. Conversely, the collection of prāṇa in the body brings about inner peace and true understanding. The free flow of prāṇa in the suṣumṇā is not normally possible because something blocks the passage. This block is symbolized by a coiled snake, the kuṇḍalinī.

The concept of kuṇḍalinī is confused by many imprecise definitions, and even a text such as the *Haṭha Yoga Pradīpikā* contains contradictory descriptions of it. The definition that follows is derived from what in my opinion is the best, the clearest, and the most coherent text on this subject, the *Yoga Yājñavalkya*. There kuṇḍalinī is defined unambiguously as an obstacle. What is to enter the suṣumṇā at some stage or other through your yoga practice is, according to this text, not the kuṇḍalinī itself, but simply prāṇa. Many books say that it is the kuṇḍalinī itself that rises up through the suṣumṇā, but this does not make sense if we follow the *Yoga Yājñavalkya*, one of the oldest texts that deals with this aspect of yoga. One of its central concepts is that prāṇa and the various forms it takes in the body are linked to the practice of yoga, and it says that if we are successful in our practice, the kuṇḍalinī is burned up, making the way clear for prāṇa.[3]

A snake killed while lying in a curled position unfolds and streches out, the muscles no longer able to keep it coiled. It is said that when the fire in the body, agni, has killed the snake, the kuṇḍalinī unrolls and the passage is open to the flow of prāṇa. This does not happen overnight. Even when parts of the kuṇḍalinī are destroyed, it remains capable of blocking suṣumṇā for a long time.

If you closely consider this image, it becomes clear that kuṇḍalinī is another way of depicting what we call avidyā. In the same way that avidyā can become so powerful that it totally prevents us from seeing puruṣa, kuṇḍalinī blocks the prāṇa and prevents it from rising through the suṣumṇā. The moment the kuṇḍalinī is burned is the same moment that avidyā ceases to exist. Then prāṇa is able to enter the suṣumṇā and slowly move upward. We can also understand haṭha yoga as part of rāja yoga, which is defined as the process in which prāṇa, the friend of puruṣa, gradually rises upward. When it gets to the top, puruṣa unfolds and the king within us emerges. When the emphasis is primarily on the

3. *Yoga Yājñavalkya* 12.11–12, 16.

concept of kuṇḍalinī, then we speak of the practice as kuṇḍalinī yoga. Haṭha yoga is so named when our practice focuses on removing the division between ha and ṭha.

Lastly, the term tantra yoga may be used in describing a yoga practice based on kuṇḍalinī. In tantra yoga the emphasis is on certain energies that are normally squandered being directed in such a way that they can reduce the blocks that stand in the way of the prāṇa. The practices of tantra yoga are distinctive; indeed, the word *tantra* translates as "technique" in the positive sense, meaning a skill or craft. In tantra yoga the focus is on the body, and a wide range of connections and relationships between the body and other aspects of the world and cosmos is made.

Further Thoughts on Kuṇḍalinī

Q: I have read that the moment the kuṇḍalinī is freed, it feels like a powerful electric shock running through a cable. It also said that if the cable is not strong enough for the current, it will burn out. This is dangerous and you must be prepared for it. Do you have any thoughts on this?

A: It seems to me that kuṇḍalinī must be described in this way because it is surrounded by a lot of mystery and a lot of superstition. It seems mysterious because we cannot simply cut the body open and see this power. But if we relate this power to prāṇa, there is no longer anything mysterious about it. That is the beauty of a text such as the *Yoga Yājñavalkya*. On the experience of the rising of prāṇa in the suṣumṇā, the *Yoga Yājñavalkya* quite simply says: "How could I describe what a person then becomes aware of?" There is no shock such as the one you described. When someone sees the truth, the only shock is to have to see what he or she was before. There is no question of a one-thousand-volt shock or the like.

While it is a good metaphor to describe the rising of the kuṇḍalinī like this, it makes little sense to take it literally. If we were to say that kuṇḍalinī is an energy force that leads us to the truth, then we would also have to accept that there are two different types of energy existing side by side: prāṇa and kuṇḍalinī. Many of these ideas are based on superficial and inaccurate translations, or the inability to explain unclear passages in certain texts. For this reason, these concepts and techniques must be explained by someone who has not only a great wealth of practical experience and well-founded knowledge, but also considerable proficiency in Sanskrit, the language in which the texts are written. Very often there is a lack of both.

Q: If we burn up kuṇḍalinī bit by bit, does more prāṇa gradually enter the suṣumṇā?

A: We must be careful that we do not go too far in using images to describe certain experiences. We should never forget that they are images and not the experience itself. Nevertheless, we could imagine it just exactly as you do. Sometimes we move into a state of mind which we could describe as dhyāna or samādhi; then we are back in a distracted state again. If the mind is without peace or clarity, the kuṇḍalinī is lying curled up, blocking suṣumṇā. If the mind quiets, it is less obstructed by kuṇḍalinī, and we may perhaps experience a state of being in which the mind is operating solely on the level of clear sight and true understanding. All that really means is that prāṇa is rising higher in the suṣumṇā and can now flow freely through places that were previously blocked.

Q: According to haṭha yoga, is the use of the bandha the only way of moving the kuṇḍalinī?

A: No. If you read the *Haṭha Yoga Pradīpikā*, for example, you will discover that none of the techniques given is "the only one." Various methods are described in different chapters. The same is true for the *Gheraṇḍa Saṃhitā*, the *Śiva Saṃhitā*, and other classical texts. Many different suggestions are made therein.

Q: Is it then the case that in other kinds of yoga you have the same physical experience as in kuṇḍalinī yoga? What is it like when avidyā disappears for someone who is, for example, following the path of jñāna yoga and who becomes a jñāni?

A: If the mind is restless, there is no jñāna, no knowledge. The terms *ha* and *ṭha* are used for describing the extreme states of an oscillating mind. The flow of prāṇa solely into ha (iḍā) and ṭha (piṅgalā) shows a restless mind swinging back and forth between extremes. Prāṇa in the suṣumṇā, on the other hand, represents a clear, quiet mind. So a jñāni is someone whose prāṇa flows in the suṣumṇā. With other people, the flow of prāṇa is still limited in a very imperfect way to the two opposing nāḍī, ha and ṭha. We must not let ourselves be confused by the way different schools of yoga describe the same process. Many of these things are described very clearly and explicitly in the *Yoga Sūtra*, but neither ha nor ṭha are mentioned in it. The *Yoga Sūtra* considers these questions from a fundamental position, showing us how little difference there really is between these various concepts. Primarily it is a question of our state of mind. Whatever happens to the mind and causes a change in it affects the whole person, including the body and all experiences on the physical level. This is the basis of the *Yoga Sūtra*, which is a great guide if you want to understand all these things more fully.

People often ask me if I teach āsanas, and when I answer "yes" they say: "Oh, then you are a haṭha yogi!" If I am talking about the *Yoga Sūtra* they say "Oh, you are a rāja yogi!" And if I say I recite the Vedas the comment is: "Oh, so you are a mantra yogi!" If I simply say that I practice yoga, they do not know what to make of me. Many people want to give everything and everyone a label. Unfortunately, these classifications have become much too important and give the impression that there are fundamental differences between the various forms of yoga. But really they are all dealing with the same thing, and are only looking at them from different perspectives. If we really follow *one* direction in yoga as far as we can go, then it will lead us along *all* paths of yoga.

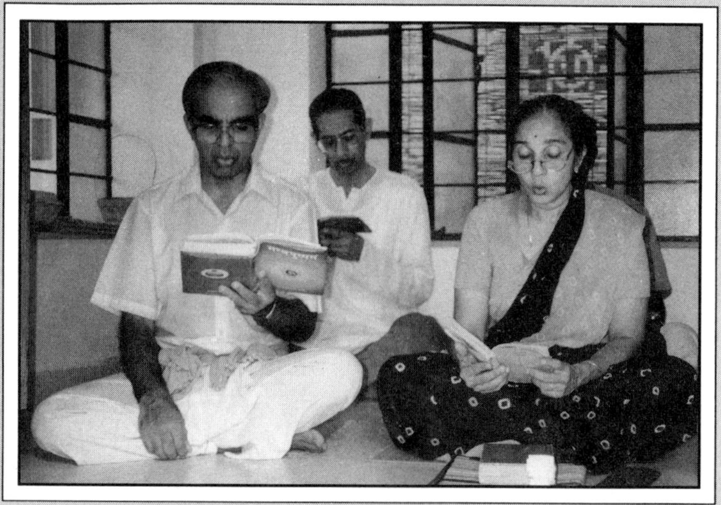

Top: Desikachar, his wife Menaka, and Chandrashakar, director of the Krishnamacharya Yoga Mandiram, chanting in the Sannadhi.

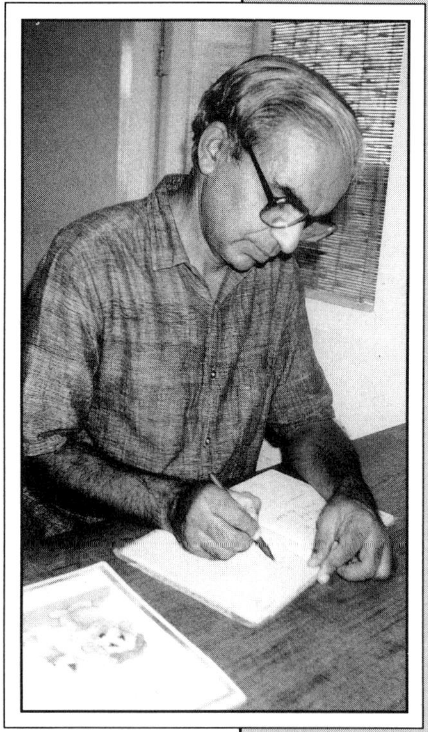

Middle: Desikachar in his study.

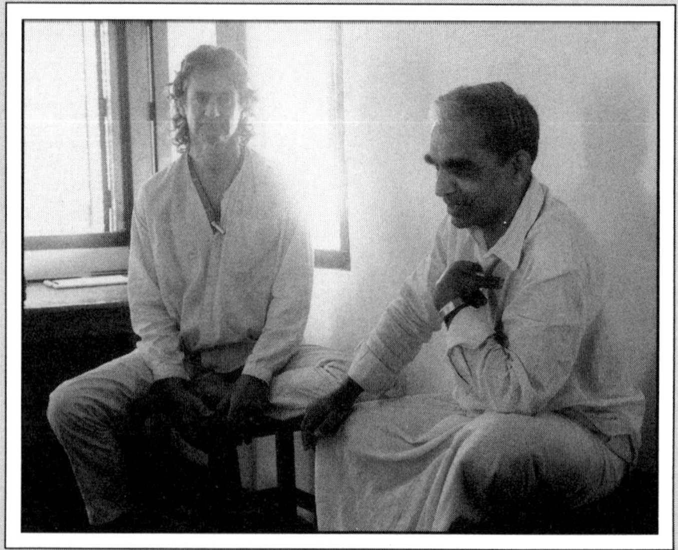

Bottom: Mark Whitwell and Desikachar.

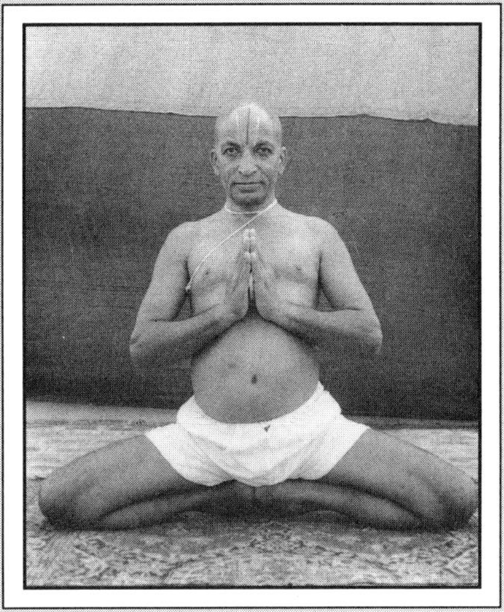

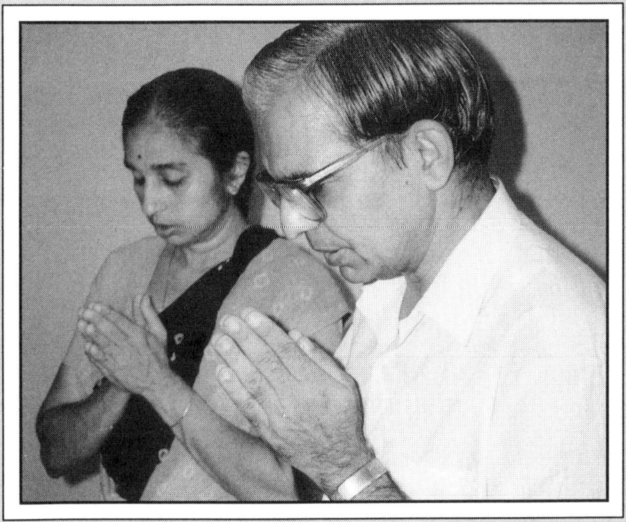

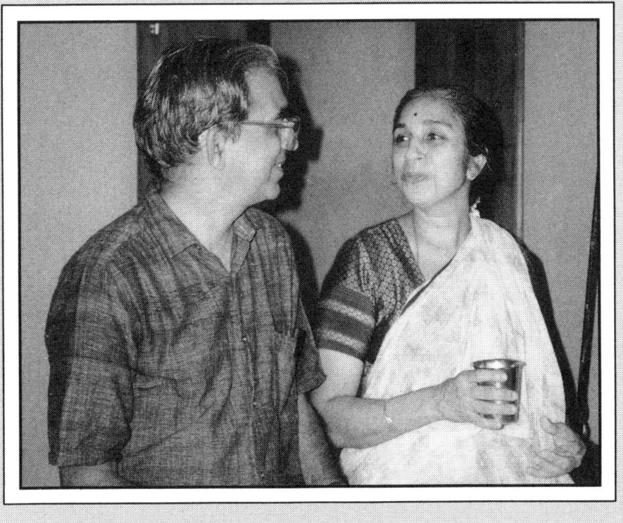

Part III

The *Yoga Sūtra* of Patañjali

with
Translation and
Commentary by
T. K. V. DESIKACHAR

Top:
Krishnamacharya in
mūlabandhāsana.

Middle and bottom:
Desikachar and Menaka.

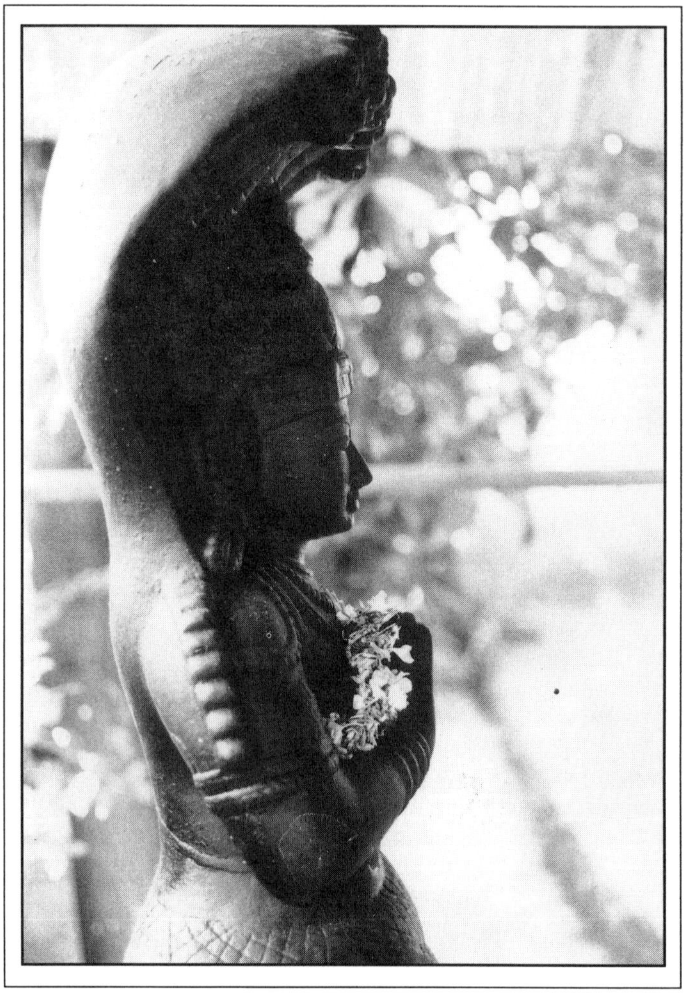

The statue of Patañjali in the courtyard of the Krishnamacharya Yoga Mandiram.

INTRODUCTION

Patañjali's *Yoga Sūtra* is *the* heart of yoga. The heart, *hṛdaya*, is that which does not change and Patañjali gave a permanent definition and form to yoga in his *Sūtra*. The heart without prāṇa, however, is not alive and is without relevance for us. Desikachar explains that the teaching relationship is the prāṇa or life of the *Yoga Sūtra*; it is the teacher who brings the heart into life. The *Yoga Sūtra* is a potent tool for the teacher who is able to make it relevant to the student and thus transmit the transformative power of the heart.

Desikachar emphasizes that what follows is an introduction because the *Yoga Sūtra* is vast in its scope. Krishnamacharya says that there is an ocean between *atha* and *iti*, the first and last syllables of the *Sūtra*. In the study of the *Sūtra* with one's teacher, meaningful and powerful insights seem to leap out of the words, sometimes in very unexpected ways. It is recommended that one study with a teacher who has likewise studied and practiced with a competent teacher, whose *tapas* (practice), *svādhyāya* (self-understanding), and *īśvarapraṇidhānā* (surrender) have produced clarity.

Patañjali presented his work in the style known as sūtra, that which has very few words, yet is free from ambiguity, full of essence, universal in context, and affirmative. The *sūtra* (from which we get *suture*) links the teacher, the teaching, and the student. As yoga study and practice develop, the message of the *Sūtra* takes on a deeper resonance and becomes more relevant, more revealing. There can be no haste or exaggerated effort to gain its understanding; it must be a natural process.

There is uncertainty as to who Patañjali was. There are some who think of him as the divine incarnation of the serpent Ananta who supports the whole universe. He is the Adhiśeṣa, "the first servant of God," who "being so close to God, knows the teaching of God best." We can assume that Patañjali did not originate the yoga teaching but inherited it from the vastness of the Vedas. On the instruction of a great teacher, he identified all the teachings in the Vedas about the mind and presented them in this precise, organized form. Yoga concepts such as *Īśvara, kleśa, karma, guṇas, puruṣa, samādhi, siddhi,* and *kaivalya* are all contained in the ancient Upaniṣads in different forms. The

Vedas, however, are presented in no particular order, making it difficult to study anything in a coherent fashion. It is a great gift therefore that Patañjali systematized the yoga teachings from the Vedas into an accessible system of development.

The short, pithy words and meanings of the *Sūtra* enabled oral transmission of the yoga understanding from teacher to student through the centuries. In our time, it was Krishnamacharya who had the privilege of learning the intricacies of these words at a very practical level from his teacher, Ramamohan Brahmachari. Likewise, Desikachar's study and practice with Krishnamacharya has resulted in clarity and the present-day relevance of every sūtra. Krishnamacharya and Desikachar are not interested in spiritual or philosophical speculation. Rather, they have brought to yoga an intellectual rigor, technical definition, and practice to determine the means by which each person may reduce duḥkha (suffering).

In contrast to other Indian systems of philosophy that state that nothing is real except God, Patañjali's position is that everything in a person's experience is *sat*, the "truth" or "reality," and cannot be denied. Even duḥkha is *sat* and is not something to be ashamed of or react against. Everyone has duḥkha. It is part of our reality and if recognized, serves to wake us up to further clarity and understanding. As Krishnamacharya would say, "Thank God for duḥkha," which he described as the "unavoidable motive for practice." Furthermore, Patañjali makes it clear that everything in our experience is changing; nothing, including duḥkha, is in a fixed condition. Therefore, if there is the desire, we can make positive changes for ourselves. Patañjali gives innumerable means within our grasp that begin with the present reality of our experience. We must begin at the beginning and Desikachar puts it simply: "If you tell a person who cannot find their own house that there is a pot of gold inside, they would be happier had they not had this information. What use is the gold if it cannot be found? It only causes pain. First they must find the house and enter it. Then there are many possibilities."

Patañjali summarizes the process and the tools for self-understanding. If the appropriate means are selected and practiced with the help of a teacher, our turbulent minds can be brought to peace and extraordinary wisdom and well-being is our potential.

This is the essential message of Patañjali communicated by Krishnamacharya and Desikachar.

—Mark Whitwell

PRONUNCIATION GUIDE

GUTTURAL *(pronounced from the throat)*

vowels	*a*	as in b<u>u</u>t
	ā	as in f<u>a</u>ther
plain	*k*	as in <u>k</u>in
	g	as in <u>g</u>ood
aspirate	*kh*	as in sin<u>kh</u>ole
	gh	as in le<u>gh</u>orn
	h	as in <u>h</u>and
nasal	*ṅ*	as in e<u>n</u>core

PALATAL *(pronounced from the palate)*

vowels	*i*	as in t<u>i</u>n
	ī	as in t<u>ee</u>th
plain	*c*	as in <u>ch</u>ur<u>ch</u>
	j	as in <u>j</u>udge
aspirate	*ch*	as in coa<u>ch</u>horse
	jh	as in hed<u>ge</u>hog
semivowel	*y*	as in <u>y</u>ou
sibilant	*ś*	as in <u>s</u>ure

RETROFLEX *(pronounced with the tip of the tongue curled up)*

vowels	*ṛ*	as in sab<u>re</u>
	ṝ	as in cha<u>gr</u>in
plain	*ṭ*	as in car<u>t</u>
	ḍ	as in ar<u>d</u>ent
aspirate	*ṭh*	as in car<u>th</u>orse
	ḍh	as in for<u>dh</u>am
nasal	*ṇ*	as in frie<u>n</u>d
semivowel	*r*	as in <u>r</u>ib
sibilant	*ṣ*	as in hu<u>sh</u>

DENTAL *(pronounced with the tip of the tongue against upper teeth)*

vowels	*ḷ*	as in ab<u>le</u>
plain	*t*	as in <u>th</u>eatre
	d	as in <u>th</u>ey
aspirate	*th*	as in wi<u>thh</u>eld
	dh	as in bud<u>dh</u>a
nasal	*n*	as in boo<u>n</u>
semivowel	*I*	as in <u>l</u>ip
sibilant	*s*	as in <u>s</u>un

LABIAL *(pronounced with the lips)*

vowel	*u*	as in bull
	ū	as in rule
plain	*p*	as in pat
	b	as in bee
aspirate	*ph*	as in uphill
	bh	as in abhor
nasal	*m*	as in man

GUTTURAL AND PALATAL

vowels	*e*	as in prey
	ai	as in aisle

GUTTURAL AND LABIAL

vowels	*o*	as in go
	au	as in cow

DENTAL AND LABIAL

semivowel	*v*	as in van

NASAL

ṁ (ṃ) or ṅ makes preceding vowel nasal

ASPIRATE

ḥ makes preceeding vowel aspirate

1

समाधिपाद :

SĀMADHIPĀDAḤ

The sūtras of Patañjali are presented in four chapters. The first chapter is called *samādhipāda* (the chapter on samādhi). This chapter defines Yoga and its characteristics and discusses the problems encountered in reaching the state of Yoga and ways in which these problems can be handled. Each sūtra is presented in the original Devanāgarī script with a transliteration of the Sanskrit, a translation in italics, and commentary.

1.1 अथ योगानुशासनम् ।

atha yogānuśāsanam

The first sūtra introduces the subject matter, as the oral tradition requires. In the convention of ancient Sanskrit literature, the first word, *atha*, carries the connotation of a prayer, both for an auspicious beginning and a successful conclusion to the work that follows.

Here begins the authoritative instruction on Yoga.

Patañjali indicates that while the subject matter is of ancient origin and he is not the originator, he has studied it to an appropriate depth under his own teacher and is now competent to share his understanding with his disciples. His style will be in a manner suitable for them to transmit it in turn directly to their disciples through the traditional oral methods.

1.2 योगश्चित्तवृत्तिनिरोधः ।

yogaśgcittavṛttinirodhaḥ

What is Yoga? It is a word with many interpretations and connotations. Patañjali defines his understanding of the word.

Yoga is the ability to direct the mind exclusively toward an object and sustain that direction without any distractions.

The object can be a concrete one either external to ourselves or part of ourselves. It can be an area of interest, a concept, or something beyond the level of the senses, such as God.

1.3 तदा द्रष्टुः स्वरूपेऽवस्थानम् ।

tadā draṣṭuḥ svarūpe 'vasthānam

Then the ability to understand the object fully and correctly is apparent.

In a state of Yoga the different preconceptions and products of the imagination that can prevent or distort understanding are controlled, reduced, or eliminated. The tendency not to be open to a fresh comprehension and the inability to comprehend are overcome.

1.4 वृत्तिसारूप्यमितरत्र ।

vṛttisārūpyamitaratra

In the absence of the state of mind called Yoga,

The ability to understand the object is simply replaced by the mind's conception of that object or by a total lack of comprehension.

A disturbed mind can rarely follow a direction. If it ever does, comprehension of the object will be faulty.

1.5 वृत्तयः पञ्चतय्यः क्लिष्टाक्लिष्टाः ।

vṛttayaḥ pañcatayyaḥ kliṣṭākliṣṭāḥ

What is the mind? Patañjali defines it as the activities that occupy it. It cannot be perceived except in terms of these activities.

There are five activities of the mind. Each of them can be beneficial and each can cause problems.

Whether these activities are beneficial or create problems cannot be immediately seen. Time alone will confirm their effects.

1.6 प्रमाणविपर्ययविकल्पनिद्रास्मृतयः ।

pramāṇaviparyayavikalpanidrāsmṛtayaḥ

The five activities are comprehension, misapprehension, imagination, deep sleep, and memory.

Each mental activity has its own characteristics and although not always apparent, they can be individually recognized. Their dominance and effects on our behavior and attitudes combine to make up our personalities.

1.7 प्रत्यक्षानुमानागमाः प्रमाणानि ।

pratyakṣānumānāgamāḥ pramāṇāni

The activities are each defined.

Comprehension is based on direct observation of the object, inference, and reference to reliable authorities.

The mind can register an object directly through the senses. When the available information is inadequate or incomplete for sensual perception, other faculties, such as logic and memory, may enable a more complete comprehension of the object to be inferred. When no direct comprehension is possible, reference to reliable authorities, such as a written text or a trusted individual, can enable comprehension indirectly. In such a way do we understand places, people, or concepts outside our direct experiences. In a state of Yoga, comprehension is different from comprehension at other times. It is closer to the true nature of the object.

1.8 विपर्ययो मिथ्याज्ञानमतद्रूपप्रतिष्ठम् ।

viparyayo mithyājñānamatadrūpapratiṣṭham

Misapprehension is that comprehension that is taken to be correct until more favorable conditions reveal the actual nature of the object.

This is considered to be the most frequent activity of the mind. It may occur through faulty observation or the misinterpretation of what is seen. It is due to our inability to understand in depth what we see, often as a result of past experiences and conditioning. The error may be recognized later or never at all. The aim of Yoga practice is to recognize and control the causes of misapprehension (see chapter 2 of the *Sūtra*).

1.9 शब्दज्ञानानुपाती वस्तुशून्यो विकल्पः ।

śabdajñānānupātī vastuśūnyo vikalpaḥ

Imagination is the comprehension of an object based only on words and expressions, even though the object is absent.

This happens in the absence of any direct perception. Reference to the meaning, connotations, or implications of descriptive words guides imagination toward comprehension. It may be further helped if the words are used poetically or oratorically. It can also arise through other means such as dreams, feelings, and emotions. Past experiences, stored in the memory, often contribute to this mental activity.

1.10 अभावप्रत्ययालम्बना तमोवृत्तिर्निद्रा ।

abhāvapratyayālambanā tamovṛttirnidrā

Deep sleep is when the mind is overcome with heaviness and no other activities are present.

Sleep is a common, regular activity for the mind and there is a time for it. But heaviness can also occur through boredom or exhaustion resulting in sleep. Sleep is a regular condition for all living beings.

1.11 अनुभूतविषयासंप्रमोषः स्मृतिः ।

anubhūtaviṣayāsaṁpramoṣaḥ smṛtiḥ

Memory is the mental retention of a conscious experience.

All conscious experiences leave an impression on the individual and are stored as memory. It is not possible to tell if a memory is true, false, incomplete or imaginary.

All and each of these activities of the mind are confirmation of the mind's existence. They are interrelated and complex so that each one, except perhaps sleep, should be considered as a matrix or genus of activity rather than a distinct entity with exclusive and limited characteristics. Each can, at different times and in different circumstances, be both beneficial or harmful. Their effects may be direct and immediate or they may be indirect as a later consequence of their manifestation.

1.12 अभ्यासवैराग्याभ्यां तन्निरोधः ।

abhyāsavairāgyābhyāṁ tannirodhaḥ

How do we arrive at a state of Yoga? What should we do and what should we not do?

The mind can reach the state of Yoga through practice and detachment.

1.13 तत्र स्थितौ यत्नोऽभ्यासः ।

tatra sthitau yatno 'bhyāsaḥ

What are the essential features of this practice and detachment? Even though the techniques involved are not specified here, the following two sūtra indicate their qualities.

Practice is basically the correct effort required to move toward, reach, and maintain the state of Yoga [see 1.2].

The practices chosen must be correctly learned from and guided by a competent teacher who understands the personal and social character of the student. If the appropriate practice for a particular student is not provided and followed, there can be little hope of achieving success.

1.14 स तु दीर्घकालनैरन्तर्यसत्कारादरासेवितो दृढभूमिः ।

sa tu dīrghakālanairantaryasatkārādarāsevito
dṛḍhabhūmiḥ

It is only when the correct practice is followed for a long time, without interruptions and with a quality of positive attitude and eagerness, that it can succeed.

There will always be a tendency to start practice with enthusiasm and energy, and a desire for sudden results. But the continuing pressures of everyday life and the enormous resistance of the mind encourages us to succumb to human weaknesses. All this is understandable, we all have these tendencies. This sūtra emphasizes the need to approach practice soberly with a positive, self-disciplined attitude and with a long-term view toward eventual success.

1.15 दृष्टानुश्रविकविषयवितृष्णस्य वशीकारसंज्ञावैराग्यम् ।

drṣtānuśravikavisayavitṛṣṇasya
vaśīkārasaṁjñāvairāgyam

As we develop our practice along the correct lines, we find that our ability to discipline ourselves and reject intrusive influences grows. Eventually we may reach a state of detachment when

> *At the highest level there is an absence of any cravings, either for the fulfillment of the senses or for extraordinary experiences.*

There are benefits from practice such as physical strength and dexterity, heightened awareness and sensitivity. There may also be the temptation to use our new skills to prove our higher state. But these are incidental benefits and diversionary temptations and if we place too much importance on them, we are in danger of losing sight of the path to Yoga.

1.16 तत्परं पुरुषख्यातेर्गुणवैतृष्ण्यम् ।

tatparaṁ puruṣakhyātergunavaitṛṣṇyam

Further

> *When an individual has achieved complete understanding of his true self, he will no longer be disturbed by the distracting influences within and around him.*

Detachment develops with self-understanding. The inevitable desires for diversion cannot be suppressed for, if they are, they will surely surface again later.

1.17 वितर्कविचारानन्दास्मितारूपानुगमात्संप्रज्ञातः ।

vitarkavicārānandāsmitārūpānugamātsaṁprajñātaḥ

> *Then the object is gradually understood fully. At first it is at a more superficial level. In time, comprehension becomes deeper. And finally it is total. There is pure joy in reaching such a depth of understanding. For then the individual is so much at one with the object that he is oblivious to his surroundings.*

Such a level of perception of the nature of the object is only possible in a state of Yoga. Frequently we are able to understand the superficial and more obvious elements. But comprehension is incomplete until we have achieved perception at the deepest level without any errors.

1.18 विरामप्रत्ययाभ्यासपूर्वः संस्कारशेषोऽन्यः ।

virāmapratyayābhyāsapūrvaḥ
saṃskāraśeṣo 'nyaḥ

When the mind rises to the state of Yoga and remains so,

> The usual mental disturbances are absent. However, memories of the past continue.

Then perception is immediate, not gradual. The memories remain to help us live in the day-to-day world, but not to create distractions.

1.19 भवप्रत्ययो विदेहप्रकृतिलयानाम् ।

bhavapratyayo videhaprakṛtilayānām

Inevitably, because of the many millions who share the world with us,

> *There will be some who are born in a state of Yoga. They need not practice or discipline themselves.*

But these are rare persons who cannot be copied and should not be emulated. Indeed some may succumb to wordly influences and lose their superior qualities.

1.20 श्रद्धावीर्यस्मृतिसमाधिप्रज्ञापूर्वक इतरेषाम् ।

śraddhāvīryasmṛtisamādhiprajñāpūrvaka
itareṣām

But what of the rest of us? Is there really a chance of achieving this state of Yoga?

> *Through faith, which will give sufficient energy to achieve success against all odds, direction will be maintained. The realization of the goal of Yoga is a matter of time.*

The goal is the ability to direct the mind toward an object without any distraction, resulting, in time, in a clear and correct understanding of that object.

Faith is the unshakable conviction that we can arrive at that goal. We must not be lulled by complacency in success or discouraged by failure. We must work hard and steadily through all distractions, whether seemingly good or bad.

1.21 तीव्रसंवेगानामासन्नः ।

tīvrasaṁvegānāmāsannaḥ

The more intense the faith and the effort, the closer the goal.

1.22 मृदुमध्याधिमात्रत्वात्ततोऽपि विशेषः ।

mṛdumadhyādhimātratvāttato 'pi viśeṣaḥ

Do we and can we all have the same chance to reach the goal?

Inevitably the depth of faith varies with different individuals and at different times with the same individual. The results will reflect these variations.

Such variations are a part of the human condition. They are a product of the individual's cultural background and capability.

1.23 ईश्वरप्रणिधानाद्वा ।

Īśvarapraṇidhānādvā

Patañjali recognizes that attempts to change our state of mind to Yoga are fraught with obstacles that vary in potency. But for those who have either an inborn faith in God or are able to develop it over the years,

Offering regular prayers to God with a feeling of submission to his power, surely enables the state of Yoga to be achieved.

In the following sūtra, Patañjali gives his definition of God.

1.24 क्लेशकर्मविपाकाशयैरपरामृष्टः पुरुषविशेष ईश्वरः ।

kleśakarmavipākāśayairaparāmṛṣṭaḥ
puruṣaviśeṣa īśvaraḥ

God is the Supreme Being whose actions are never based on misapprehension.

1.25 तत्र निरतिशयं सर्वज्ञबीजम् ।

tatra niratiśayaṁ sarvajñabījam

How can God be so extraordinary?

He knows everything there is to be known.

His comprehension is beyond any human comparisons.

1.26 स एष पूर्वेषामपि गुरुः कालेनानवच्छेदात् ।

sa eṣa pūrveṣāmapi guruḥ
kālenānavacchedāt

Is God, according to Patañjali, timebound or timeless?

God is eternal. In fact he is the ultimate teacher. He is the source of guidance for all teachers: past, present, and future.

1.27 तस्य वाचकः प्रणवः ।

tasya vācakaḥ praṇavaḥ

How should we refer to God? How should we address him?

In the way most appropriate to the qualities of God.

In different cultures and different religions different words are used to describe God and his qualities. It is more important that we express God with the greatest respect and without any conflicts. In this a teacher can be a great help.

1.28 तज्जपस्तदर्थभावनम् ।

tajjapastadarthabhāvanam

How do we relate to God?

In order to relate to God it is necessary to regularly address him properly and reflect on his qualities.

Patañjali suggests that it is necessary to reflect constantly on the qualities of God. This might be aided by the repeated recitation of his name together with prayer and contemplation. But mechanical repetition and prayer is worthless, it must be accompanied by conscious thought and consideration, and by profound respect.

1.29 ततः प्रत्यक्चेतनाधिगमोऽप्यन्तरायाभावश्च ।

tataḥ pratyakcetanādhigamo 'pyantarāyābhāvaśca

For those who have faith in God, such reflections will inevitably be beneficial.

The individual will in time perceive his true nature. He will not be disturbed by any interruptions that may arise in his journey to the state of Yoga.

1.30 व्याधिस्त्यानसंशयप्रमादालस्याविरतिभ्रान्तिदर्शनालब्ध-
भूमिकत्वानवस्थितत्वानि चित्तविक्षेपास्तेऽन्तरायाः ।

vyādhistyānasaṁśayapramādālasyāvirati-
bhrāntidaśsanālabdhabhūmikatvāna-
vasthitatvāni cittavikṣepāste 'ntarāyāḥ

What, if any, are the interruptions?

There are nine types of interruptions to developing mental clarity: illness, mental stagnation, doubts, lack of foresight, fatigue, overindulgence, illusions about one's true state of mind, lack of perseverance, and regression. They are obstacles because they create mental disturbances and encourage distractions.

The more we are vulnerable to these interruptions the more difficult it is to reach a state of Yoga.

1.31 दुःखदौर्मनस्याङ्गमेजयत्वश्वासप्रश्वासा विक्षेपसहभुवः ।

duḥkhadaurmanasyāṅgamejayatvaśvāsapraśvāsā
vikṣepasahabhuvaḥ

Can we tell when these interruptions are having an effect and taking root?

All these interruptions produce one or more of the following symptoms: mental discomfort, negative thinking, the inability to be at ease in different body postures, and difficulty in controlling one's breath.

Any of these symptoms can have further consequences. The following eight sūtras give some suggestions for controlling these interruptions and their symptoms. These suggestions are useful both for those with great faith in God and for those with no faith.

1.32 तत्प्रतिषेधार्थमेकतत्त्वाभ्यासः ।

tatpratiṣedhārthamekatattvābhyāsaḥ

If one can select an appropriate means to steady the mind and practice this, whatever the provocations, the interruptions cannot take root.

1.33 मैत्रीकरुणामुदितोपेक्षाणां सुखदुःखपुण्यापुण्यविषयाणां भावनाताश्चित्तप्रसादनम् ।

maitrīkaruṇāmuditopekṣānāṁ
sukhaduhkhapun̄yāpuṇyaviṣayāṇāṁ
bhāvanātaścittaprasādanam

In daily life we see people around who are happier than we are, people who are less happy. Some may be doing praiseworthy things and others causing problems. Whatever may be our usual attitude toward such people and their actions, if we can be pleased with others who are happier than ourselves, compassionate toward those who are unhappy, joyful with those doing praiseworthy things, and remain undisturbed by the errors of others, our mind will be very tranquil.

1.34 प्रच्छर्दनविधारणाभ्यां वा प्राणस्य ।

pracchardanavidhāraṇābhyaṁ vā prāṇasya

When we find interruptions or the symptoms of interruptions

The practice of breathing exercises involving extended exhalation might be helpful.

The techniques, however, must be correctly taught and guided.

1.35 विषयवती वा प्रवृत्तिरुत्पन्ना मनसः स्थितिनिबन्धिनी ।

viṣayavatī vā pravṛttirutpannā manasaḥ sthitinibandhinī

The role of the senses, such as sight and hearing, in providing information to the mind has far-reaching effects. They are the doors of perception and we are often their slaves. But can we not examine what is even more powerful in us than our senses? Can we not make them sharper and at our disposal?

> *By regular inquiry into the role of the senses we can reduce mental distortions.*

1.36 विशोका वा ज्योतिष्मती ।

viśokā vā jyotiṣmatī

One of the great mysteries of life is life itself.

> *When we inquire into what life is and what keeps us alive, we may find some solace for our mental distractions.*

Consideration of things greater than our individual selves helps us put ourselves in perspective.

1.37 वीतरागविषयं वा चित्तम् ।

vītarāgaviṣayaṁ vā cittam

> *When we are confronted with problems, the counsel of someone who has mastered similar problems can be a great help.*

Such counsel can come directly from a living person or from the study of someone alive or dead.

1.38 स्वप्ननिद्राज्ञानालम्बनं वा ।

svapnanidrājñānālambanaṁ vā

When we believe we know a lot, we may become arrogant in our knowledge. The consequences can be disturbing. In fact even the most ordinary, day-to-day occurrences are not always clear to us.

Inquiry into dreams and sleep and our experiences during or around these states can help to clarify some of our problems.

How refreshing it is after a good night's sleep! How disturbing a bad dream can be!

1.39 यथाभिमतध्यानाद्वा ।

yathābhimatadhyānādvā

Any inquiry of interest can calm the mind.

Sometimes the most simple objects of inquiry, such as the first cry of an infant, can help relieve mental disturbances. Sometimes complex inquiries, such as into mathematical hypotheses, will help. But such inquiries should not replace the main goal, which remains to change our state of mind gradually from distraction to direction.

1.40 परमाणुपरममहत्त्वान्तोऽस्य वशीकारः ।

paramāṇuparamamahattvānto 'sya vaśīkāraḥ

What are the consequences of developing this state of Yoga?

When one reaches this state, nothing is beyond comprehension. The mind can follow and help understand the simple and the complex, the infinite and the infinitesimal, the perceptible and the imperceptible.

The actual process of this comprehension is explained below.

1.41 क्षीणवृत्तेरभिजातस्येव मणेर्ग्रहीतृग्रहणग्राह्येषु तत्स्थतदञ्जनता समापत्तिः ।

kṣīṇavṛtterabhijātasyeva
maṇergrahītṛgrahaṇagrāhyeṣu
tatsthatadañjanatā samāpattiḥ

When the mind is free from distraction, it is possible for all the mental processes to be involved in the object of inquiry. As one remains in this state, gradually one becomes totally immersed in the object. The mind then, like a flawless diamond, reflects only the features of the object and nothing else.

In the beginning all mental activities, except sleep, are involved in the comprehension of an object. But, gradually only those needed for correct, flawless comprehension remain.

1.42 तत्र शब्दार्थज्ञानविकल्पैः संकीर्णा सवितर्का समापत्तिः ।

tatra śabdārthajñānavikalpaiḥ saṅkīrṇā savitarkā samāpattiḥ

However this does not happen spontaneously. It is gradual.

Initially, because of our past experiences and ideas, our understanding of the object is distorted. Everything that has been heard, read, or felt may interfere with our perception.

Some of these influences may have no validity. Others may now be redundant.

1.43 स्मृतिपरिशुद्धौ स्वरूपशून्येवार्थमात्रनिर्भासा निर्वितर्का ।

smṛtipariśuddhau svarūpaśūnyevārthamātranirbhāsā nirvitarkā

When the direction of the mind toward the object is sustained, the ideas and memories of the past gradually recede. The mind becomes crystal clear and one with the object. At this moment there is no feeling of oneself. This is pure perception.

1.44 एतयैव सविचारा निर्विचारा च सूक्ष्मविषया व्याख्याता ।

etayaiva savicārā nirvicārā ca sūkṣmaviṣayā vyākhyātā

But this phenomenon is not limited in scope.

This process is possible with any type of object, at any level of perception, whether superficial and general or in-depth and specific.

1.45 सूक्ष्मविषयत्वं चालिङ्गपर्यवसानम् ।

sūkṣmaviṣayatvaṁ cāliṅgaparyavasānam

Except that the mind cannot comprehend the very source of perception within us, its objects can be unlimited.

1.46 ता एव सबीजः समाधिः ।

tā eva sabījaḥ samādhiḥ

Can the mind arrive at a state of Yoga unilaterally?

All these processes of directing the mind involve an object of inquiry.

They also involve preparation, gradual progression, and sustained interest. For without this interest, there will be distraction. Without preparation, there can be no foundation. And without gradual progression, the human system may react and rebel.

1.47 निर्विचारवैशारद्येऽध्यात्मप्रसादः ।

nirvicāravaiśāradye 'dhyātmaprasādaḥ

What are the consequences of achieving this ability to direct the mind?

Then the individual begins to truly know himself.

As the correct comprehension of the object begins to enrich us, we also begin to understand our very being.

1.48 ऋतंभरा तत्र प्रज्ञा ।

ṛtaṁbharā tatra prajñā

Then, what he sees and shares with others is free from error.

1.49 श्रुतानुमानप्रज्ञाभ्यामन्यविषया विशेषार्थत्वात् ।

śrutānumānaprajñābhyāmanyaviṣayā viśeṣārthatvāt

His knowledge is no longer based on memory or inference. It is spontaneous, direct, and at both a level and an intensity that is beyond the ordinary.

In such circumstances, our mind reflects the object of our inquiry simply, like a clear and perfect mirror.

1.50 तज्जः संस्कारोऽन्यसंस्कारप्रतिबन्धी ।

tajjaḥ saṁskāro 'nyasaṁskārapratibandhī

As this newly acquired quality of the mind gradually strengthens, it dominates the other mental tendencies that are based on misapprehensions.

1.51 तस्यापि निरोधे सर्वनिरोधान्निर्बीजः समाधिः ।

tasyāpi nirodhe sarvanirodhānnirbījaḥ samādhiḥ

Finally, if ever,

The mind reaches a state when it has no impressions of any sort. It is open, clear, simply transparent.

Such comprehension is not sought. It comes inevitably and nothing can stop it.

This is the highest state of Yoga, but it cannot be described in words. Only those who have reached this state can comprehend its nature.

2

साधनपादः

SĀDHANAPĀDAḤ

The second chapter is called *sādhanapāda*. It describes the qualities necessary to change the mind effectively and gradually from a state of distraction to one of attention and why these qualities are important and what the practice of them entails.

2.1 तपःस्वाध्यायेश्वरप्रणिधानानि क्रियायोगः ।

tapaḥsvādhyāyeśvarapraṇidhānāni kriyāyogaḥ

The practice of Yoga must reduce both physical and mental impurities. It must develop our capacity for self-examination and help us to understand that, in the final analysis, we are not the masters of everything we do.

If the practice of Yoga does not help us to remove the symptoms and causes of our physical and mental problems, it cannot lead us on to discovering our inner being and does not lead us to understanding the nature and quality of actions. In such circumstances the practices will be of doubtful validity. The more we refine ourselves through Yoga the more we realize that all our actions need to be reexamined systematically and we must not take the fruits of our actions for granted.

2.2 समाधिभावनार्थः क्लेशतनूकरणार्थश्च ।

samādhibhāvanārthaḥ kleśatanūkaranārthaśca

Then such practices will be certain to remove obstacles to clear perception.

We are all inherently capable of clear perception. But something or the other frequently seems to come in its way. What sort of things are they?

2.3 अविद्यास्मितारागद्वेषाभिनिवेशाः क्लेशाः ।

avidyāsmitārāgadveṣābhiniveśāḥ kleśāḥ

The obstacles are misapprehensions, confused values, excessive attachments, unreasonable dislikes, and insecurity.

2.4 अविद्या क्षेत्रमुत्तरेषां प्रसुप्ततनुविच्छिन्नोदाराणाम् ।

avidyā kṣetramuttareṣāṁ prasuptatanuvicchinnodārāṇām

The following sūtra explains the interrelationships between the above obstacles:

Misapprehension is the source of all the other obstacles. They need not appear simultaneously and their impact varies. Sometimes they are obscure and barely visible; at other times they are exposed and dominant.

It is only when they are completely exposed, that the effects of these obstacles are evident to other people, although not necessarily to the individual concerned.

2.5 अनित्याशुचिदुःखानात्मसु नित्यशुचिसुखात्मख्याति-
रविद्या ।

anityāśuciduḥkhānātmasu nityaśucisukhātmakhyātiravidyā

The following sūtras describe the five obstacles listed above:

Misapprehension leads to errors in comprehension of the character, origin, and effects of the objects perceived.

What at one time may appear to be a great help, later turns out to be a problem. What we seek as a source of pleasure may turn out to have the opposite effect. Fool's gold is assumed to be gold. Things that must change, like the beauty of youth, may be considered everlasting. What might be considered as the most important learning may, in time, prove useless.

2.6 दृग्दर्शनशक्त्योरेकात्मतेवास्मिता ।

drgdarśanaśaktyorekātmatevāsmitā

False identity results when we regard mental activity as the very source of perception.

Mental attitudes and activities change. They modify themselves according to influences such as moods, habits, and surroundings. Yet, somehow we often assume that they are a constant, unchanging source of perception (see 2.20).

2.7 सुखानुशयी रागः ।

sukhānuśayī rāgaḥ

Excessive attachment is based on the assumption that it will contribute to everlasting happiness.

When an object satisfies a desire, it provides a moment of happiness. Because of this experience, the possession of objects can become very important, even indispensable, whatever the cost. The result may be future unhappiness and the loss of some essentials of life.

2.8 दुःखानुशयी द्वेषः ।

duḥkhānuśayī dveṣaḥ

Unreasonable dislikes are usually the result of painful experiences in the past connected with particular objects and situations.

These dislikes continue to persist even after the circumstances that caused the unpleasant experiences have changed or disappeared.

2.9 स्वरसवाही विदुषोऽपि समारूढोऽभिनिवेशः ।

svarasavāhī viduṣo 'pi samārūḍho 'bhiniveśaḥ

Insecurity is the inborn feeling of anxiety for what is to come. It affects both the ignorant and the wise.

This syndrome may have a reasonable base in past experiences. It may be completely irrational. It does not disappear even when we know that death is imminent. It is, perhaps, the most difficult obstacle to overcome.

2.10 ते प्रतिप्रसवहेयाः सूक्ष्माः ।

te pratiprasavaheyāḥ sūkṣmāḥ

Having described the obstacles that prevent clear perception, Patañjali indicates what should be the attitude of one who is keen to reduce them.

> *When the obstacles do not seem to be present, it is important to be vigilant.*

A temporary state of clarity should not be confused with a permanent state. To assume then that everything will be free from now on can be fraught with danger. It is now even more important to be careful. The fall from clarity to confusion is more disturbing than a state with no clarity at all.

2.11 ध्यानहेयास्तद्वृत्तयः ।

dhyānaheyāstadvṛttayaḥ

When there is evidence that obstacles are reappearing, however, immediately

> *Advance toward a state of reflection to reduce their impact and prevent them from taking over.*

Any means that will help us free ourselves from the consequences of these obstacles is acceptable. It could be a prayer, a discussion with a teacher, or a diversion. Patañjali has suggested a number of means in the first chapter (1.23, 1.30–39) and more follow.

2.12 क्लेशमूलः कर्माशयो दृष्टादृष्टजन्मवेदनीयः ।

kleśamūlaḥ karmāśayo dṛṣṭādṛṣṭajanmavedanīyaḥ

Why should we be so concerned about these obstacles?

> *Our actions and their consequences are influenced by these obstacles. The consequences may or may not be evident at the time of the action.*

These obstacles are based in the mind and in the body as well. All our actions emanate from them. Those actions that are initiated when the obstacles are dominant will certainly produce undesirable results, for the obstacles are based on misapprehension. When we mistake what we see, the conclusions drawn from what we see must be incorrect. The next sūtra goes into this further.

2.13 सति मूले तद्विपाको जात्यायुर्भोगाः ।

sati mūle tadvipāko jātyāyurbhogāḥ

As long as the obstacles prevail they will affect action in every respect: in its execution, its duration, and its consequences.

Obstacles may lead to the faulty execution of actions. They may influence our mental attitude during the process of taking actions and perhaps reduce or extend their time span. And finally the fruits of actions may be such that they contribute to existing problems or create new ones.

2.14 ते ह्लादपरितापफलाः पुण्यापुण्यहेतुत्वात् ।

te hlādaparitāpaphalāḥ puṇyāpuṇyāhetutvāt

Does it follow that all our actions can lead to problems of some sort?

The consequences of an action will be painful or beneficial depending on whether the obstacles were present in the concept or implementation of the action.

If the obstacles are dormant during the initiation and execution of an action, there is enough clarity to perceive the correct attitude and means of acting and thus avoid mistakes. If they are active, however, there cannot be enough clarity and the consequences can be undesirable or painful.

2.15 परिणामतापसंस्कारदुःखैर्गुणवृत्तिविरोधाच्च दुःखमेव सर्वं विवेकिनः ।

pariṇāmatāpasaṁskāraduḥkhairguṇavṛttivirodhācca duḥkhameva sarvaṁ vivekinaḥ

What is the cause of unpleasant or painful effects?

Painful effects from any object or situation can be a result of one or more of the following: changes in the perceived object, the desire to repeat pleasurable experiences, and the strong effect of conditioning from the past. In addition, changes within the individual can be contributing factors.

There is constant change of some sort in ourselves and in the objects of our senses. These changes may be unrecognized. Thus, we may have an urge to seek for more of the same, when there is no possibility of achieving this. The effects of past conditioning can create strong reactions if what we are used to is not forthcoming. We must add to this the complexity of patterns in ourselves and the world around us. Thus, there is potential in any object or situation to contribute to painful or unpleasant effects. What can we do?

2.16 हेयं दुःखमनागतम् ।

heyaṁ duḥkhamanāgatam

Painful effects that are likely to occur should be anticipated and avoided

Whatever helps us to anticipate or reduce painful effects must be done. Patañjali goes on to present the causes of such painful effects and what we can do to develop within ourselves the capacity to anticipate, prevent, reduce, or accept them. In brief, the practice of Yoga has as its purpose the reduction of effects that are painful to us by increasing our clarity. This means we must learn to contain and control the obstacles listed in sūtra 2.3.

2.17 द्रष्टृदृश्ययोः संयोगो हेयहेतुः ।

draṣṭṛdṛśyayoḥ saṁyogo heyahetuḥ

The primary cause of the actions that produce painful effects is now presented.

The cause of actions that produce painful effects is the inability to distinguish what is perceived from what perceives.

In each of us there exists an entity that perceives. This is quite distinct from what is perceived, such as the mind, body, senses, and objects. But, we do not often make this distinction. What is perceived is subject to changes, but we do not recognize these changes. This lack of clear understanding can produce painful effects, even without our recognizing them.

2.18 प्रकाशक्रियास्थितिशीलं भूतेन्द्रियात्मकं भोगापवर्गार्थं दृश्यम् ।

prakāśakriyāsthitiśīlaṁ bhūtendriyātmakaṁ bhogāpavargārthaṁ dṛśyam

What distinguishes the objects of perception from that which perceives? The following sūtras explain:

All that is perceived includes not only the external objects but also the mind and the senses. They share three qualities: heaviness, activity, and clarity. They have two types of effects; to expose the perceiver to their influences, or to provide the means to find the distinction between them and itself.

All that is perceived has the capacity to display the three qualities mentioned above but they vary in intensity and degree. The nature of their effects on us is explored further in the next few sūtras.

2.19 विशेषाविशेषलिङ्गमात्रालिङ्गानि गुणपर्वाणि ।

viśeṣāviśeṣaliṅgamātrāliṅgāni guṇaparvāṇi

All that is perceived is related by the common sharing of the three qualities.

In addition they affect each other. For instance, what we eat influences our state of mind. Our state of mind affects our attitude to our bodies and to our environment.

2.20 द्रष्टा दृशिमात्रः शुद्धोऽपि प्रत्ययानुपश्यः ।

draṣṭā dṛśimātraḥ śuddho 'pi pratyayānupaśyaḥ

What is it that perceives?

That which perceives is not subject to any variations. But, it always perceives through the mind

Consequently, the quality of perception is affected by the state of the mind which is the instrument of perception. Whether there is perception or not, whether it is correct or incorrect, depends on the state of mind. In the same way, the color of an object is affected by the color of glass through which it is seen.

2.21 तदर्थ एव दृश्यस्यात्मा ।

tadartha eva dṛśyasyātmā

All that can be perceived has but one purpose: to be perceived.

In this way they serve the perceiver but have no individuality of their own. Their purpose comes from their perception by a perceiver. In the same way food on the table is there for the guest, not for its own sake.

2.22 कृतार्थं प्रति नष्टमप्यनष्टं तदन्यसाधारणत्वात् ।

kṛtārthaṁ prati naṣṭamapyanaṣṭam tadanyasādhāraṇatvāt

Does this mean that without a perceiver the objects of perception do not exist?

The existence of all objects of perception and their appearance is independent of the needs of the individual perceiver. They exist without individual reference, to cater for the different needs of different individuals.

The needs of an individual may only be defined at a particular time. Some needs may be periodic or spasmodic. And the needs of one individual cannot be considered more important, in terms of quality and justification, than those of another. A car may not be required by the owner, but by the owner's spouse. The food may not be needed now, but in a few hours may be essential. Does the food on the table vanish if the guest does not arrive?

2.23 स्वस्वामिशक्त्योः स्वरूपोपलब्धिहेतुः संयोगः ।

svasvāmiśaktyoḥ svarūpopalabdhihetuḥ saṁyogaḥ

In addition,

All that is perceived, whatever it is and whatever its effect may be on a particular individual, has but one ultimate purpose. That is to clarify the distinction between the external that is seen and the internal that sees.

However powerful or disturbing something may appear to be, it is our reaction to it that determines its effects. Therefore, we can, by distinguishing between what perceives and what is perceived, what sees and what is seen, put the object into its correct perspective and ensure that we determine its effect and influence on us.

2.24 तस्य हेतुरविद्या ।

tasya heturavidyā

Why, on occasion, does the clarity not exist?

The absence of clarity in distinguishing between what perceives and what is perceived is due to the accumulation of misapprehension.

2.25 तदभावात्संयोगाभावो हानं तद्दृशेः कैवल्यम् ।

tadabhāvātsaṁyogābhāvo hānaṁ taddṛśeḥ kaivalyam

As misapprehension is reduced there is a corresponding increase in clarity. This is the path to freedom.

Yes, this is the ultimate goal of Yoga practice. Freedom is the absence of the consequences of obstacles and the avoidance of actions that have distracting or disturbing effects.

2.26 विवेकख्यातिरविप्लवा हानोपायः ।

vivekakhyātiraviplavā hānopāyaḥ

How do we achieve this freedom? Is it really possible?

Essentially the means must be directed toward developing clarity so that the distinction between the changing qualities of what is perceived and the unchanging quality of what perceives becomes evident.

This requires constant effort. This effort must reduce the persistent intrusion of the obstacles listed in sūtra 2.3 and eventually completely eliminate their effects. Once a beginning is made, the foundation of Yoga is laid.

2.27 तस्य सप्तधा प्रान्तभूमिः प्रज्ञा ।

tasya saptadhā prāntabhūmiḥ prajñā

The attainment of clarity is a gradual process.

The first step is to recognize that certain tendencies of our mind are responsible for producing painful effects. If these tendencies are not curtailed, we may reach a point of no return.

2.28 योगाङ्गानुष्ठानादशुद्धिक्षये ज्ञानदीप्तिराविवेकख्यातेः ।

yogāṅgānuṣṭhānādaśuddhikṣaye
jñānadīptirāvivekakhyāteḥ

Can something be done to recognize and correct these tendencies? Patañjali proposes some definitive means for reducing the accumulation of obstacles such as misapprehension. For only the reduction of these obstacles can reverse our tendencies responsible for producing undesirable effects.

> *The practice and inquiry into different components of Yoga gradually reduce the obstacles such as misapprehension [2.3]. Then the lamp of perception brightens and the distinction between what perceives and what is perceived becomes more and more evident. Now everything can be understood without error.*

If the mind is cleared of the obstacles that cloud real perception there can be no errors or flaws in perception. Actions are freed from regrettable consequences.

Patañjali presents the components of Yoga:

2.29 यमनियमासनप्राणायामप्रत्याहारधारणाध्यानसमाध-
योऽष्टावङ्गानि ।

yamaniyamāsanaprāṇāyāmapratyāhāra-
dhāraṇadhyānasamādhayo 'ṣṭavaṅgāni

There are eight components of Yoga. These are:

1. yama, our attitudes toward our environment.

2. niyama, our attitudes toward ourselves.

3. āsana, the practice of body exercises.

4. prāṇāyāma, the practice of breathing exercises.

5. pratyāhāra, the restraint of our senses.

6. dhārāna, the ability to direct our minds.

7. dhyāna, the ability to develop interactions with what we seek to understand.

8. samādhi, complete integration with the object to be understood.

The order of presentation is from the external relationship to a very intense and refined state of introspection. This order, however, is not necessarily the sequence for practice. There are no set rules or definitive routes. Whatever is the route most suited for the individual to reach the state described in sūtra 1.2 should be followed. They all develop simultaneously as the individual progresses.

2.30 अहिंसासत्यास्तेयब्रह्मचर्यापरिग्रहा यमाः ।

ahiṁsāsatyāsteyabrahmacaryāparigrahā yamāḥ

The eight components of Yoga are discussed in the following sūtras.

Yama comprises:

1. Consideration for all living things, especially those who are innocent, in difficulty, or worse off than we are.

2. Right communication through speech, writings, gesture, and actions.

3. Noncovetousness or the ability to resist a desire for that which does not belong to us.

4. Moderation in all our actions.

5. Nongreediness or the ability to accept only what is appropriate.

How we exhibit these qualities and how we strive for them depends inevitably on our social and cultural background, our religious beliefs, and our individual character and potential. But their representation in an individual is a reflection of the extent to which the obstacles in the mind are at work. How we behave toward others and our environment reveals our state of mind and our personalities. The knock at the door tells the character of the visitor!

2.31 जातिदेशकालसमयानवच्छिन्नाः सार्वभौमा महाव्रतम् ।

jātideśakālasamayānavacchinnāḥ sārvabhaumā mahāvratam

When the adoption of these attitudes in our environment is beyond compromise, regardless of our social, cultural, intellectual or individual station, it approaches irreversibility.

We cannot begin with such attitudes. If we adopt them abruptly we cannot sustain them. We can always find excuses for not maintaining them. But if we seek to identify the reasons why we hold contrary views, isolate the obstacles that permit such views and our attitudes will gradually change. The obstacles will give way and our behavior toward others and our environment will change for the better.

2.32 शौचसंतोषतपःस्वाध्यायेश्वरप्रणिधानानि नियमाः ।

śaucasaṅtoṣatapaḥsvādhyāyeśvara-praṇidhānāni niyamāḥ

Niyama comprises:

1. Cleanliness, or keeping our bodies and our surroundings clean and neat.

2. Contentment, or the ability to be comfortable with what we have and what we do not have.

3. The removal of impurities in our physical and mental systems through the maintenance of such correct habits as sleep, exercise, nutrition, work, and relaxation.

4. Study and the necessity to review and evaluate our progress.

5. Reverence to a higher intelligence or the acceptance of our limitations in relation to God, the all-knowing.

As with our attitudes to others and our environment, these priorities establish themselves and the correct attitudes develop concurrently with our rectification of errors and actions that cause problems.

2.33 वितर्कबाधने प्रतिपक्षभावनम् ।

vitarkabādhane pratipakṣabhāvanam

How can we examine and reexamine our attitudes to others?

When these attitudes are questioned, self-reflection on the possible consequences of alternative attitudes may help.

This means we must find a way to examine intellectually the consequences of the different attitudes possible at a given time or in given circumstances: To look before we leap!

2.34 वितर्का हिंसादयः कृतकारितानुमोदिता लोभक्रोध-
मोहपूर्वका मृदुमध्याधिमात्रा दुःखाज्ञानानन्तफला इति
प्रतिपक्षभावनम् ।

vitarkā hiṁsādayaḥ kṛtakāritānumoditā
lobhakrodhamohapūrvakā mṛdumadhyādhimātrā
duḥkhājñānantaphalā iti pratipakṣabhāvanam

Patañjali explains this further:

> *For example, a sudden desire to act harshly, or encourage or approve of harsh actions can be contained by reflecting on the harmful consequences. Often such actions are the results of lower instincts such as anger, possessiveness, or unsound judgment. Whether these actions are minor or major, reflection in a suitable atmosphere can contain our desires to act in this way.*

Often some of our attitudes toward people, situations, and ideas are not very clear. Then a hasty step may land us in situations we do not want to be in. In such circumstances any opportunity to have second thoughts is worth considering. Prevention is better than cure.

2.35 अहिंसाप्रतिष्ठायां तत्संनिधौ वैरत्यागः ।

ahimsāpratiṣṭhāyāṁ tatsaṅnidhau vairatyāgaḥ

We must remember that there are individual variations. Some of us may be quite comfortable examining our motives and attitudes. Others may find it very difficult to reflect upon themselves. Patañjali now indicates signs of progress in each of the ten attitudes listed in sūtras 2.30 and 2.32.

> *The more considerate one is, the more one stimulates friendly feelings among all in one's presence.*

Even those who are unfriendly at other times and among other people may show a different aspect and be friendly in our presence.

2.36 सत्यप्रतिष्ठायां क्रियाफलाश्रयत्वम् ।

satyapratiṣṭhāyām kriyāphalāśrayatvam

> *One who shows a high degree of right communication will not fail in his actions.*

The ability to be honest in communication with sensitivity, without hurting others, without telling lies, and with the necessary reflection requires a very refined state of being. Such persons cannot make mistakes in their actions.

2.37 अस्तेयप्रतिष्ठायां सर्वरत्नोपस्थानम् ।

asteyapratiṣṭhāyām sarvaratnopasthānam

One who is trustworthy, because he does not covet what belongs to others, naturally has everyone's confidence and everything is shared with him, however precious it might be.

2.38 ब्रह्मचर्यप्रतिष्ठायां वीर्यलाभः ।

brahmacaryapratiṣṭhāyām vīryalābhaḥ

At its best, moderation produces the highest individual vitality.

Nothing is wasted by us if we seek to develop moderation in all things. Too much of anything brings problems. Too little may be inadequate.

2.39 अपरिग्रहस्थैर्ये जन्मकथंतासंबोधः ।

aparigrahasthairye janmakathaṁtāsaṁbodhaḥ

One who is not greedy is secure. He has time to think deeply. His understanding of himself is complete.

The more we have, the more we need to take care of it. The time and energy spent on acquiring more things, protecting them, and worrying about them cannot be spent on the basic questions of life. What is the limit to what we should possess? For what purpose, for whom, and for how long? Death comes before we have had time to begin to consider these questions.

2.40 शौचात्स्वाङ्गजुगुप्सा परैरसंसर्गः ।

śaucātsvāṅgajugupsā parairasaṁsargaḥ

When cleanliness is developed it reveals what needs to be constantly maintained and what is eternally clean. What decays is the external. What does not is deep within us.

Our overconcern with and attachment to outward things, which is both transient and superficial, is reduced.

2.41 सत्त्वशुद्धिसौमनस्यैकाग्र्येन्द्रियजयात्मदर्शनयोग्यत्वानि च ।

sattvaśuddhisaumanasyaikāgryendriya-
jayātmadarśanayogyatvāni ca

In addition one becomes able to reflect on the very deep nature of our individual selves, including the source of perception, without being distracted by the senses and with freedom from misapprehension accumulated from the past.

To take outward things as the most valuable and to guard them at all costs is not the most important part of living. There is much more to look into. Dirty clothes may make a person look ugly. But they can be changed. If there is dirt deep inside, however, it cannot be changed so easily.

2.42 संतोषादनुत्तमः सुखलाभः ।

saṁtoṣādanuttamaḥ sukhalābhaḥ

The result of contentment is total happiness.

The happiness we get from acquiring passions is only temporary. We need to find new ones and acquire them to sustain this sort of happiness. There is no end to it. But true contentment, leading to total happiness and bliss, is in a class by itself.

2.43 कायेन्द्रियसिद्धिरशुद्धिक्षयात्तपसः ।

kāyendriyasiddhiraśuddhikṣayāttapasaḥ

The removal of impurities allows the body to function more efficiently.

Both physical and mental illness and disabilities are contained.

2.44 स्वाध्यायादिष्टदेवतासंप्रयोगः ।

svādhyāyādiṣṭadevatāsaṁprayogaḥ

Study, when it is developed to the highest degree, brings one close to higher forces that promote understanding of the most complex.

The more effective our study, the more we understand our weaknesses and our strengths. We learn to nullify our weaknesses and use our strengths to the utmost. Then there is no limit to our understanding.

2.45 समाधिसिद्धिरीश्वरप्रणिधानात् ।

samādhisiddhirīśvarapraṇidhānāt

Reverence to God promotes the ability to completely understand any object of choice.

We gain a feeling of confidence from such reverence to the highest intelligence. Then, to direct the mind toward any object of any complexity is not a problem.

2.46 स्थिरसुखमासनम् ।

sthirasukhamāsanam

Āsana and prāṇāyāma, the next two aspects of Yoga (see sūtra 2.29), are now presented as they help us to understand and use correctly and appropriately our bodies and our breath. They are easier to begin with, unlike changing our attitudes. With them it is possible for most of us to begin reducing the obstacles to Yoga. The instructions given here are brief because the practices must be learnt directly from a competent teacher.

Āsana must have the dual qualities of alertness and relaxation.

Āsana practice involves body exercises. When they are properly practiced there must be alertness without tension and relaxation without dullness or heaviness.

2.47 प्रयत्नशैथिल्यानन्तसमापत्तिभ्याम् ।

prayatnaśaithilyānantasamāpattibhyām

These qualities can be achieved by recognizing and observing the reactions of the body and the breath to the various postures that comprise āsana practice. Once known, these reactions can be controlled step-by-step.

2.48 ततो द्वंद्वानभिघातः ।

tato dvaṅdvānabhighātaḥ

When these principles are correctly followed, āsana practice will help a person endure and even minimize the external influences on the body such as age, climate, diet, and work.

This is the beginning of the reduction of the effect of obstacles such as misapprehension; for the body expresses what is in the mind. Practices such as āsana begin to rectify the harmful consequences of the obstacles at the level of the body. The well-being so developed opens us up to the possibilities of further understanding of ourselves. If we have a back pain, the need for relief from this pain dominates our thoughts. If, through our efforts at āsana practice, we reduce this back pain, we can then begin to explore the causes of the pain.

2.49 तस्मिन्सतिश्वासप्रश्वासयोर्गतिविच्छेदः प्राणायामः ।

tasminsatiśvāsapraśvāsayorgativicchedaḥ prāṇāyāmaḥ

Through āsana practices we can also understand how the breath behaves. Breathing patterns are very individual. They can vary as a result of our state of mind or bodily changes as a result of both internal and external forces. This knowledge of breath, gained through āsana practice, is the foundation for beginning prāṇāyāma practice.

Prāṇāyāma is the conscious, deliberate regulation of the breath replacing unconscious patterns of breathing. It is possible only after a reasonable mastery of āsana practice.

This practice is usually done in a comfortable, but erect, seated position.

2.50 बाह्याभ्यन्तरस्तम्भवृत्तिर्देशकालसंख्याभिः परिदृष्टो दीर्घसूक्ष्मः ।

bāḥyābhyantarastambhavṛttirdeśakāla-
saṁkhyabhiḥ paridṛṣṭo dīrghasūkṣmaḥ

What are the components of prāṇāyāma?

It involves the regulation of the exhalation, the inhalation, and the suspension of the breath. The regulation of these three processes is achieved by modulating their length and maintaining this modula-

tion for a period of time, as well as directing the mind into the process. These components of breathing must be both long and uniform.

Many combinations are possible in the practice of prāṇāyāma. Many techniques are available, but details about them are beyond the scope of this text.

2.51 बाह्याभ्यन्तरविषयाक्षेपी चतुर्थः ।

bāhyābhyantaraviṣayākṣepī caturthaḥ

An entirely different state of breathing appears in the state of yoga.

Then the breath transcends the level of the consciousness.

It is not possible to be more specific.

2.52 ततः क्षीयते प्रकाशावरणम् ।

tataḥ kṣīyate prakāśāvaraṇam

The results of prāṇāyāma practice are indicated:

The regular practice of prāṇāyāma reduces the obstacles that inhibit clear perception.

2.53 धारणासु च योग्यता मनसः ।

dhāraṇāsu ca yogyatā manasaḥ

And the mind is now prepared for the process of direction toward a chosen goal.

2.54 स्वविषयासंप्रयोगे चित्तस्य स्वरूपानुकार इवेन्द्रियाणां प्रत्याहारः ।

svaviṣayāsaṁprayoge cittasya svarūpānukāra ivendriyāṇāṁ pratyāhāraḥ

The restraint of the senses, *pratyāhāra*, which is the fifth aspect of yoga (see 2.29), is now defined:

> *The restraint of senses occurs when the mind is able to remain in its chosen direction and the senses disregard the different objects around them and faithfully follow the direction of the mind.*

2.55 ततः परमा वश्यतेन्द्रियाणाम् ।

tataḥ paramā vaśyatendriyāṇām

> *Then the senses are mastered.*

They cooperate in the chosen inquiry instead of being a cause of distraction. The restraint of the senses cannot be a strict discipline. It develops as the obstacles to perception within us are cleared up.

3

विभूतिपादः

VIBHŪTIPĀDAḤ

In this chapter, *vibhūtipāda*, Patañjali describes the capacity of the mind, which through the various practices described in the eariler two chapters can achieve a state free from distractions. Such a mind can probe deeply into objects and concepts; indeed, there are innumerable possibilities for it. Then there arises in the individual a knowledge of the objects of a dimension previously unknown. Such a knowledge, however, can itself be a source of distraction and prevent a person from reaching the highest state of being. This highest state is freedom from disturbance of any sort and at any time. The next three sūtras describe the sixth, seventh, and eighth components of Yoga first mentioned in sūtra 2.29. The first five components are described in chapter 2.

3.1 देशबन्धश्चित्तस्य धारणा ।

deśabandhaścittasya dhāraṇā

The mind has reached the ability to be directed [dhāraṇā] when direction toward a chosen object is possible in spite of many other potential objects within the reach of the individual.

The object is chosen by the individual regardless of the attraction of alternatives. The chosen object may be sensual or conceptual, simple or complex, tangible or beyond touch, in favorable conditions or against all odds. The ability to maintain direction in this way is not possible if our minds are immersed in distractions or strongly affected by obstacles such as misapprehension (see sūtra 2.3).

3.2 तत्र प्रत्ययैकतानता ध्यानम् ।

tatra pratyayaikatānatā dhyānam

Once the direction is fixed, a link develops between the mind's activities and the chosen object.

Then the mental activities form an uninterrupted flow only in relation to this object.

Initially our understanding is influenced by misapprehension, our imaginations, and our memories. But as the process of comprehension intensifies it freshens and deepens our understanding of the object.

3.3 तदेवार्थमात्रनिर्भासं स्वरूपशून्यमिव समाधिः ।

tadevārthamātranirbhāsaṁ svarūpaśūnyamiva samādhiḥ

Soon the individual is so much involved in the object that nothing except its comprehension is evident. It is as if the individual has lost his own identity. This is the complete integration with the object of understanding [samādhi].

When we reach this state all that is evident is the object itself. We are not even aware that we are distinct beings separate from the object. Our mental activities are integrated with the object and nothing else.

3.4 त्रयमेकत्र संयमः ।

trayamekatra saṁyamaḥ

The three processes described in sūtras 3.1, 3.2, and 3.3 can be employed with different objects at different times or they can all be directed for an indefinite period of time on the same object.

When these processes are continuously and exclusively applied to the same object it is called saṁyama.

3.5 तज्जयात्प्रज्ञालोकः ।

tajjayātprajñālokaḥ

What results from this continuous and exclusive practice of saṁyama?

Saṁyama on a chosen object leads to a comprehensive knowledge of the object in all its aspects.

3.6 तस्य भूमिषु विनियोगः ।

tasya bhūmiṣu viniyogaḥ

Can any object be selected for directing the mind into the process of saṁyama? What is the basis of our choice?

Saṁyama must be developed gradually.

The object of saṁyama must be chosen with due appreciation of our potential for such inquiry. We should begin with the less complicated objects and with those that can be inquired into in several different ways. Then there is a greater chance of successful development. It is implied that a teacher who knows us well is a great help in choosing our objects.

3.7 त्रयमन्तरङ्गं पूर्वेभ्यः ।

trayamantaraṅgaṁ pūrvebhyaḥ

To specify what is easy for one individual is not possible in saṁyama or any other practice. Patañjali presents the idea of relativity. Everything is relative.

Compared to the first five components of Yoga [sūtra 2.29] the next three [sūtras 3.1, 2, 3] are more intricate.

The first five components are our attitudes toward our environment, our attitudes toward ourselves, the practice of body exercises (āsana), the practice of breathing exercises (prāṇāyāma), and the restraint of the senses (pratyāhāra). They are easier to understand and attempt than the next three aspects. These are the ability to direct our minds (dhāraṇā), the ability to develop, faultlessly, our interactions with what we seek to understand (dhyāna), and complete integration with the object of our understanding (samādhi).

3.8 तदपि बहिरङ्गं निर्बीजस्य ।

tadapi bahiraṅgaṁ nirbījasya

If we develop our capacities, we can, through sustained discipline, refine and adapt our minds sufficiently to facilitate the process of directing them without difficulty.

The state where the mind has no impressions of any sort and nothing is beyond its reach [nirbījah samādhi] is more intricate than the state of directing the mind towards an object [samādhi].

Sūtra 1.51 defines this, the highest state of Yoga. The mind in this state is simply transparent, devoid of any resistance to inquiry and free from past impressions of any sort.

The message of sūtras 3.7 and 3.8 is that saṁyama is only possible at our own individual level. There can be no universal gradation in choosing the direction of inquiry. It cannot be at the same level for all of us at all times. This is the relative aspect of saṁyama, for it is based on each and everyone's individual capacity and needs. Some of us may, in other ways, have developed capacities that enable us to begin saṁyama at a higher level than others. An expert on human anatomy does not need to study much to understand the vertebral column of a horse. But an expert in finance might have to begin with the study of basic anatomy.

3.9 व्युत्थाननिरोधसंस्कारयोरभिभवप्रादुर्भावौ निरोधक्षणचित्तान्वयो निरोधपरिणामः ।

vyutthānanirodhasaṁskārayorabhibhavaprādurbhāvau nirodhakṣaṇacittānvayo nirodhapariṇāmaḥ

How can our minds, which are used to one way of operating, be changed? Patañjali tackles this question by showing that everything that we perceive is subject to modification. More than this, everything can be modified in a chosen way.

The mind is capable of having two states based on two distinct tendencies. These are distraction and attention. At any one moment, however, only one state prevails, and this state influences the individual's behavior, attitudes, and expressions.

When the state of attention prevails, our pose is serene, our breathing quiet, and our concentration on our object is such that we are completely absorbed in it and oblivious to our surroundings. But when we are in the state of distraction, our poise is far from serene, our breathing is irregular, and our attitudes give little indication of any capacity to be attentive.

3.10 तस्य प्रशान्तवाहिता संस्कारात् ।

tasya praśāntavāhitā saṁskārāt

Can we develop the state of attention?

By constant and uninterrupted practice the mind can remain in a state of attention for a long time.

But if we do not attempt to sustain this state, then the state of distraction takes over.

3.11 सर्वार्थतैकाग्रतयोः क्षयोदयौ चित्तस्य समाधिपरिणामः ।

sarvārthataikāgratayoḥ kṣayodayau cittasya samādhipariṇāmaḥ

Even the quality of distraction can vary and be modified. The mind can be chaotic, or it can be so heavy it cannot be disturbed or it can be very susceptible to disturbance. These variations depends upon our past tendencies and how we have responded to them. There is another, intermediate state of being.

The mind alternates between the possibility of intense concentration and a state where alternative objects can attract attention.

The difference between the previous situation and this one is that while in the former our mind alternated between two quite different, opposite states, in this case the difference between the two alternating states is much less. There is, therefore, a greater chance to return to the fixed direction of inquiry without too much loss of time and without the lasting effects of the distracted state of mind.

3.12 ततः पुनः शान्तोदितौ तुल्यप्रत्ययौ चित्तस्यैकाग्रता-
परिणामः ।

tataḥ punaḥ śāntoditau tulyapratyayau
cittasyaikāgratāpariṇāmaḥ

With further refinements:

The mind reaches a stage where the link with the object is consistent and continuous. The distractions cease to appear.

Then our relationship with the object is no longer disrupted by the other tendencies of the mind. Complete comprehension of the object is definite.

3.13 एतेन भूतेन्द्रियेषु धर्मलक्षणावस्थापरिणामा
व्याख्याताः ।

etena bhūtendriyeṣu dharmalakṣaṇāvasthāpariṇāmā
vyākhyātāḥ

Thus it is clear that our minds can have different characteristics. These characteristics are also subject to change. The mind, the senses and the objects of the senses, share three basic characteristics: heaviness, activity, and clarity. In some ways most of the changes in our mind are possible because these three qualities are in a state of constant flux. How they change, when they change, and what combinations produce the different characteristics of the mind is a complex subject. However,

As it has been established that the mind has different states [corre-

sponding to which there arose different attitudes, possibilities, and behavior patterns in the individual] it can also be said that such changes can occur in all the objects of perception and in the senses. These changes can be at different levels and influenced by external forces such as time or our intelligence.

Time can change a fresh flower into a few dry petals. A goldsmith can change a nugget of gold into a delicate pendant. A metallurgist can convert it yet again to a compound capable of storing very corrosive fluids. Those characteristics that are apparent in one moment cannot be the whole story of the object. But if all the potential of, for instance, gold is known, then many products can be produced even though they may have quite different properties. The same is true of the body and the senses. The manual skills of an artist are quite different from those of a car mechanic, the reasoning of a philosopher from that of a businessman.

3.14 शान्तोदिताव्यपदेश्यधर्मानुपाती धर्मी ।

śāntoditāvyapadeśyadharmānupātī dharmī

All these different characteristics must be housed somewhere, in some form or other.

A substance contains all its charateristics and, depending on the particular form it takes, those characteristics conforming to that form will be apparent. But whatever the form, whatever the characteristics exhibited, there exists a base that comprises all characteristics. Some have appeared in the past, some are currently apparent, and others may reveal themselves in the future.

The significance of sūtras 3.9 to 3.14 is that everything that we perceive is fact and not fiction. But these facts are subject to change. These two rules of Patañjali, known as *satvāda* and *pariṇāmavāda*, are the foundation of his teaching.

3.15 क्रमान्यत्वं परिणामान्यत्वे हेतुः ।

kramānyatvaṁ pariṇāmanyatve hetuḥ

Can these changes in the characteristics of substances be influenced?

By changing the order or sequence of change, characteristics that are of one pattern can be modified to a different pattern

Change has a sequence, but this sequence can be altered. A river following a valley can be diverted through a tunnel. The intelligence to grasp this possibility is what produces the different patterns of change.

3.16 परिणामत्रयसंयमादतीतानागतज्ञानम् ।

pariṇāmatrayasaṁyamādatītānāgatajñānam

In a way saṁyama is the process of changing our mental potential from incomplete, erroneous comprehension of an object, or no comprehension at all, to total comprehension. When this potential is developed the individual can choose any object for developing a deep knowledge about it. These objects can be external, within the limits of sensual perception or concepts like change, time, or communication. In the following sūtras examples are given of such knowledge resulting from different saṁyamas. Whether we are interested in using our highly developed minds to acquire deep knowledge of a specific nature, or whether we are more concerned with true freedom, is our individual choice. True freedom is more than an expertise, it is a state in which all our actions are such that they do not bring repentance or regret. Patañjali cautions about the misuse of saṁyama elsewhere.

The first example of directing the mind through saṁyama follows:

Saṁyama on the process of change, how it can be affected by time and other factors, develops knowledge of the past and the future.

In sūtras 3.9 to 3.14, the changes that occur in objects and senses as well as in the mind were explained. If we pursue this idea in depth we will be in a position to anticipate what may happen in a particular situation and what has happened in the past. Astronomy is the classic example of this.

3.17 शब्दार्थप्रत्ययानामितरेतराध्यासात्संकरस्तत्प्रवि-
भागसंयमात्सर्वभूतरुतज्ञानम् ।

śabdārthapratyayānāmitaretarādhyāsāts-
aṅkarastatpravibhāgasaṁyam-
atsarvabhūtarutajñānam

Patañjali takes up the process of communication for saṁyama. Different symbols and languages exist for relating to other people. These symbols and languages are affected by use, abuse, and misinterpretations. Languages serve to explain something that was experienced, is being experienced, or may be experienced. An object is an entity in itself. Our ability to see an object is based on our interests and our potential. Our memories and imaginations can influence our comprehension. Therefore, there is ample scope for us to communicate improperly, however hard we try.

Saṁyama on the interactions between language, ideas, and object is to examine the individual features of the objects, the means of describing them, and the ideas and their cultural influences in the minds of the describers. Through this, one can find the most accurate and effective way of communication regardless of linguistic, cultural, and other barriers.

3.18 संस्कारसाक्षात्करणात्पूर्वजातिज्ञानम् ।

samskārasākṣātkaraṇātpūrvajātijñānam

In all areas of human activity there is the potential to develop individual habits and tendencies. Some will be more obvious than others.

Saṁyama on one's tendencies and habits will lead one to their origins. Consequently one gains deep knowledge of one's past.

We learn how our behavior and personal characteristics developed and what events in the past influenced our attitudes, likes, and dislikes. We learn to what degree they are related to our heredity, tradition, social requirements, and so on. When these roots are known we can reexamine our lifestyle for the better.

3.19 प्रत्ययस्य परचित्तज्ञानम् ।

pratyayasya paracittajñānam

Every mental activity produces distinct physical effects. For example, our physical features, posture, and breathing are different from those when we are sleeping or when we are angry.

Saṁyama on the changes that arise in an individual's mind and their consequences develops in one the ability to acutely observe the state of mind of others.

Then we can see how others' states of mind are developing. Physical expressions, rates of breathing, and other indicators will reveal turbulence, confusion, doubt, fear, and so on.

3.20 न च तत्सालम्बनं तस्याविषयीभूतत्वात् ।

na ca tatsālambanaṁ tasyāviṣayībhūtatvāt

But, can we see from this what is the origin of the state of mind?

No. The cause of the state of mind of one individual is beyond the scope of observation by another.

This is because different objects produce different responses in different individuals. Our field of observation is limited to the symptoms, and cannot extend to the causes.

3.21 कायरूपसंयमात्तद्ग्राह्यशक्तिस्तम्भे चक्षुःप्रकाशा-
संप्रयोगेऽन्तर्धानम् ।

kāyarūpasaṁyamāttadgrāhyaśaktistambhe

cakṣuḥprakāśāsaṁprayoge 'ntardhānam

The physical features of one individual are distinguishable because of their difference from their surroundings. In the same way a white patch is obvious on a black wall, but a black patch is not.

> *Saṁyama on the relationship between the features of the body and what affects them can give one the means to merge with one's surroundings in such a way that one's form is indistinguishable.*

This is comparable to the camouflage principles employed by chameleons and other wild animals. Thus, an experienced stalker can merge his human form into an environment, however featureless it is, by developing an acute awareness of what it is that differentiates him from his environment and minimizing its effects by the careful placing, moving and shaping of his human form.

3.22 सोपक्रमं निरुपक्रमं च कर्म तत्संयमादपरान्तज्ञान-
मरिष्टेभ्यो वा ।

sopakramaṁ nirupakramaṁ ca karma
tatsaṁyamadaparāntajñānamariṣṭebhyo vā

Our actions are influenced by the purpose of the action, the state of mind of the actor, the clarity at our disposal, and the circumstances.

> *The results of actions may be immediate or delayed. Saṁyama on this can give one the ability to predict the course of future actions and even his own death.*

3.23 मैत्र्यादिषु बलानि ।

maitryādiṣu balāni

> *Different qualities such as friendliness, compassion, and contentment can be inquired into through saṁyama. Thus, one can learn how to strengthen a chosen quality.*

In the same way specific physical and mental skills can be obtained.

3.24 बलेषु हस्तिबलादीनि ।

baleṣu hastibalādīni

For example,

> *Saṁyama on the physical strength of an elephant can give one the strength of an elephant*

This does not mean, of course, that we can acquire the same strength as an elephant, but we can acquire comparable strength proportionate to the limits of the human form.

3.25 प्रवृत्त्यालोकन्यासात्सूक्ष्मव्यवहितविप्रकृष्टज्ञानम् ।

pravṛttyālokanyāsātsūkṣmavyavahitaviprakṛṣṭajñānam

> *Directing the mind to the life-force itself and sustaining that direction through saṁyama, results in the ability to observe fine subtleties and understand what is preventing deep observation.*

In the absence of such fine abilities, our observation is distinctly limited.

3.26 भुवनज्ञानं सूर्ये संयमात् ।

bhuvanajñānaṁ sūrye saṁyamāt

Saṁyama can be directed toward the cosmos. A few examples follow:

> *Saṁyama on the sun gives wide knowledge of the planetary system and the cosmic regions.*

3.27 चन्द्रे ताराव्यूहज्ञानम् ।

candre tārāvyūhajñānam

> *Saṁyama on the moon gives a thorough knowledge of the position of the stars at different times.*

Observation of the different phases of the moon, its eclipses, and the path it travels, takes us all over the sky and thus encompasses all the visible stars and their constellations.

3.28 ध्रुवे तद्गतिज्ञानम् ।

dhruve tadgatijñānam

For us on earth everything seems to revolve around Polaris, the North Star, thus,

> *Saṁyama on Polaris gives knowledge about the relative movements of the stars.*

3.29 नाभिचक्रे कायव्यूहज्ञानम् ।

nābhicakre kāyavyūhajñānam

Even the different parts of the body can be the objects of saṁyama.

> *Saṁyama on the navel gives knowledge about the different organs of the body and their dispositions.*

Because of its location in the midabdomen around which so many vital organs are found, as well as it being the channel through which the body received its vital needs while it was in the womb, the navel is considered the seat of some bodily forces.

3.30 कण्ठकूपे क्षुत्पिपासानिवृत्तिः ।

kaṇṭhakūpe kṣutpipāsānivṛttiḥ

> *Using the throat as the point of inquiry for saṁyama provides an understanding of thirst and hunger. This enables one to control their extreme symptoms.*

Like the navel, the throat is a vital area. Our appetite for certain foods, our hunger, and our thirst are all felt there.

3.31 कूर्मनाड्यां स्थैर्यम् ।

kūrmanāḍyāṁ sthairyam

> *Saṁyama on the chest area and inquiry into the sensations felt there in different physical and mental states gives one the means to remain stable and calm even in very stressful situations.*

Many of the symptoms of stress and anxiety are felt in the chest area. Physical postures can be affected by mental states, for instance, a permanent stoop can be the result of a lack of self-confidence.

3.32 मूर्धज्योतिषि सिद्धदर्शनम् ।

mūrdhajyotiṣi siddhadarśanam

Saṁyama on the source of high intelligence in an individual develops supernormal capabilities.

Through this, we may receive support and greater vision from the divine forces and consequently,

3.33 प्रातिभाद्वा सर्वम् ।

prātibhādvā sarvam

Anything can be understood. With each attempt fresh and spontaneous understanding arises.

3.34 हृदये चित्तसंवित् ।

hṛdaye cittasaṁvit

The heart is considered to be the seat of the mind.

Saṁyama on the heart will definitely reveal the qualities of the mind.

It is only when we are quiet and calm that this is possible. We cannot see the color of the water in a lake if the lake is turbulent.

3.35 सत्त्वपुरुषयोरत्यन्तासंकीर्णयोः प्रत्ययाविशेषो भोगः
परार्थत्वात्स्वार्थसंयमात्पुरुषज्ञानम् ।

sattvapuruṣayoratyantāsaṅkīrṇayoḥ pratyayāviśeṣobhogaḥ
parārthatvātsvārthasaṁyamātpuruṣajñānam

The mind, which is subject to change, and the Perceiver, which is not, are in proximity but are of distinct and different characters. When the mind is directed externally and acts mechanically toward objects there is either pleasure or pain. When at the appropriate time, however, an individual begins inquiry into the very nature of the link between the Perceiver and perception the mind is disconnected from external objects and there arises the understanding of the Perceiver itself.

Under the influence of external stimuli the mind is a mechanical instrument. The results can be unpleasant. This happens in spite of the central force of the perceiver. However good the eye, if the glass is clouded, the object is blurred. Through saṁyama inquiry and the practice of Yoga on the basis of sūtra 2.1, we can look into the mechanics of mental activity. Our minds gradually rise to a level where they can be disconnected from the external objectives. In this silent moment the understanding of the very source of perception is apparent.

3.36 ततः प्रातिभश्रावणवेदनादर्शास्वादवार्ता जायन्ते ।

tataḥ prātibhaśrāvaṇavedanādarśāsvādavārtā jāyante

What are the consequences of such a moment?

Then one begins to acquire extraordinary capacities for perception.

3.37 ते समाधावुपसर्गा व्युत्थाने सिद्धयः ।

te samādhāvupasargā vyutthāne siddhayaḥ

But the mind is like a double edged sword. These special faculties, acquired through saṁyama, may produce an illusion of freedom as opposed to the highest state, free from error.

For an individual who may revert to a state of distraction, this extraordinary knowledge and the capabilities acquired through saṁyama are worth possessing. But for one who seeks nothing less than a sustained state of Yoga the results of saṁyama are obstacles in themselves.

Incidental benefits along the way should not be confused with the eventual goal. However pleasurable our experiences are as we travel on a journey, they cannot substitute for our chosen destination. It would be as if on the way to the snowcapped peaks, we were to settle down by the shore of a lake to watch the beautiful swans, and forget forever our original destination.

Having warned about the limitations of saṁyama, Patañjali continues with other possibilities for it.

3.38 बन्धकारणशैथिल्यात्प्रचारसंवेदनाच्च चित्तस्य परशरीरावेशः ।

bandhakāranaśaithilyātpracārasaṁvedanācca cittasya paraśarīrāveśaḥ

The mind is a storehouse of experiences, although distinct for each individual. In addition, its function is limited to the individual to whom it belongs. Thus the mind becomes an isolated fortress resisting all entry.

> *By inquiring into the cause of this rigid situation binding the mind to the individual and examining the means of relaxing this rigidity there is great potential for an individual to reach beyond the confines of himself.*

The mind must have the ability to see the results of past actions that are preventing clear perception. Through the systematic practice of prāṇāyāma and other disciplines the range of mental activity can be extended to influence others. A teacher who seeks to transform a stupid or confused student must have this capacity.

3.39 उदानजयाज्जलपङ्ककण्टकादिष्वसङ्ग उत्क्रान्तिश्च ।

udānajayājjalapaṅkakaṇṭakādiṣvasaṅga utkrāntiśca

Physical pain is closely linked to the mind. A child completely absorbed in play may not be aware of hunger. But later he may cry violently for food. Physical manifestations of sensations like pain are linked to the mind through vital forces that run through the body. These forces can be directed by certain practices like prāṇāyāma and different effects can be produced by specific modifications.

> *By mastering the forces that transmit sensations from the body to the mind it is possible to master the external stimuli. For instance, one can tolerate water of any temperature or the effects of thorns or one can walk on unstable surfaces and even feel as light as a balloon.*

Cold, heat, sharp thorns, all these have relative effects. A summer in the Arctic may still feel wintery for someone used to the tropics, and someone used to the Arctic may find a tropical winter unbearably hot. A farm worker in India may find walking through a paddyfield as comfortable as a New Yorker finds concrete pavement.

3.40 समानजयाज्ज्वलनम् ।

samānajayājjvalanam

The life forces, *prāṇa*, have different roles and differing areas of activity. For example, *samāna* is responsible for digestion. It is based in the navel area.

> *By mastering samāna one can experience sensations of excessive heat.*

Digestion occurs when the gastric juices process the food that enters the stomach. If samāna is stimulated the feeling of heat increases. The prāṇāyāma technique which emphasizes the retention of breath after inhalation is suggested. Other techniques can be considered.

3.41 श्रोत्राकाशयोः संबन्धसंयमाद्दिव्यं श्रोत्रम् ।

śrotrākāśayoḥ saṁbandhasaṁyamāddivyaṁ śrotram

We know that sound travels through space.

Saṁyama on the relationship between the sense of hearing and space develops an extraordinary sense of hearing.

3.42 कायाकाशयोः संबन्धसंयमाल्लघुतूलसमापत्तेश्चा-
काशगमनम् ।

kāyākāśayoḥ saṁbandhasaṁyamāllaghu-
tūlasamāpatteścākāśagamanam

Man has long been interested in the relationship between physical objects and space. Why can birds fly but a stone falls?

By saṁyama on the relationship between the body and space, and examining the properties of objects that can float such as cotton fluff, the knowledge to move about in space can be achieved.

Again, this does not mean that we can learn how to physically float, but we can acquire the understanding of what it is to float. In the same way, the properties of a cotton seed prevent it from floating, but the same seed when changed to cotton fluff floats easily.

3.43 बहिरकल्पिता वृत्तिर्महाविदेहा ततः
प्रकाशावरणक्षयः ।

bahirakalpitā vṛttirmahāvidehā tataḥ prakāśāvaraṇakṣayaḥ

The mind influences our perception through memory, imagination, and other characteristics such as heaviness. But the same mind can be altered to a state in which the mind does not color perception of an object. When this happens, our perception of the object is correct. Further, it is possible to completely withhold the mind from perception of an object, no matter how attractive and tempting it might be.

> *By examining these phenomena and developing conditions when the mind does not confuse perception, there arises an extraordinary faculty with which one can probe other minds. In addition the clouds that obscure correct perception are minimized.*

Such developments are only possible in stages. The obscuring clouds are the obstacles described in sūtra 2.3.

3.44 स्थूलस्वरूपसूक्ष्मान्वयार्थवत्त्वसंयमाद्भूतजयः ।

sthūlasvarūpasūkṣmānvayārthavattvasaṁyamādbhūtajayaḥ

> *Saṁyama on the origin of matter in all its forms, appearances, and uses can develop into mastery of the elements.*

Matter consists of elements in different but mutually related forms. Each element has a distinct existence. They comprise the body as well as things outside the body, and their characteristics change. They form the very basis of the objects we perceive and if we are ignorant of their nature we face problems.

3.45 ततोऽणिमादिप्रादुर्भावः कायसंपत्तद्धर्मानभिघातश्च ।

tato 'ṇimādiprādurbhāvaḥ
kāyasaṁpattaddharmānabhighātaśca

Thus,

> *When the elements are mastered one is no longer disturbed by them. The body reaches perfection and extraordinary capabilities become possible.*

These capabilities include the ability to change our body to great heaviness, great lightness, and so on.

3.46 रूपलावण्यबलवज्रसंहननत्वानि कायसंपत् ।

rūpalāvaṇyabalavajrasaṁhananatvāni kāyasaṁpat

> *Perfection in the body means good features, attractiveness to others, physical firmness, and unusual physical strength.*

3.47 ग्रहणस्वरूपास्मितान्वयार्थवत्त्वसंयमादिन्द्रियजयः ।

grahaṇasvarūpāsmitānvayārthavattvasaṁyamādindriyajayaḥ

Mastery over the senses is achieved through samyama on the ability of the senses to observe their respective objects, how such objects are understood, how the individual identifies with the object, how the object, the senses, the mind, and the Perceiver are interrelated, and what results from such perception.

The senses, the object, and the mind have to be interlinked for an observation to materialize. This is possible because of the power of the Perceiver as well as the power of the mind and the senses to register the object. In addition, the three common characteristics possessed by the mind, the senses, and the object in different combinations (i.e., heaviness, activity, and clarity) assist perception as much as they affect perception.

3.48 ततो मनोजवित्वं विकरणभावः प्रधानजयश्च ।

tato manojavitvaṁ vikaraṇabhāvaḥ pradhānajayaśca

Then the response of the senses will be as swift as that of the mind. They will perceive acutely and the individual will have the capacity to influence the characteristics of the elements.

Through this saṁyama the changes that the elements undergo can be controlled at will. And we gain the necessary knowledge to determine such changes in the same way that a chemist can convert seawater into its component chemicals.

3.49 सत्त्वपुरुषान्यताख्यातिमात्रस्य सर्वभावाधिष्ठातृत्वं सर्वज्ञातृत्वं च ।

sattvapuruṣānyatākhyātimātrasya sarvabhāvādhiṣṭhātṛtvam sarvajñātṛtvaṁ ca

When there is clear understanding of the difference between the Perceiver and the mind, all the various states of mind and what affects them become known. Then, the mind becomes a perfect instrument for the flawless perception of everything that need be known.

3.50 तद्वैराग्यादपि दोषबीजक्षये कैवल्यम् ।

tadvairāgyādapi doṣabījakṣaye kaivalyam

These extraordinary capabilities that can be gained through *saṁyama* should not be the final goal. In fact,

> *Freedom, the last goal of Yoga, is attained only when the desire to acquire extraordinary knowledge is rejected and the source of obstacles is completely controlled.*

3.51 स्थान्युपनिमन्त्रणे सङ्गस्मयाकरणं
पुनरनिष्टप्रसङ्गात् ।

sthānyupanimantraṇe saṅgasmayākaraṇaṁ
punaraniṣṭaprasaṅgāt

> *The temptation to accept the respectful status as a consequence of acquiring knowledge through samyama should be restrained. Otherwise, one is led to the same unpleasant consequences that arise from all obstacles to Yoga.*

These obstacles include confused values. When respect for high learning is given more value than everlasting freedom from the painful consequences of our action, a fall is certain.

3.52 क्षणतत्क्रमयोः संयमाद्विवेकजं ज्ञानम् ।

kṣaṇatatkramayoḥ saṁyamādvivekajaṁ jñānam

> *Saṁyama on time and its sequence brings about absolute clarity.*

Clarity is the ability to see distinctly the difference between one object and another and to see each object in its totality without impediments. Time is relative, it exists by comparison of one moment with another. A unit of time is in fact a representation of change. Change is the replacement of one characteristic by another. This link between time and change is what needs to be examined in this saṁyama.

3.53 जातिलक्षणदेशैरन्यतानवच्छेदात्तुल्ययोस्ततः प्रतिपत्तिः ।

jātilakṣaṇadeśairanyatānavacchedāttulyayostataḥ pratipattiḥ

This clarity makes it possible to distinguish objects even when the distinction is not apparently clear. Apparent similarity should not deter one from the distinct perception of a chosen object.

3.54 तारकं सर्वविषयं सर्वथाविषयमक्रमं चेति विवेकजं ज्ञानम् ।

tārakaṁ sarvaviṣayaṁ sarvathāviṣayamakramaṁ ceti vivekajaṁ jñānam

Further,

Such clarity is not exclusive of any object, any particular situation, or any moment. It is not the result of sequential logic. It is immediate, spontaneous, and total.

3.55 सत्त्वपुरुषयोः शुद्धिसाम्ये कैवल्यम् ।

sattvapuruṣayoḥ śuddisāmye kaivalyam

What is freedom?

Freedom is when the mind has complete identity with the Perceiver.

And nothing less. Then the mind has no color or features of its own.

4

कैवल्यपादः

KAIVALYAPĀDAḤ

In this, the final chapter of the *Yoga Sūtra*, *kaivalyapāda*, Patañjali presents the possibilities for a person with a highly refined mind. The mind is basically a servant and not a master. If the mind is allowed to play the role of master, whatever the achievements of the individual there are bound to be problems ultimately and serenity will be beyond that individual's reach.

4.1 जन्मौषधिमन्त्रतपःसमाधिजाः सिद्धयः ।

janmauṣadhimantratapaḥsamādhijāḥ siddhayaḥ

Exceptional mental capabilities may be achieved by: genetic inheritance, the use of herbs as prescribed in the Vedas, reciting incantations, rigorous austerities, and through that state of mind that remains with its object without distractions [samādhi].

Some people are born with extraordinary capabilities. The Vedas describe various rituals whereby the taking of herbal preparations in a prescribed way can change one's personality. Different types of incantations, appropriately initiated by competent teachers, can bring positive changes. The ancient scriptures record the great achievements of those who went through severe austerities. Finally, there are the possibilities for those who gradually change their minds from a state of distraction to one of sustained direction. These are mentioned in abundance in the third chapter and elsewhere. Whether any particular one of these alternatives is to be preferred will be examined in sūtras 4.6, 7, and 8.

4.2 जात्यन्तरपरिणामः प्रकृत्यापूरात् ।

jātyantarapariṇāmaḥ prakṛtyāpūrāt

How does the change resulting in the appearance of exceptional and supernormal possibilities come about?

Change from one set of characteristics to another is essentially an adjustment of the basic qualities of matter.

All that we perceive, including the mind, have three basic qualities: clarity, activity, and heaviness. Different characteristics arise at different times as a result of different combinations of these qualities. Every characteristic that is possible is the combination of these three qualities. It is one of the changes in the characteristics of the mind that result in the supernormal capabilities that Patañjali speaks about in sūtra 4.1.

4.3 निमित्तमप्रयोजकं प्रकृतीनां वरणभेदस्तु ततः क्षेत्रिकवत् ।

nimittamaprayojakaṁ prakṛtīnāṁ varaṇabhedastu tataḥ kṣetrikavat

How can change in the characteristics of matter or mind be achieved? By profound intelligence.

But such intelligence can only remove obstacles that obstruct certain changes. Its role is no more than that of a farmer who cuts a dam to allow water to flow into the field where it is needed.

This profound intelligence is the ability to perceive the role of the basic qualities in producing different characteristics. For example, the farmer who knows his field and the requirements of his crop will adjust the flow of the water to achieve the best yield. On the other hand, an ignorant novice who embarks on farming will fail in spite of having potentially good soil, water, climate, and equipment.

4.4 निर्माणचित्तान्यस्मितामात्रात् ।

nirmāṇacittānyasmitāmātrāt

What are the possibilities for someone with supernormal capabilities?

With exceptional mental faculties an individual can influence the mental state of other beings.

4.5 प्रवृत्तिभेदे प्रयोजकं चित्तमेकमनेकेषाम् ।

pravṛttibhede prayojakaṁ cittamekamanekeṣām

Are these influences consistent or variable?

This influence also depends on the state of the recipient.

How receptive is the person? What capabilities does he have? What does he lack? This decides the outcome of the influence of another. The same rain can relieve a drought-stricken farmer, worry a mother with inadequate shelter for the child, and have no effect on the open ocean.

4.6 तत्र ध्यानजमनाशयम् ।

tatra dhyānajamanāśayam

Is it only the state of the recipient that decides the final outcome of the effect a person can have?

Influence on another by one whose mind is in a state of dhyāna can never increase anxiety or other obstacles. In fact, they are reduced.

Those who have reached this state of dhyāna through the gradual elimination of obstacles (see 2.3) are not blind to the conditions of human suffering. They know where the shoe pinches.

4.7 कर्माशुक्लाकृष्णं योगिनस्त्रिविधमितरेषाम् ।

karmāśuklākṛṣṇaṁ yoginastrividhamitareṣām

And they act without any motivation while others who also have exceptional capabilities act with some motivation or other.

In sūtra 4.1 Patañjali lists the different means of achieving an exceptional or supernormal state of mind. Of them all, only those who have reached a state of Yoga in the correct way and through it have reached the highest state of clarity and detachment can be beyond motivation. They are naturally and unambiguously concerned. Therefore they can help others to emulate their living examples. Others may appear to be in a state of Yoga, but their clarity and degree of detachment is less complete and everlasting. Besides, they may be unaware of the limitations of man to follow their advice.

4.8 ततस्तद्विपाकानुगुणानामेवाभिव्यक्तिर्वासनानाम् ।

tatastadvipākānuguṇānāmevābhivyaktirvāsanānām

How can these differences exist?

> *Because the tendency of the mind to act on the basis of the five obstacles, such as misapprehension, has not been erased, they will surface in the future to produce their unpleasant consequences.*

Only the practices described in earlier chapters to reduce and render the five obstacles ineffective can guarantee the end of these tendencies. Genetic inheritance, the use of herbs, and other means cannot be as effective.

4.9 जातिदेशकालव्यवहितानामप्यानन्तर्यं स्मृतिसंस्कार-
योरेकरूपत्वात् ।

jātideśakālavyavahitānāmapyānantaryaṁ
smṛtisaṁskārayorekarūpatvāt

In addition,

> *Memory and latent impressions are strongly linked. This link remains even if there is an interval of time, place, or context between similar actions.*

This link between impressions and memory is an important contribution to most of our actions and their consequences.

4.10 तासामनादित्वं चाशिषो नित्यत्वात् ।

tāsāmanāditvaṁ cāśiṣo nityatvāt

What is the origin of those impressions that influence our actions unpleasantly?

> *There is a strong desire for immortality in all men at all times. Thus these impressions cannot be ascribed to any time.*

One of the strange but ever present states of affairs in all beings is the desire to live forever. Even those in the presence of death every day have this illogical impulse. This is what inspires the instinct for self-preservation in all of us.

4.11 हेतुफलाश्रयालम्बनैः संगृहीतत्वादेषामभावे तदभावः ।

hetuphalāśrayālambanaiḥ saṅgrhītatvādeṣāmabhāve tadabhāvaḥ

Is there absolutely no hope at all of ending the effect of these undesirable impressions?

> *These tendencies are both maintained and sustained by misapprehensions, external stimuli, attachment to the fruits of actions, and the quality of mind that promotes hyperactivity. Reduction of these automatically makes the undesirable impressions ineffective.*

Various ways of reducing and eliminating these protective obstacles by regulated, progressive practices have already been indicated. There are many ways, including the help of God. For those who do not appreciate God, there are many other ways described in the first three chapters. Conversely, it can also be said that impressions free from the five obstacles are in turn maintained and sustained by a discriminating mind.

4.12 अतीतानागतं स्वरूपतोऽस्त्यध्वभेदाद्धर्माणाम् ।

atītānāgataṁ svarūpato 'styadhvabhedāddharmāṇām

Whatever will appear in the future or has appeared in the past is essentially in a dormant state. What is past has not disappeared forever.

> *The substance of what has disappeared as well as what may appear always exists. Whether or not they are evident depends upon the direction of change.*

Patañjali again stresses that nothing can be annihilated. What is replaced in the process of change remains in a dormant state.

4.13 ते व्यक्तसूक्ष्मा गुणात्मानः ।

te vyaktasūkṣmā guṇātmānaḥ

> *Whether or not particular characteristics appear depends on the mutations of the three qualities.*

These qualities are heaviness, activity, and clarity. All apparent characteristics are simply different combinations of these three basic qualities that comprise all things (sūtra 2.18).

4.14 परिणामैकत्वाद्वस्तुतत्त्वम् ।

parināmaikatvādvastutattvam

The characteristics of a substance at one moment in time is in fact a single change in these qualities.

Change itself is a continuous process based on many factors (sūtras 3.9–12). The required change in objects and in the mind can be achieved by knowing the potential combinations of these three qualities and what can influence them. There are many possible examples such as that given in sūtra 4.3. Food and the environment provide others.

4.15 वस्तुसाम्ये चित्तभेदात्तयोर्विभक्तः पन्थाः ।

vastusāmye cittabhedāttayorvibhaktaḥ panthāḥ

But are the characteristics that appear to one observer the real characteristics?

The characteristics of an object appear differently, depending upon the different mental states of the observer.

This applies to one observer with various states of mind at different times as well as various observers with different states of mind observing the object at the same time. Thus, a Hindu temple is a place of worship to a devoted believer, an artistic monument to a tourist, a place of solicitation to a beggar, and even a place of ridicule to an atheist.

4.16 न चैकचित्ततन्त्रं चेद्वस्तु तदप्रमाणकं तदा किं स्यात् ।

na caikacittatantraṁ cedvastu tadapramāṇakaṁ tadā kiṁ syāt

Does this not raise doubts about the common reality of any object? Can an object simply be in the imagination of a person without having independent reality?

If the object were indeed the conception of a particular individual's mind, then in the absence of his perception, would it exist ?

Patañjali asks a rhetorical question. The answer is obvious. The existence of an object cannot depend solely on any one person's observation. The river does not stop flowing because no one is looking at it.

4.17 तदुपरागापेक्षित्वाच्चित्तस्य वस्तु ज्ञाताज्ञातम् ।

taduparāgāpekṣitvāccittasya vastu jñātājñātam

On what does the perception of an object depend?

Whether an object is perceived or not depends on its accessibility as well as the individual's motivation.

The object must exist. It must be observable and it must motivate the observer and stimulate a desire to see it.

4.18 सदा ज्ञाताश्चित्तवृत्तयस्तत्प्रभोः
पुरुषस्यापरिणामित्वात् ।

sadā jñātāścittavṛttayastatprabhoḥ puruṣasyāpariṇāmitvāt

What is it that sees? Is it the mind?

Mental activities are always known to the Perceiver that is nonchanging and master of the mind.

The mind cannot function without the power of the Perceiver. The mind changes, the Perceiver does not. The mind has the quality of heaviness but not so the Perceiver. All mental activities are therefore observed by the Perceiver.

4.19 न तत्स्वाभासं दृश्यत्वात् ।

na tatsvābhāsaṁ dṛśyatvāt

In addition, the mind is a part of what is perceived and has no power of its own to perceive.

The mind is seen through its activities in the same way that external objects, the body, and the senses are seen. Its very existence is dependent upon the Perceiver.

4.20 एकसमये चोभयानवधारणम् ।

ekasamaye cobhayānavadhāraṇam

Let us suppose the mind itself could function in two roles, as the fabricator of what is observed and as the observer.

> *The premise that the mind can play two roles is untenable because it cannot simultaneously fabricate and see what it fabricates.*

An object existing independently of an observer can be perceived. However, the concept of the mind creating an object and, at the same time, observing that object, is impossible to maintain. Another agency, independent of the mind, and with the ability to perceive, is essential.

4.21 चित्तान्तरदृश्ये बुद्धिबुद्धेरतिप्रसङ्गः स्मृतिसंकरश्च ।

cittāntaradṛśye buddhibuddheratiprasaṅgaḥ
smṛtisaṅkaraśca

If we then postulate the concept of a succession of minds that exist momentarily to create images and in turn recognize and observe them,

> *In an individual with such a series of minds of momentary existence there would be disorder and the difficulty of maintaining consistency of memory.*

What is suggested in sūtras 4.20 and 4.21 is that there must be an independent source of perception. The mind can of course influence the perception of an object. This object has an independent existence apart from the source of perception. If we insist on the concept of the mind from moment to moment being the source, the means, and the object of perception, we face problems in comprehending the possibility of one person remembering what he saw in the past, sharing what he has seen, and reconciling the fact that one object seen by one person is not necessarily seen by another or in the same way.

4.22 चितेरप्रतिसंक्रमायास्तदाकारापत्तौ स्वबुद्धिसंवेदनम् ।

citerapratisaṅkramāyāstadākārāpattau
svabuddhisaṁvedanam

Is the role of the mind limited to helping to see extemal objects?

When the mind is not linked to external objects and it does not respect an external form to the Perceiver, then it takes the form of the Perceiver itself.

When there are no external stimuli and interests to extrapolate, there are no impressions in the mind relating to them. Then the mind is in total contact with and identical to the Perceiver. Then cognition of the Perceiver is possible. This cognition is not by the mind. This is related to the concept of freedom in sūtra 3.55. It is assumed that the heaviness that causes sleep is not in operation.

4.23 द्रष्टृदृश्योपरक्तं चित्तं सर्वार्थम् ।

draṣṭṛdṛśyoparaktaṁ cittaṁ sarvārtham

Thus the mind serves a dual purpose. It serves the Perceiver by presenting the external to it. It also repects or presents the Perceiver to itself for its own enlightenment.

4.24 तदसंख्येयवासनाभिश्चित्रमपि परार्थं
संहत्यकारित्वात् ।

tadasaṅkhyeyavāsanābhiścitramapi parārthaṁ
saṁhatyakāritvāt

The role of the mind to serve the Perceiver in every way is further reiterated:

Even though the mind has accumulated various impressions of different types it is always at the disposal of the Perceiver. This is because the mind cannot function without the power of the Perceiver.

The mind has no purpose of its own. It cannot act on its own (see sūtra 2.21).

4.25 विशेषदर्शिन आत्मभावभावनानिवृत्तिः ।

viśeṣadarśina ātmabhāvabhāvanānivṛttiḥ

Patañjali now suggests the qualities of one who has reached the highest state of clarity:

> *A person of extraordinary clarity is one who is free from the desire to know the nature of the Perceiver.*

One has no curiosity to speculate on the Perceiver, the quality of the mind, the "Where-was-I? What-will-I be?" because he has felt his true nature. Such persons have reached the level that is free from obstacles (sūtra 2.3) because one of the products of obstacles is the question "Who am I?"

4.26 तदा विवेकनिम्नं कैवल्यप्राग्भारं चित्तम् ।

tadā vivekanimnaṁ kaivalyaprāgbhāraṁ cittam

> *And their clarity takes them to their only concern; to reach and remain in a state of freedom.*

4.27 तच्छिद्रेषु प्रत्ययान्तराणि संस्कारेभ्यः ।

tacchidreṣu pratyayāntarāṇi saṁskārebhyaḥ

Is such a person now beyond regression?

> *In the unlikely possibility of distraction from this aim, disturbing past impressions are able to surface.*

Since our actions are influenced by such impressions, regression, unlikely as it may be, is still possible.

4.28 हानमेषां क्लेशवदुक्तम् ।

hānameṇām kleśavaduktam

> *One must never accommodate even small errors because they are as detrimental as the five obstacles.*

Even at such a refined state of being, help from a teacher, who can see us through, is essential. In the first chapter (sūtra 1.30) regression is considered to be one of the impediments to progress, as serious as disease and doubt.

4.29 प्रसंख्यानेऽप्यकुसीदस्य सर्वथा विवेकख्यातेर्धर्ममेघः समाधिः ।

prasaṅkhyāne 'pyakusīdasya sarvathā
vivekakhyāterdharmameghaḥ samādhiḥ

When we have crossed the last hurdle

There arises a state of mind full of clarity concerning all things at all times. It is like a rainfall of pure clarity.

Life is full of contentment. Vision is never dimmed. The extraordinary capabilities are never misused.

4.30 ततः क्लेशकर्मनिवृत्तिः ।

tataḥ kleśakarmanivṛttiḥ

This is, indeed, the state free from actions based on the five obstacles.

But it is not a life without action. It is a life devoid of errors or selfish interests.

4.31 तदा सर्वावरणमलापेतस्य ज्ञानस्यानन्त्याज्ज्ञेयमल्पम् ।

tadā sarvāvaraṇamalāpetasya
jñānasyānantyājjñeyamalpam

When the mind is free from the clouds that prevent perception, all is known, there is nothing to be known.

The sun shines. All is evident. There is no need for artificial light.

4.32 ततः कृतार्थानां परिणामक्रमसमाप्तिर्गुणानाम् ।

tataḥ kṛtārthānāṁ pariṇāmakramasamāptirguṇānām

With this highest potential at our disposal,

> *The three basic qualities cease to follow the sequence of alternating pain and pleasure.*

With the high intelligence at our disposal, the objects of perception are in our control. Their mutation through the combination of the three qualities are no more. We are able to influence them to serve our immediate needs, without ever producing or provoking regrettable actions. Changes in the mind, the senses, and the body no longer create trouble.

4.33 क्षणप्रतियोगी परिणामापरान्तनिर्ग्राह्यः क्रमः ।

kṣaṇapratiyogī pariṇāmāparāntanirgrāhyaḥ kramaḥ

What is a sequence?

> *A sequence is the replacement of one characteristic by one that follows it. This is linked to moment. A replacement of characteristics is also the basis of a moment.*

Moment, which is the basic unit of time, and sequence are related. The change in the characteristics of an object is their common basis. The sequence is affected by the changes. Therefore time is essentially relative in that it is the essential of change. The order of change is the variation in the characteristics that follow one after the other (see sūtras 3.15 and 3.52).

In the context of sūtra 4.32 the changes that now arise in the objects of perception follow a different sequence from that of the past when it was both unpredictable and liable to bring regrets. Now the individual can command the changes.

4.34 पुरुषार्थशून्यानां गुणानां प्रतिप्रसवः कैवल्यं स्वरूपप्रतिष्ठा वा चितिशक्तिरिति ।

puruṣārthaśunyānāṁ guṇānāṁ pratiprasavaḥ kaivalyaṁ
svarūpapratiṣṭhā vā citiśaktiriti

What is the final state of Yoga?

> *When the highest purpose of life is achieved the three basic qualities do not excite responses in the mind. That is freedom. In other words, the Perceiver is no longer colored by the mind.*

It is serenity in action as well as in inaction. There is no sense of obligation, whether to take responsibility or to reject it. The three qualities can no longer combine to disrupt the individual. He is fully conscious of his own state of pure clarity and it remains at the highest level throughout his lifetime. The mind is a faithful servant to the master, the Perceiver.

Top:
Krishnamacharya at the completion of his university studies, 1925.

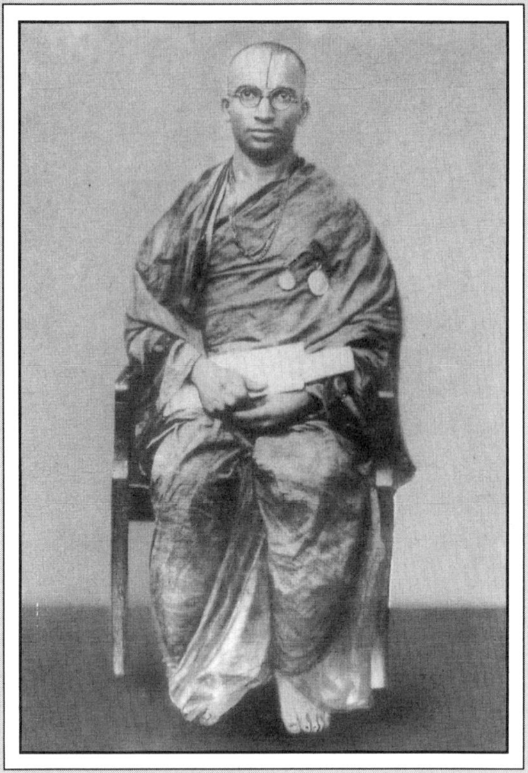

Middle: Śri Vageesa Brahmatantra Parakala Swami, one of Krishnamacharya's preceptors.

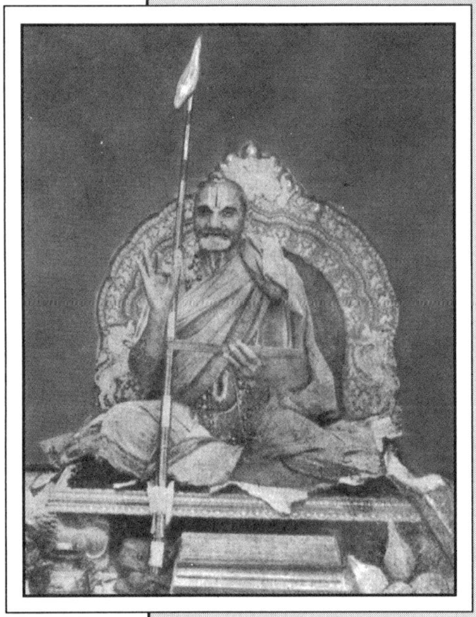

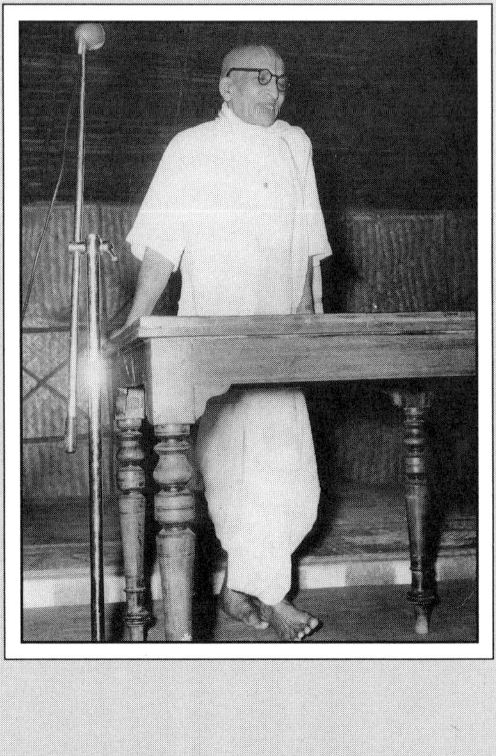

Bottom:
Krishnamacharya lecturing in Madras.

PART IV
A Life of Yoga

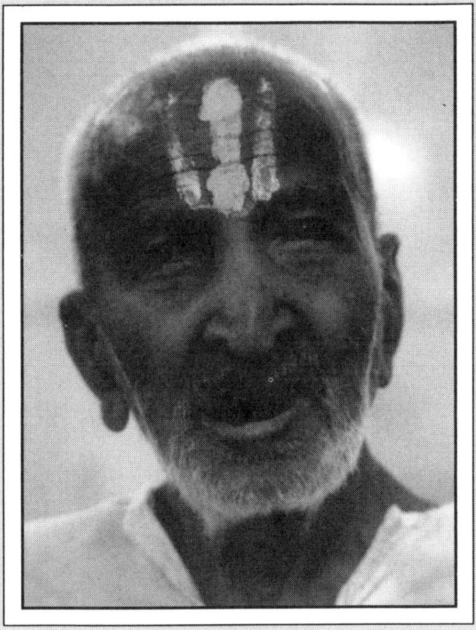

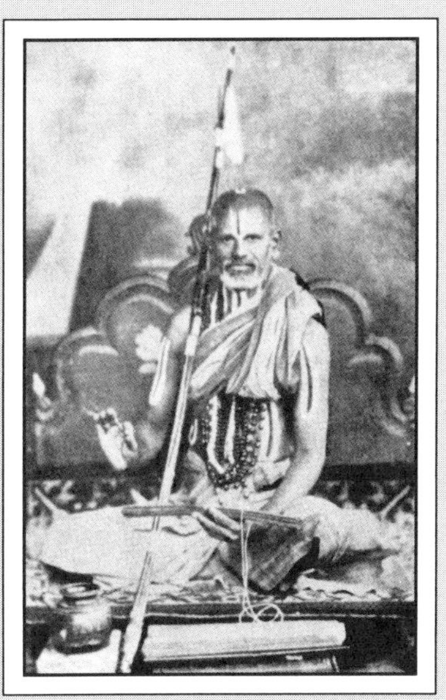

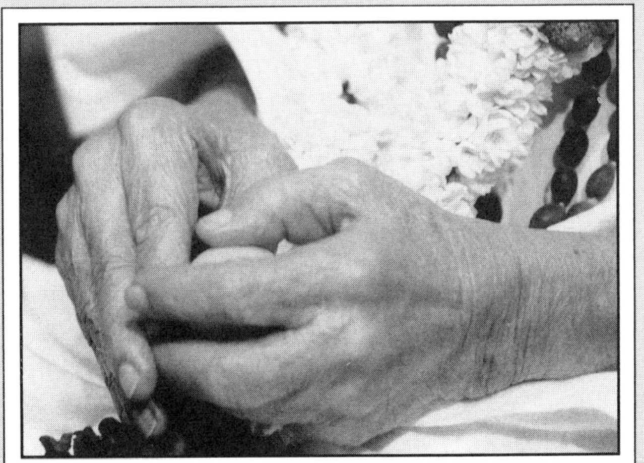

Top: Krishnamacharya at 100 years.

Middle: Śrī Krishna Brahmatantra Swami, another of Krishnamacharya's preceptors.

Bottom: Krishnamacharya's healing hands.

The Life and Yoga of Śrī T. Krishnamacharya

AN INTERVIEW WITH T. K. V. DESIKACHAR

Tirumalai Krishnamacharya was born on November 18, 1888, in a village in the state of Mysore, South India. He was born into a family that traces its roots back to the famous ninth-century South Indian sage Nathamuni, author of the *Yoga Rahasya* and the first teacher in the line of Vaishnava gurus.

Krishnamacharya received his first instruction in Sanskrit and yoga from his father before becoming a pupil at the Brahmatantra Parakala Mutt in Mysore, one of the best known and most respected Brahmin schools. Enrolled at the age of twelve, he studied the Vedic texts and learned the Vedic rituals while simultaneously attending the Royal College of Mysore. At the age of eighteen he moved to Banaras, where he studied Sanskrit, logic, and grammar at the university. Back in Mysore, he received a thorough grounding in the philosophy of the Vedānta from Śrī Krishna Brahmatantra Swami, the director of the Parakala Mutt. Then he went north again to study the Sāṃkhya, India's oldest philosophical system and the one on which yoga is fundamentally based. In 1916 he went to the Himalayas where, at the foot of Mount Kailash, he met his teacher, Śrī Ramamohan Brahmachari, a learned yogi who was living with his family near Lake Manasarovar in Tibet.

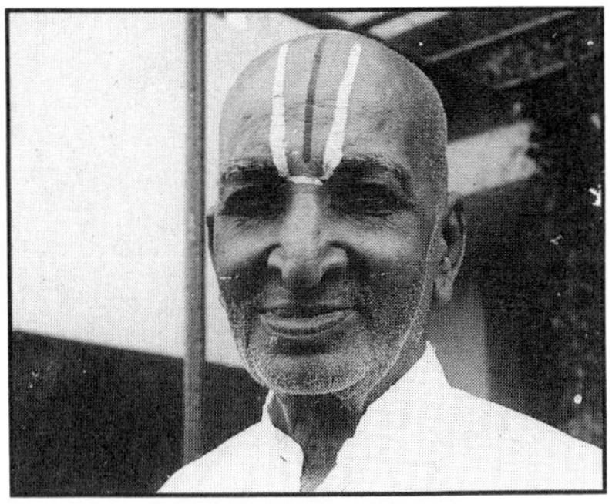

Krishnamacharya at age 84.

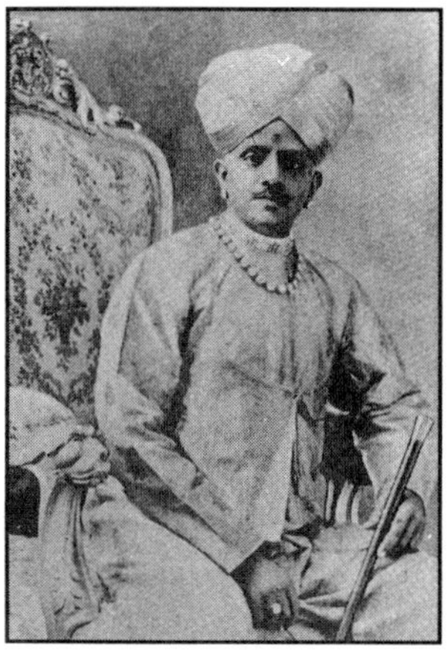

Krishnamacharya patron and student, Krishnarajendra Wodoyar IV, the mahārājah of Mysore.

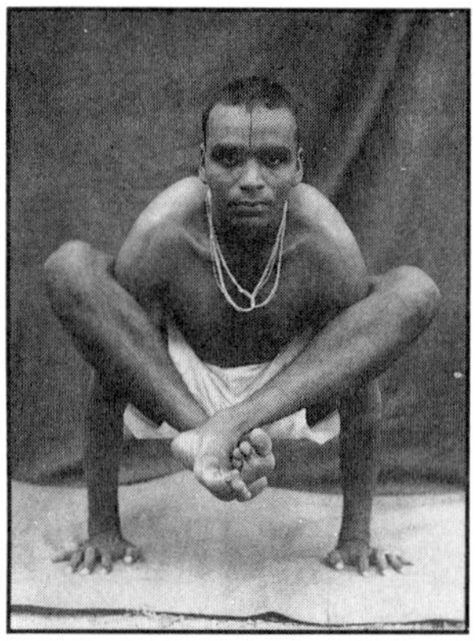

B. K. S. Iyengar at age 24 demonstrating bhujapīdāsana.

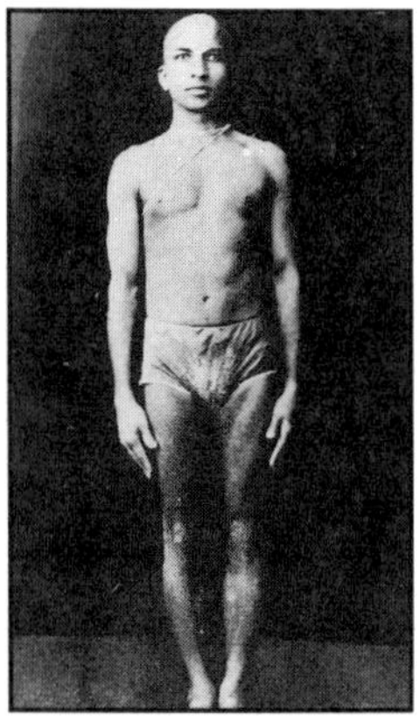

Krishnamacharya at age 46 in samasthiti.

Krishnamacharya spent more than seven years with this teacher, who exercised considerable influence over the direction he took in life, giving him the great task of spreading the message of yoga and using his abilities as a healer and helper of sick people. Consequently, Śrī Krishnamacharya did not embark upon an academic career, but returned to the south where he studied Āyurveda, the traditional Indian healing system, as well as the philosophy of Nyāya, a Vedic school of logic recognized for its tools of inquiry and emphasis on discrimination gained by valid knowledge. In 1924 he returned to Mysore, where the rājah, a progressive ruler, gave him the opportunity to open a yoga school. The rājah himself was one of Krishnamacharya's most enthusiastic students. From 1933 to 1955 Krishnamacharya taught yoga at the school and wrote his first book, *Yoga Makarandam* (Secrets of Yoga).

By this time his reputation was spreading throughout South India and beyond. Krishnamacharya's first Western students came to study yoga with him in 1937. Indra Devi was among them. B. K. S. Iyengar, who was to become Krishnamacharya's brother-in-law, received his first yoga instruction with the acclaimed teacher. In 1939 and 1940, Krishnamacharya was visited by a French medical team who wanted to verify that an experienced yogi could deliberately stop his heartbeat. For Śrī Krishnamacharya, this much-marvelled-at examination was a rather bothersome demonstration, one that he undertook out of feeling responsible to validate yoga in the eyes of the skeptical scientific world.

Soon Krishnamacharya's interest and work turned toward treating the sick, using Āyurveda and yoga as healing agents. He became increasingly well known, and in 1952 was summoned to Madras to treat a popular politician who had suffered a heart attack. Finally, Krishnamacharya settled in Madras with his family.

As well as his Indian students, more Westerners came to Madras to study. Gerard Blitz, who brought these teachings to Europe, was one of the first to seek out Krishnamacharya, as was Jean Klein, the Advaita teacher. In 1976, T. K. V. Desikachar, Krishnamacharya's son and one of his closest disciples, founded the Krishnamacharya Yoga Mandiram, an institution where yoga is used to treat sick people, and is taught to both Indian and foreign students. Śrī Krishnamacharya was teaching and inspiring those around him until six weeks prior to his death in 1989.

Q: As both son and student of Śrī Krishnamacharya, you must have been one of the people closest to him and one of those who knew him best. Can you please tell us something about Krishnamacharya, the Sanskrit scholar, healer, and yogi?

A: The foremost reason my father became a scholar of Sanskrit was because of his family tradition. In the old days, people like my father's forebears were well known as advisors, even to the kings. Nowadays we would call my father's grandfather something like prime minister, for example, but at that time the position of prime minister was not a political one in the way that we now know it. He was rather an advisor who told the rulers what was right and what was wrong. For this purpose, these scholars naturally studied the old texts, which are all written in Sanskrit. So at that time it was perfectly normal for someone who grew up in the milieu in which my father did to become versed in Sanskrit; it was the language of these circles, just as today English is the language of technology.

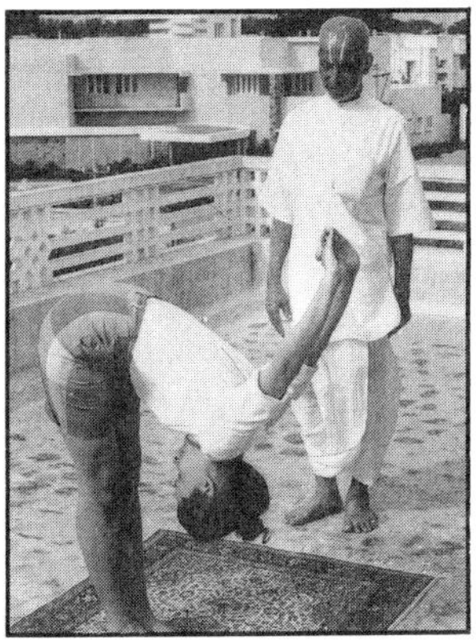
Krishnamacharya teaching a Western student, 1954.

In his formal education he had to learn Sanskrit well enough to be able to read and study the classic texts that describe the branches of the Vedas. Yoga is just one of those branches, but my father developed a special interest in yoga because his family was historically involved with yoga. One of his ancestors was the famous yogi Nathamuni. The interest in yoga is like a thread going right through the history of this family, and my father simply picked it up. His first teacher was his own father.

He pursued this interest further when he studied with great masters in the north of India, and he found his own special teacher, Ramamohan Brahmachari, in the region of Lake Manasarovar in the Himalayas. Krishnamacharya stayed with his teacher for nearly eight years. Ramamohan Brahmachari instructed him in the *Yoga Sūtra* and taught him how to help the sick by means of yoga. Much of what is seen as the uniqueness of my father's work comes from this teacher.

It is normal for someone with a family tradition like this to become a great Sanskrit scholar and to be versed in the literature and religion given to us in the Vedas. But because his teacher said to him, "You must spread the message of yoga," Krishnamacharya decided to become a yoga teacher. He turned down many offers of professorships—in Sanskrit, in logic, in Vedānta and other subjects. He immersed himself in everything he had been taught and finally became a guru. It was no easy matter—indeed there were inner struggles for him—but he did it.

Another important point was that, through his interest in religion, especially his own tradition of the Vaishnava, Krishnamacharya came across the teachings of some great yogis of South India. These people are called *alvar*, which means "someone who has come to us to rule." Alvar direct the minds of other people and are regarded as an incarnation of God. Their greatness is bestowed upon them as babies, and many of them are not from Brahmin families but sometimes come from simple peasant families. They were born into the world as extraordinary people. Śrī Krishnamacharya studied the writings of these masters, which are in our language of Tamil, and so discovered the meaning of yoga as it is understood in the south of India. This is how he could combine the great teachings from the north, learned from his teacher in the Himalayas, with the great teachings of the south, which come from our Tamil masters, the alvar.

Q: Was it required at that time that someone taking this path should go to the Himalayas and live there with a master?

A: No, this was Krishnamacharya's personal decision. He decided that he wanted to learn everything about the Vedic darśanas—the various systems of Indian thought—because some of his views were not accepted by his teachers. When he was attending lectures on Sāṃkhya and Mīmāṃsā in

Mysore, he vowed he would go to the best universities in India and learn all there was to learn about various schools of Indian thought. In those days, the best place for studying these was Kashi, now known as Varanasi or Banaras so he went there. He was lucky to have the opportunity to go there, because the teachers there recognized his special abilities. It was in Banaras, where Krishnamacharya met a teacher named Ganganath-Jha who recommended he go to a great yoga teacher in the north. That is how he went to Tibet. It was not a requirement, but instead almost chance.

Q: And the healer Krishnamacharya?

A: For most people yoga is purely a spiritual discipline, but it is clear that for my father, yoga included other things as well. One of the biographies written about him relates how he was concerned with the sick even as a student. My father himself told me that once he was asked to come to the British governor, who suffered from diabetes. My father was able to help him, then left to continue his studies in the north, at Mount Kailash.

The ability to heal must have come from his own background. Probably it was his father who first gave him tips on how to treat diabetes and other illnesses, for in Nathamuni's *Yoga Rahasya* we find many remarks about the use of yoga in the treatment of sick people. Illness is an obstacle on the road to spiritual enlightenment; that is why you have to do something about it. There are many ways of treating sickness through yoga: sometimes a mantra is needed, sometimes a change of diet, sometimes certain āsanas, and sometimes prāṇāyāma. Probably Krishnamacharya had heard about all of this early in life and wanted to learn more about it. It became clear to him that if he wanted to learn more about healing, he would have to learn about Āyurveda. So he went to a well-known teacher named Krishna Kumar in Bengal and stayed with him in order to learn Āyurveda. Eventually, as well as knowing Nathamuni's teachings about how to use yoga to promote good health, my father had all the knowledge of Āyurveda at his fingertips. This is how he knew the importance of the pulse for giving information about a person's condition. He learned this from masters as well as by studying the old texts on the subject. Krishnamacharya always took the pulse of anyone who came to him; one of the first things he taught me was how to take someone's pulse. Being able to diagnose a condition through taking the pulse and using Āyurveda and Nathamuni's yogic health system were the means Krishnamacharya used when he gave advice on physical, mental, and spiritual wellness. So it is not surprising that he sometimes performed real miracles.

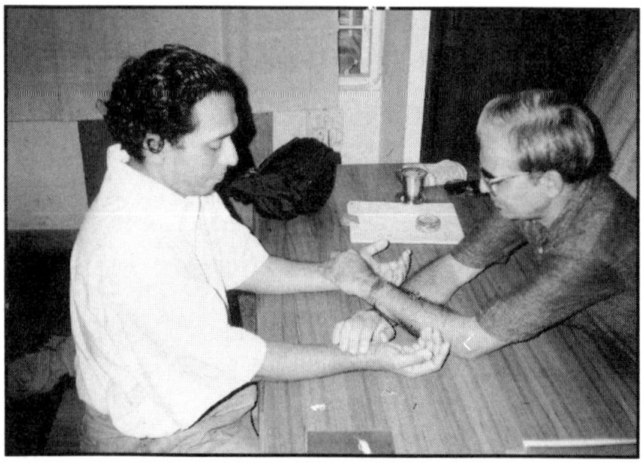

Desikachar making a diagnosis based on the pulse.

Q: What makes Krishnamacharya's yoga so unique?

A: What makes my father's yoga teachings unique is his insistence on attending to each individual and to his or her uniqueness. If we respect each person individually, it naturally means we will always start from where each person currently is. The starting point is never the teacher's needs but those of the student. This requires many different approaches; there is not just one approach for everybody. The way yoga is taught nowadays often gives the impression that there is *one* solution to everyone's problems and *one* treatment for every illness. But yoga affects the mind, primarily, and each person's mind is different. Indeed the culture and background of each person is different as well. In every case, my father chose what seemed necessary and useful: sometimes it might be āsanas, sometimes it was a prayer, sometimes he even told people to stop a certain yoga practice: then the healing occurred. There are many stories I could tell, all of which show the necessity for an individual approach to yoga. By this I do not mean that I have to give only private lessons, but I must create an atmosphere in my classes in which each student can find his or her own way to yoga. I have to realize that each of my students is not the same person today as they were yesterday, and not at all the same as when they came last week, perhaps with similar questions. This is the most important message my father passed on, and it is essentially the opposite of what is currently being taught in most places.

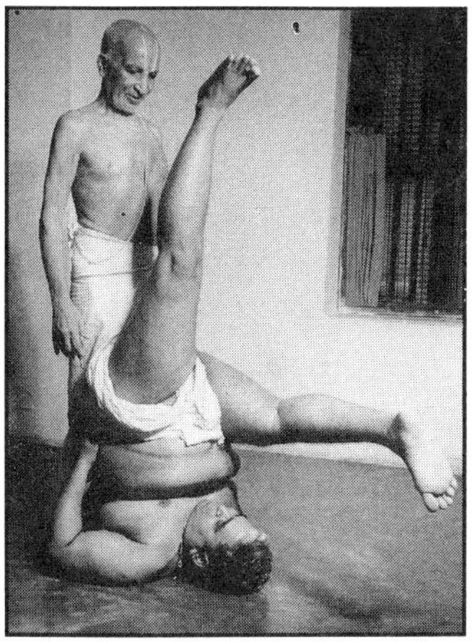

Krishnamacharya and student performing eka pāda sarvāngāsana.

The essence of my father's teachings is this: it is not that the person needs to accommodate him- or herself to yoga, but rather the yoga practice must be tailored to fit each person. I would even go so far as to say that this is what makes my father's approach different from most of the others around today, where everything is well organized and you have to fit into a certain structure. With Krishnamacharya's yoga there is no organization, and the individual must find her or his own structure.

This implies that progress on the path of yoga means different things for different people. We must not obstruct this progress by deliberately setting certain goals. Yoga serves the individual, and does so through inviting transformation rather than by giving information. These are two very different things. For instance, this book gives information about various topics, but in order to bring about transformation, I would explain each topic in a different way to each person. My father taught us more ways to approach a person in yoga than I have found anywhere else. Who should teach whom? When? And what? These are the important questions to be asked in beginning a practice. But underlying all these is the most important question of all: How can the power of the breath be utilized? That is something quite exceptional; nowhere else is the breath given so much importance, and our work has proven that the breath is a wonder drug, if I may use this term.

Q: As well as the breath, you, like your father, use many sounds and mantra. Mantra belong to the Indian tradition. Can we in the West relate to this aspect of Krishnamacharya's yoga?

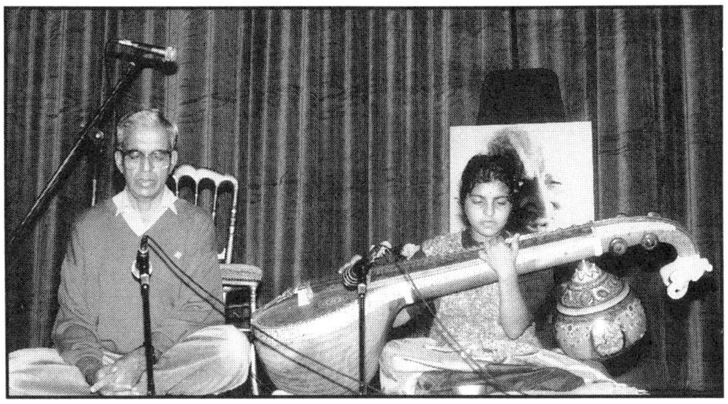

Desikachar chanting with daughter Mekhala, age 10, accompanying on the vīnā, Germany, 1992.

A: You must understand the word *mantra* correctly. It is not a Hindu symbol but rather something much more universal: it is something that can bring a person's mind to a higher plane. Sound has a lot of power; the voice has a tremendous influence. Just think about how an orator can capture an audience just by the way he speaks. In our Indian tradition we have made use of these qualities of sound. We use Sanskrit words, but your language too is made up of sounds. In India we use mantra because, by virtue of their religious tradition, they mean something to many people. But I would never use a mantra indiscriminately. We can always work within an individual's tradition. What is universally true is that sounds can have a powerful influence on us. Our work proves this again and again.

Q: Can you say something about the concept of structuring your yoga practice intelligently—the concept of viṅyāsa krama?

A: First I must ask: What do you mean by "intelligently"? You are probably familiar with the argument that doing the headstand brings more blood into the head. Somebody who has the feeling that the blood supply to the head is not good enough then comes to the conclusion that the headstand is the best āsana for them. But first we should think this through. Do we all suffer from a deficient supply of blood to the head simply because we stand and walk upright? Suppose that someone is haunted by this idea so much that he begins to practice the headstand every day, if possible first thing in the morning, perhaps as the first or only āsana. Our experience in working with all kinds of people has taught us that people who do this eventually suffer from enormous problems in the neck, that then result in great tension and stiffness in that area and a decreased supply of blood to the whole musculature of the neck—precisely the opposite of what they hoped they would achieve.

An intelligent approach to yoga practice means that, before you begin, you are clear about the various aspects of the āsana you wish to practice, and know how to prepare for them in such a way that you reduce or negate any undesired effects. With regard to the headstand, for example, the questions are: Is my neck prepared for this? Can I breathe well in the āsana? Is my back strong enough to raise the entire weight of my legs? To approach your practice intelligently means to know all the implications of what you want to do, whether that be āsana or prāṇāyāma, and to make appropriate preparations and adjustments. It is not enough to jump if you want to reach the sky. Taking an intelligent approach means working toward your goal step by step. If you want to travel overseas, the first thing you need is a passport. Then you need visas for the countries you intend to visit, and so forth. The simple fact that you want to go there does not make the trip possible. All learning follows this pattern.

Q: How did Krishnamacharya see the significance of āsanas in the practice of yoga?

A: My father never saw yoga simply as a physical practice. Yoga was much more about reaching the highest, which for him was God. So for Krishnamacharya, yoga meant taking steps that would lead to God in order to become one with God. This path demands much from those who follow it: a strong will, trust, and the ability keep up one's efforts constantly. Illness is definitely not a good companion on the way, for it can distract the attention; instead of being devoted to God we can think only of our physical pains. The steps in yoga that are concerned with the physical body are steps that should enable us to go the whole way, not the other way around. It is not a matter of making the body the center of all activities, nor of depriving it altogether. Yoga for one person can mean becoming healthy again through the practice of āsanas; for someone else it can mean finding help in preparing for death—certainly not through practicing āsanas, but rather by finding a way of reaching a peaceful state of mind where there are no feelings of guilt or blame. Perhaps in this case I would teach the person to pray. For a child it is interesting and meaningful to have a lot of physical exertion—but why should I teach an eighty-year-old person to do a headstand or sit in the lotus posture?

Yoga is primarily a practice intended to make someone wiser, more able to understand things than they were before. If āsanas help in this, terrific! If not, then some other means can be found instead. The goal is always bhakti or, to put it in my father's words, to approach the highest intelligence, namely, God.

Q: When Śrī Krishnamacharya was teaching, his explanations were always closely linked to the old texts. There was scarcely one explanation that did not contain a reference to an appropriate quotation from one of the writings of the sages of old. Was there one work that was most central to his teaching?

A: The most important yoga text as far as my father was concerned was always Patañjali's *Yoga Sūtra*. The other texts were certainly useful, but there was no doubt in his mind concerning the relevance of the *Yoga Sūtra*. Another text that was important to him was Nathamuni's *Yoga Rahasya*. In that text there are hints on practical procedures; it is a book much concerned with the question of how yoga can be adapted to each individual. There is a lot of detailed information about breathing in the āsanas, for example. The *Yoga Rahasya* contains a wealth of information that is not given in the *Yoga Sūtra*. Furthermore, Nathamuni's text places great emphasis on bhakti, devotion to God. The *Bhagavad Gītā* is also a great yoga text. It emphasizes the thought that the way to the highest power does not mean that we should neglect or refuse to carry out our duties in life. This is what makes the *Bhagavad Gītā* unique. It tells us that our search should not be a flight from life. For anyone to whom the Vedas is important, the *Bhagavad Gītā* is a significant text. It relates many of the things from the Upaniṣads in a way that is easy to understand, and surprisingly enough, it contains important hints on things like breathing techniques and nutrition. In details like this the *Bhagavad Gītā* is much clearer and more precise than the *Yoga Sūtra*. A text like the *Haṭha Yoga Pradīpikā* contains a lot of good information, yet the essential text is still Patañjali's *Yoga Sūtra*. Understanding the *Yoga Sūtra* is a lifelong task. Each time you read it you can see something more, something different. I studied it eight times with my father, and I think my father went on studying it throughout his life. Each time he went through the *Yoga Sūtra* with me he could say something new about it. His last commentary on this text, written from 1984–1986, contained thoughts that he had never expressed before. In 1961 I studied the verse regarding *nābhicakra* with him,[1] but how much more information about the human body he put in his later commentary on this same verse! The *Yoga Sūtra* is an inspired text on all levels, whether about the body, the breath, or the mind.

[1] *Yoga Sūtra* 3.29.

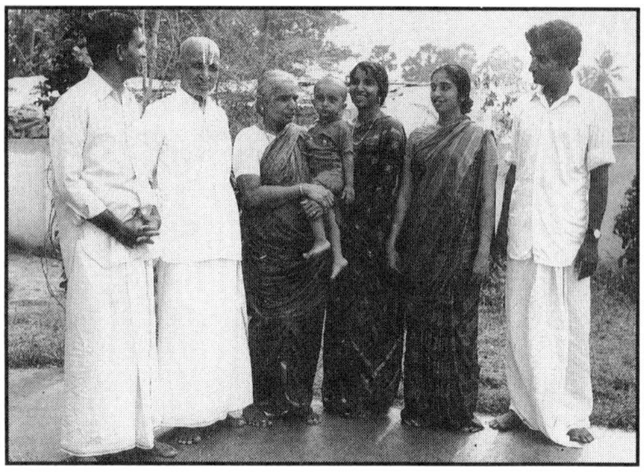

Krishnamacharya and his family.

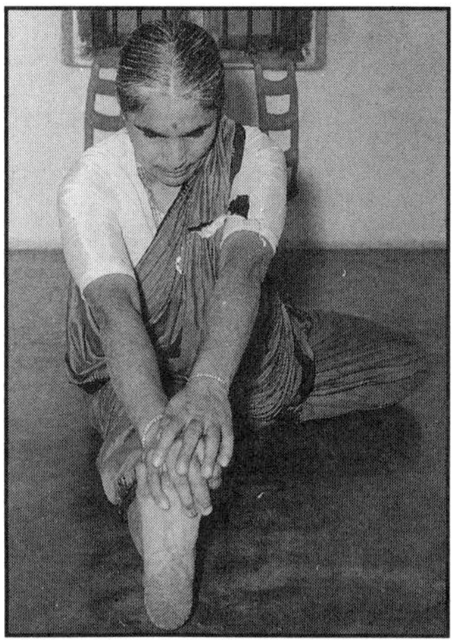

Namagiriamma, Krishnamacharya's wife, demonstrating mahāmudrā.

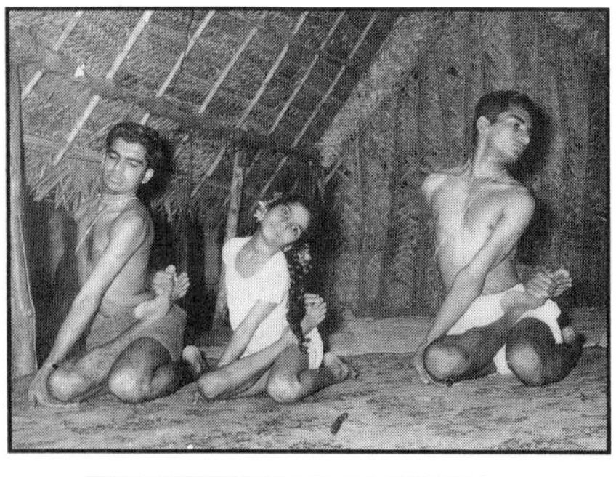

A young Desikachar with his sister and brother demonstrating bharadvājāsana at a public lecture.

Besides Nathamuni's *Yoga Rahasya*, which goes into more detail and emphasizes the theme of bhakti, the *Yoga Sūtra* was the seminal text for Krishnamacharya.

Q: Śrī Krishnamacharya was a family man and had six children. Can you say a few words about his family life?

A: My father was a very concerned person. He wanted all of us to do yoga and know everything he knew. At the same time, he found time to take care of our needs. I remember him taking us to the cinema when I was eight years old. But somehow we children were much closer to our mother. She was the one we usually went to when we needed something.

Q: What part did yoga play in the family?

A: Whether we liked it or not, we all did yoga. Everyone, including my mother and my three sisters, practiced āsanas. I remember seeing my mother doing āsanas, prāṇāyāma, and meditation when she was expecting my younger sister. I was the least interested, I must confess. When my father was around, though, I pretended to practice āsanas. My elder brother was the expert.

Q: Contrary to the trends of the time, your father did a lot to promote yoga for women, and your mother practiced regularly.

A: Yes. How she learned so much, I do not know. She must have picked it up from Father, who taught at home. I never saw him actually teach her, but she was able to correct all our practices. She knew all the texts by heart, even though she did not have much schooling. Her sister was adept at yoga too. She used to accompany Father on his lecture tours. And my sisters helped Father in his classes; my youngest sister now teaches yoga. Some of our women teachers are former students of his, including my wife. The well-known American yoga teacher Indra Devi studied yoga with my father in 1937.

Q: It is interesting that your father chose family life rather than the life of a sannyāsin. What was his attitude toward sannyāsin?

A: To be a sannyāsin means to give yourself totally to a higher power, to God. I think my father was a great example of that. There was never any doubt that he felt that it was not he himself who did things. He regarded himself as powerless, and it was always the power of his teacher or God that worked through him. He always claimed that everything he said and did came from his teacher and from God. He never claimed to have discovered anything, but always said: "Nothing is mine; it all comes from my teacher or from God." To me, that is sannyāsa. You cannot be a sannyāsin and at the same time say you discovered something yourself. To be a sannyāsin means to lay all that you do at the feet of your teacher or God. My father was an example of this. Those who met him often saw him take his teacher's sandals and lay them on his head as a way of saying that he felt he was small, smaller than the feet of his teacher. I think my father was a sannyāsin par excellence, and yet he was also a family man; he never experienced any contradiction between living with his family and living in the true spirit of a sannyāsin.

Sannyāsa in the sense of wearing orange robes, never staying long in one place but wandering about and begging for food was, in my father's opinion, no longer appropriate for our times. Manu, one of our great scholars, used to say that in these times of kaliyuga, sannyāsa has become impossible. My father's teacher told him that he must lead a family life, and Nathamuni says that family life is the most important part of one's existence. By that he does not just mean having children, but living as others do and having responsibilities. Even the Upaniṣads do not insist on sannyāsa in the formal sense of the word. The *Bhagavad Gītā* places no great value on sannyāsa. In it, Arjuna comes to see that he should involve himself in life and not run away from his tasks. Perhaps it is appropriate for those who have carried out all the tasks they have to do in the world to choose the way of sannyāsa, but there are not many like this. What was traditionally understood by the term *sannyāsa* is nowadays no longer possible.

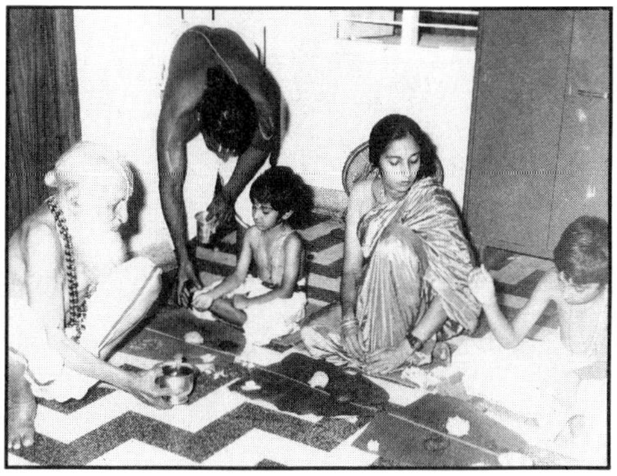

Krishnamacharya with his grandsons Bhushan and Kausthub and their mother Mrs. Menaka Desikachar on the occasion of their bhramhoupadesham *or sacred thread ceremony, 1983.*

Q: You studied with your father for more than twenty-five years. How did you come to be a student of your father's?

A: First of all, it is not quite accurate to say that I studied with him for twenty-five years. To say that gives the impression that I was like a student at university where the whole day is filled with studying. No, I lived with him for twenty-five adult years and during that time I also studied with him. In this way, studying with my father was like going to a foreign country and slowly becoming familiar with the language, customs, and habits of the people there. That is how I learned from him. He taught me how to understand the important texts such as the Upaniṣads. I learned how to recite these texts and how to interpret them. He told me what I had to learn and decided what I should teach. For instance, when I was wondering whether to accept an invitation from the European Union of Yoga, he said, "Go to the yoga conference in Switzerland!" and I went. He told me to go and teach Krishnamurthi, and so I did, and my father told me how I should do that.

Living with him, being with him, seeing him, eating with him, and so forth were the most important aspects of my life. I studied with him too, which is how I can now explain this and that to you from the *Yoga Sūtra*. But my explanations contain more of my experience with him, my shared life with him, than his words themselves. All that has been a great gift for me. Everything happened in our house: his treatments, his teaching, our family life, everything. That was the essential part of my "study" with him.

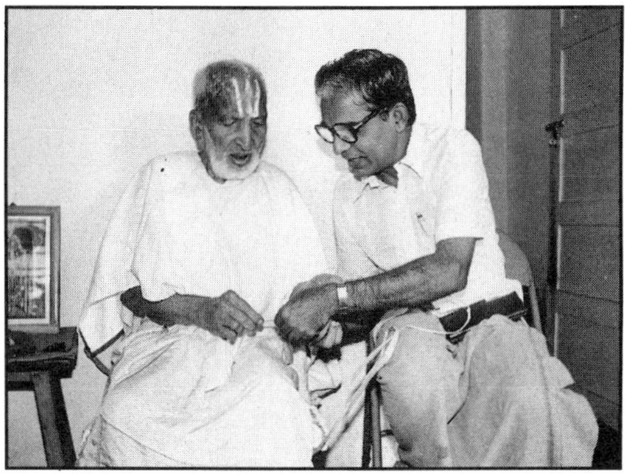

Krishnamacharya at 100 years old with Desikachar.

Q: What was his instruction like? How did he teach you and what did you learn?

A: I learned āsanas, but I only needed to work on them for six months or so. I was twenty-five and very flexible. He often took me with him to lectures and I had to demonstrate the āsanas to the audience as he explained their particular details. He told me how I had to perform them, and I did what he said.

I did not find the āsanas difficult, and my own āsana practice did not play an important part in his instruction. Much more time was taken up with the study of texts, learning to read pulses, working with sick people, and learning the important principles for teaching yoga. I had to teach first, and afterward ask questions. For example, I did not know how to teach yoga to pregnant women, so I asked him and he gave me advice. He watched my students closely and he watched my work with them closely. Even in 1989, the year in which he died, I never hesitated to ask him for advice, and he always gave me an answer.

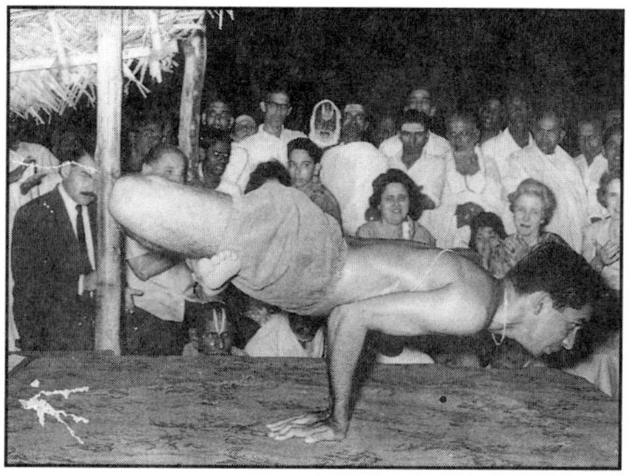

A young Desikachar demonstrating padma mayūrāsana at a public lecture.

When I first began studying with him he sometimes said: "What you are teaching at the moment is wrong." He said this in front of the students, but I did not feel any shame. On the contrary, I was happy that mistakes would thus be avoided. My students were not in the least put off by this practice. It was rather seen as good fortune to be given advice by the teacher. The well-being of the students was always central to our teaching, and I had no problem in telling them that I would have to ask my father for advice because I did not know enough myself. And my father was always very kind and told me what was to be done. This way of teaching requires kindness from the teacher and much modesty and humility on the part of the student. I can say that living with him and being able to observe and experience him working, treating himself when he was sick, preparing his meals and carrying out other rituals—all of this was the real yoga instruction that I received from him.

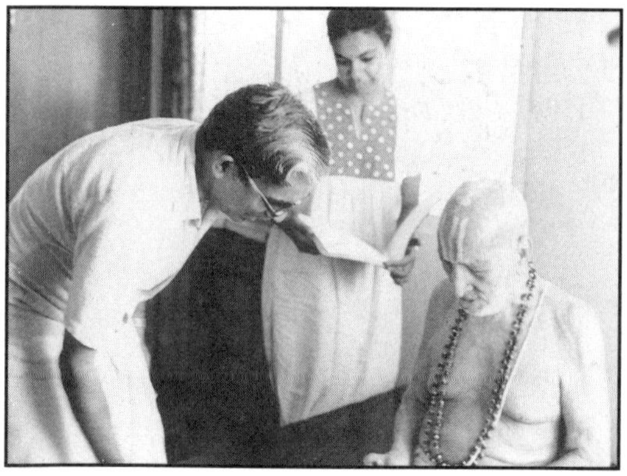

Sharing a verse from the Ramāyāna.

Of course there was the study of texts too, which took much more time than āsana technique because once you have understood this there is nothing more to say about it. The texts provide the content of your practice and make what you are doing comprehensible. The study of certain texts was compulsory, and here too the relationship between teacher and pupil was beyond question. First I had to learn the text he chose by heart. These texts are recited in a particular way. There are certain rules, and there is a game made of listening and repeating them as you learn them. Only after you have learned them by heart are they explained, and the explanations are given in the way the teacher thinks appropriate for each student. Instruction like this is only possible when you live with your teacher. In earlier days this was indeed the only way teachers could pass on the old texts at all.

Q: Nowadays it is not so easy to live in such close proximity with your teacher. What can we do?

A: I see a great difference between the struggle my father had to follow his path and the comfort I had in learning yoga. He left his home and went north into Tibet, far away from his people and culture, and stayed there for eight years. I scarcely had to take a couple of steps to receive my instruction. We lived in the same house. At first I divided my time between work and study.

Perhaps I missed out on something by doing it like this, but my father wanted it this way.

I think that we do not necessarily have to live with a teacher nowadays. We should rather work in our own environment and then meet our teacher from time to time in order to find a point of reference. Having a point of reference is absolutely necessary. We need somebody who can hold a mirror in front of us. Otherwise we very quickly begin to imagine that we are perfect and know it all. This personal connection cannot be replaced by books or videos. There must be a relationship, a real relationship, one that is based on trust.

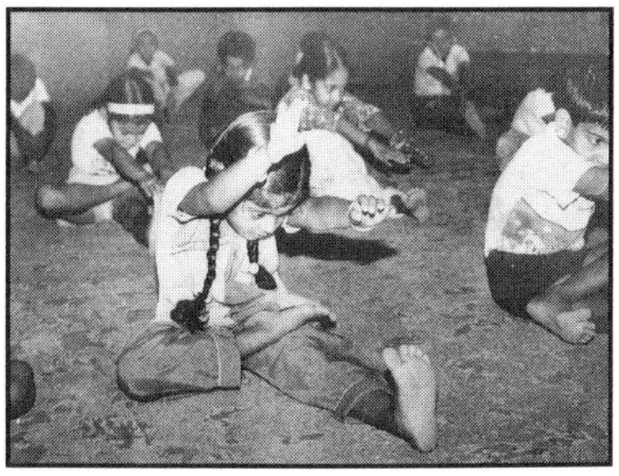

Children performing āsanas at the Krishnamacharya Yoga Mandiram.

Q: In 1976 the Krishnamacharya Yoga Mandiram was set up in Madras. What kind of work is carried out there?

A: We do essentially three things: First, we are available to anyone seeking help. Among those who come to us are people who have problems or those who are sick. This follows my father's tradition; throughout his life as a teacher he was again and again asked for advice and help by people suffering from all sorts of illnesses. It was not our intention that this focus on working with the sick should come to be such a big part of the mandiram's activities, but now we are recognized as an institution by the Department of Health.

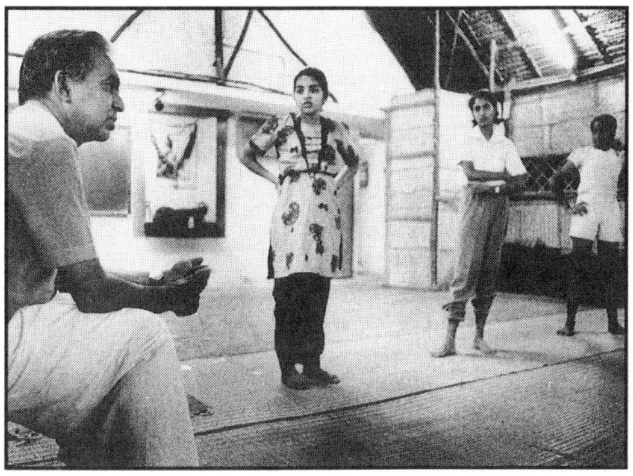

Tim Williams

Teaching the children's teachers, an important activity at the mandiram.

Second, we offer instruction to anyone who asks for it. If someone wants to know about yoga, they can come and learn here. By instruction I do not mean just instruction in āsanas. Yoga instruction at the mandiram includes learning about the whole spiritual and cultural heritage of India. We give classes in the recitation of Vedic texts and there are classes on the important ancient texts such as the Upaniṣads, the *Yoga Sūtra*, and the *Yoga Rahasya*.

The third area in which we work is in research and study projects. More by chance than anything else, we have begun asking ourselves how the various aspects of yoga can be investigated more closely. We are doing this so as to make our work in some way or other more comparable with other systems. For example, we have carried out research on the treatment of back pain and on our work with mentally handicapped people. Another project on which we are working is how to present my father's teachings to the public.

We also have publications on my father's teachings. There are more publications in the planning stages—commentaries on the *Yoga Sūtra* and a new edition of Nathamuni's *Yoga Rahasya*, for example. And this year we began publishing a quarterly journal entitled *Darśanam*. Its purpose is to make yoga better known in India and to bring traditional Indian medicine and various other aspects of Indian tradition and culture to the attention of an interested public. We are doing this as an expression of our respect for and thanks to our teacher, Śrī Krishnamacharya.

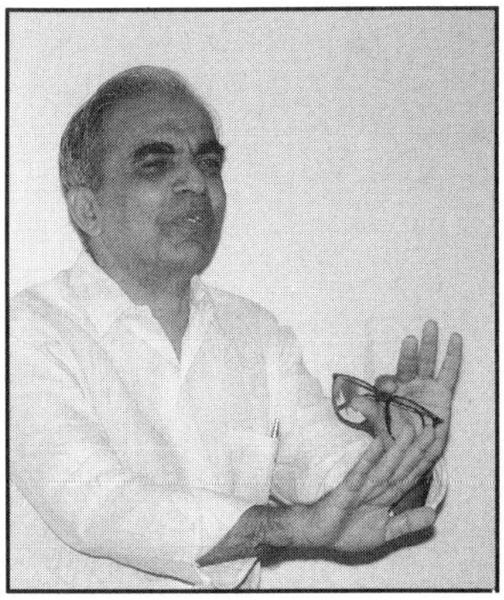

Desikachar teaching.

APPENDIX 1

The Texts Mentioned in This Book

The Yoga Sūtra

This, the most fundamental text on yoga and part 3 of this book, dates back to the period between the second and the end of the third centuries. The 195 verses (sūtras) of the text are short aphorisms, which are grouped in four chapters. The first chapter, entitled "Samādhipāda," gives us the famous definition of yoga,[1] and describes our state of mind in yoga and in nonyoga. The second chapter, "Sādhanapāda," presents yoga as a practice. Chapter three, "Vibhūtipāda," discusses the results that those who practice yoga can achieve and also discusses the dangers of these changes. The fourth chapter, entitled "Kaivalyapāda," concerns the freedom to which yoga can lead.

Various scholars have, from very early on, written commentaries on the *Yoga Sūtra.* Five of these are of significance today. The first, dating back to the fifth century, is Vyasa's *Bhāṣya.* It is available in countless English editions. (There are also many subcommentaries on this commentary.) The second, the *Vivrana*, was written by the Shankaracharya as a subcommentary on Vyasa's *Bhāṣya.* The third was written in the ninth century by Vacaspati Mishra. Entitled *Tattvaiśāradī*, this text also discusses Vyasa's commentary. The fourth, the *Rājamārtaṇḍa*, was written by Bhojadeva around the tenth century. Bhojadeva was a great king who also wrote important texts on music and dance. The fifth well-known commentary, which also includes comments on Vyasa's *Bhāṣya*, was written by Vijñānabikṣu in the sixteenth century. It is known by the title *Yogavārttika.*

[1] Yoga citta vṛtti nirodahaḥ: Yoga is the ability to direct the mind exclusively toward an object and sustain that direction without any distractions.

Yoga Yājñavalkya

This text, dating back to sometime between the second and fourth centuries, is the oldest text that talks about the concepts of prāṇāyāma, āsana, and especially kuṇḍalinī. The practices mentioned in it are not, as in many other texts, restricted to a particular caste or social group. On the contrary, in the text

Yājñavalkya explains the practice of yoga to his wife Gargi and a few other sages who have gathered around. The twelfth and final chapter, in which the writer talks about the role of kuṇḍalinī in the cleansing process of yoga, is exclusively addressed to his wife. Yājñavalkya introduces her to the "secrets" of yoga; hence the title of the chapter, "Rahasya." Yoga is defined as the link between the individual seed *(jivātma)* and the highest power *(parātman).*

Like the *Yoga Sūtra,* the *Yoga Yājñavalkya* describes eight limbs (aṅga) of yoga and describes the path of yoga practice as the development of these eight limbs. Some of the individual aṅga are, however, understood slightly differently from the way they are described in Patañjali's *Yoga Sūtra.* In contrast to later works about haṭha yoga from the tradition of the Nath yogis, there is no reference to the *shatkarma,* the special cleansing exercises of yoga. There is one critical edition of the *Yoga Yājñavalkya* written by Śrī Prabhad C. Divanji.[2]

Yoga Rahasya

One text that we do not have in written form yet, but whose existence is indicated by numerous references, is the *Yoga Rahasya* (Secrets of Yoga) by Nathamuni. Nathamuni was a ninth century South Indian sage who, like so many Indian teachers, did not belong to the monastic tradition but was fully involved with family life. His work, which is supposed to have originally consisted of twelve chapters, was handed down by word of mouth. Four of these chapters are known to us through Śrī Krishnamacharya, who dictated them to his son and pupil T. K. V. Desikachar.

For Nathamuni, the meaning and goal of yoga is devotion to God or a higher power (bhakti). In his text Nathamuni gives very precise instructions on aṣṭāṅga yoga, which partly correspond to those of Patañjali and emphasizes the need to tailor yoga to suit the particular needs of those who practice it. The text implies the absolute necessity for a teacher, and this is repeated again and again. A great number of āsanas and prāṇāyāma techniques are explained very precisely by Nathamuni. He also pays particular attention to the treatment of illness with yoga.

Nathamuni devotes many verses of the *Yoga Rahasya* to the meaning and practice of yoga for pregnant women. Like the *Yoga Yājñavalkya,* he insists that yoga is meaningful and worthwhile for women, thereby setting himself in opposition to the Brahmin teachings that wanted to completely exclude women from all spiritual practices.

Bhagavad Gītā

The *Bhagavad Gītā* ("The Song of the Lord") is *the* sacred text of India. It is the sixth section, the Bhīṣma Parva, of a great epic entitled the *Mahābhārata,* a long poem that is also a treatise on yoga. The discussion between the hero Arjuna and the god Kṛṣṇna, who appears as Arjuna's charioteer in a great battle

2. Journal of the Bombay Branch of the Royal Asiatic Society, reprint, monograph no. 3, 1954.

between two royal families, deals with the highest principles of yoga: the philosophy of action (karma), the show of discrimination, knowledge, and devotion to God (bhakti).

Haṭha Yoga Pradīpikā

This text by Yogi Svatmarama dates from the fifteenth century. It is one of the most important and most comprehensive, although sometimes contradictory, texts on haṭha yoga and presents sequentially in its four chapters the techniques of haṭha yoga: āsana, prāṇāyāma, mudrā, and nāda (external and internal sound).

In addition to these five texts, two others are mentioned in this book: the *Gheraṇḍa Saṃhitā* and the *Śiva Saṁhitā*. Like the *Haṭha Yoga Pradīpikā*, both these texts deal with yoga techniques.

APPENDIX 2

Four General Practice Sequences

An āsana practice should be planned according to the requirements of each person. The following examples of thoughtfully constructed practice sequences follow the principle of viṅyāsa krama, the step-by-step progression that can bring us to balance in body, breath, and mind. These practice sequences may not be suitable for those with no previous experience with yoga. Regardless of your background, the help of a competent teacher is important in designing the most appropriate yoga practice for you. These four sequences are shown as examples of how a practice might be planned. Variations to suit individual needs are infinite.

Make sure to allow for adequate rest between āsanas so that the heartbeat and breath can return to normal. There should also be adequate rest before beginning prāṇāyāma and upon completing prāṇāyāma.

In these practice sequences, the word *breaths* denotes static practice of an āsana, whereas *times* denotes dynamic practice. Remember: the breath is the gage to āsana practice. In each āsana practice you should work to maintain the connection between movement of the body and movement of the breath. Appropriate pauses can be placed between the in- and out-breath without compromising the length of the inhale or exhale. These retentions may increase as your practice develops. While maintaining the link of body and breath, each āsana is sustained over several breaths according to each person's capacity. Effort is appropriate to maintain the link of breath and body, but not struggle. A practice should always be designed to make you feel better and result in more equanimity and more energy.

Prāṇāyāma may be practiced by gradually increasing retentions with each breath cycle until a maximum retention is reached without struggle. Then retentions can be gradually reduced again to complete the prāṇāyāma. Likewise the length of the inhale or exhale may be progressively increased and reduced with or without retentions. As always, these variations depend on a person's requirements and capacity. It is essential that you practice prāṅāyāma only under the guidance of a competent teacher.

Practice 1

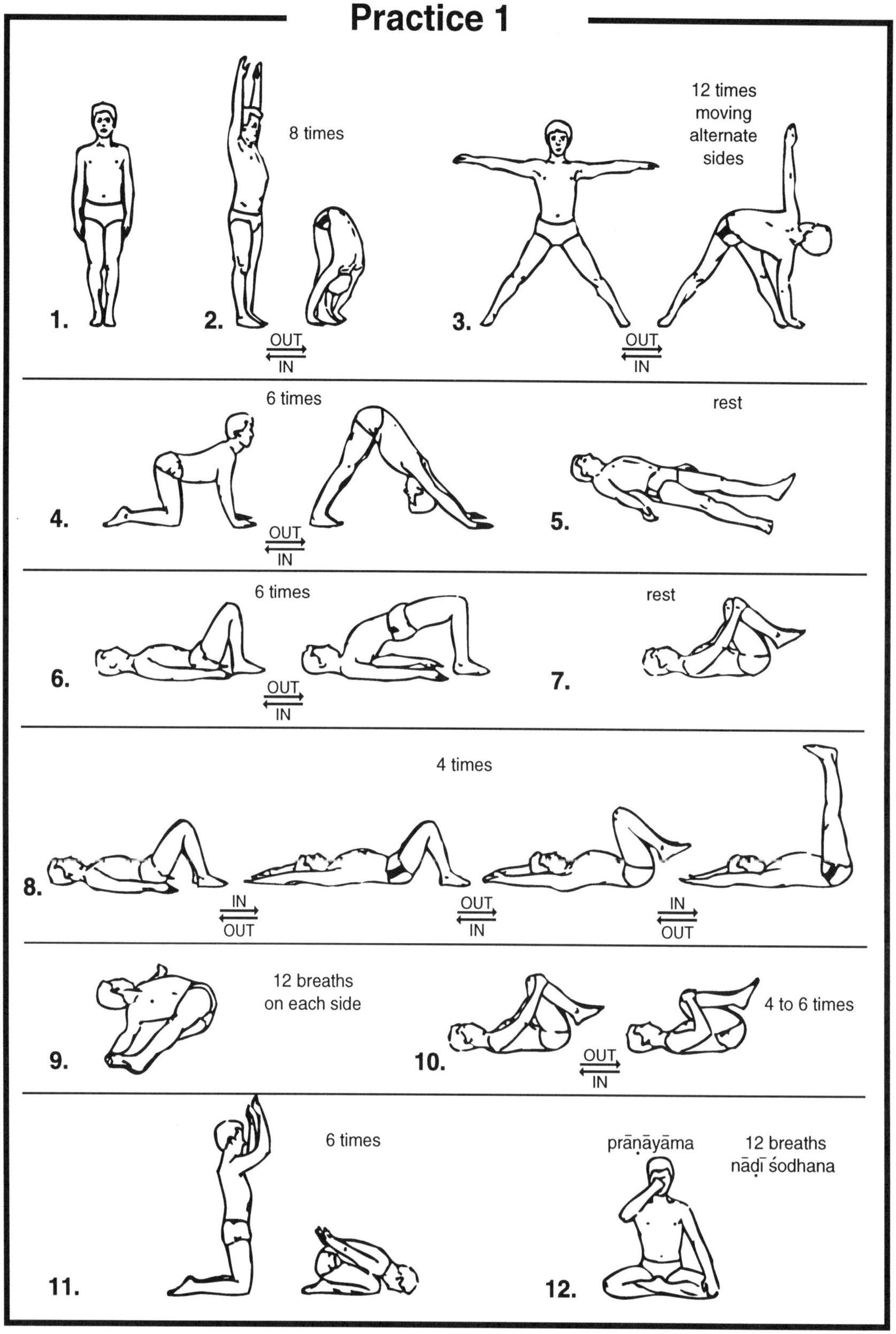
1.
2.
8 times
OUT
IN
3.
12 times moving alternate sides
OUT
IN
4.
6 times
OUT
IN
5.
rest
6.
6 times
OUT
IN
7.
rest
8.
4 times
IN
OUT
OUT
IN
IN
OUT
9.
12 breaths on each side
10.
OUT
IN
4 to 6 times
11.
6 times
12.
prāṇāyāma
12 breaths nāḍī śodhana

Practice 2

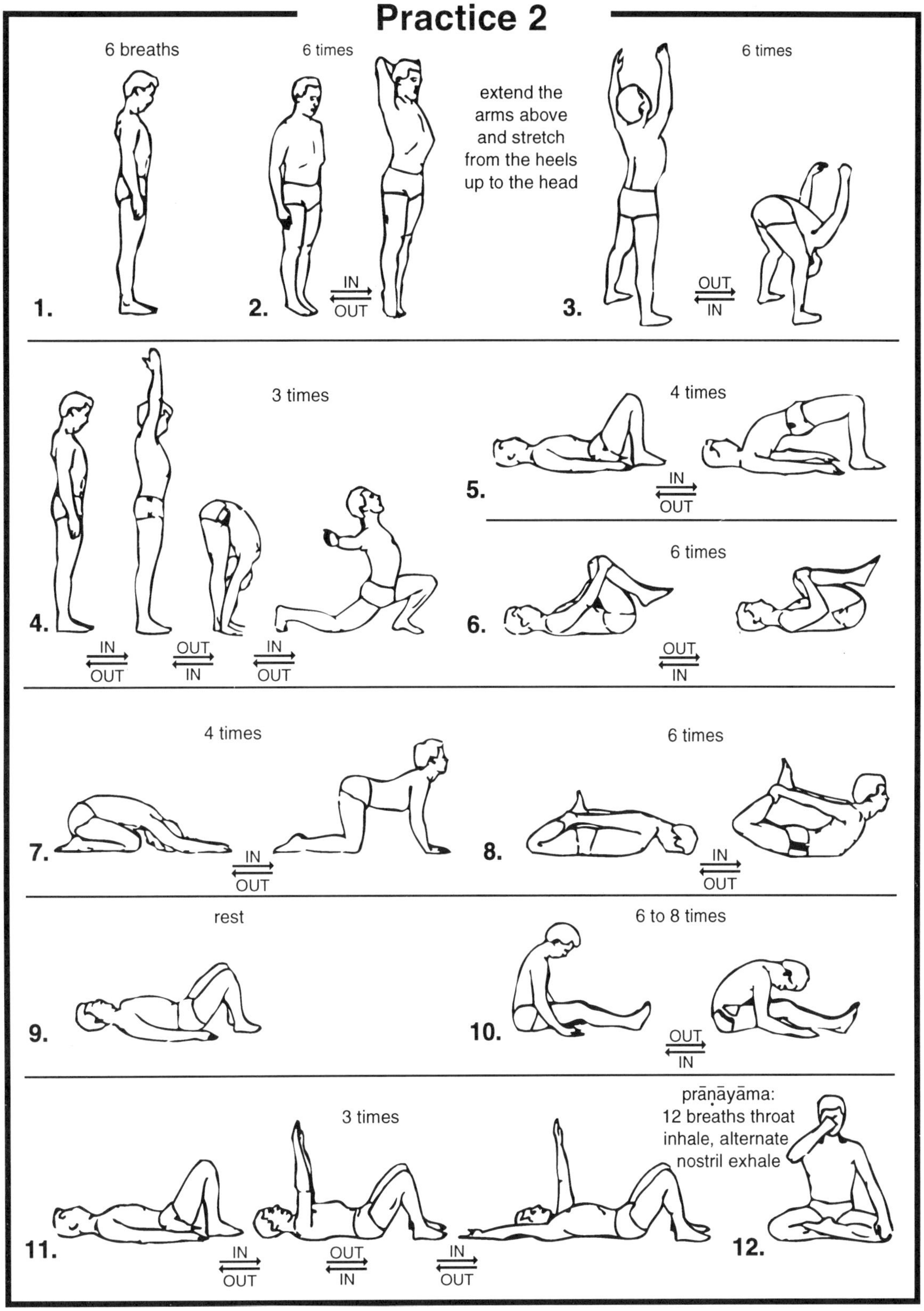
6 breaths
1.
6 times
2.
IN
OUT
extend the arms above and stretch from the heels up to the head
6 times
3.
OUT
IN
3 times
4.
IN
OUT
OUT
IN
IN
OUT
4 times
5.
IN
OUT
6 times
6.
OUT
IN
4 times
7.
IN
OUT
6 times
8.
IN
OUT
rest
9.
6 to 8 times
10.
OUT
IN
3 times
11.
IN
OUT
OUT
IN
IN
OUT
prāṇāyāma:
12 breaths throat inhale, alternate nostril exhale
12.

Practice 3

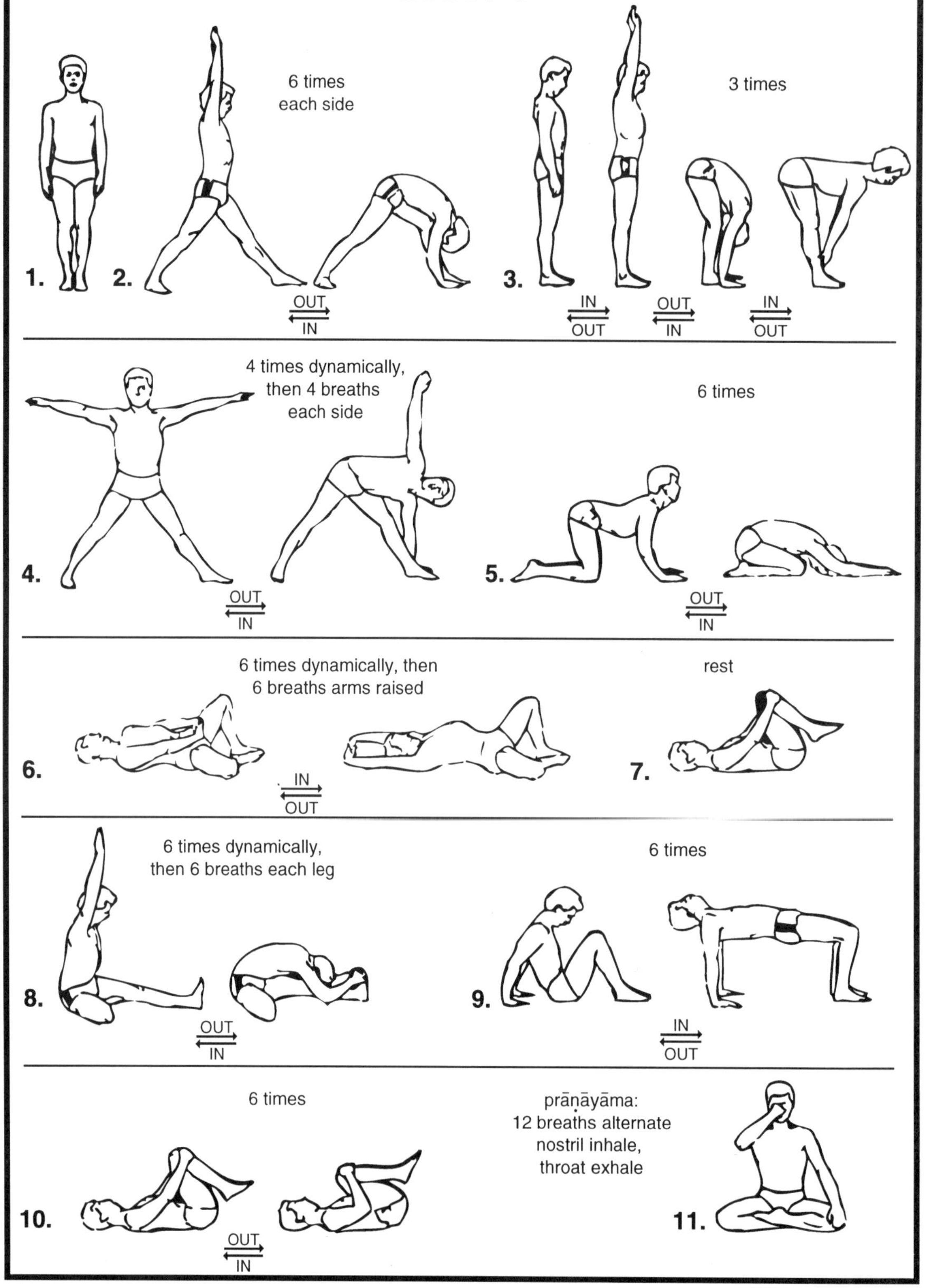
1.
2.
6 times
each side
OUT
IN
3.
3 times
IN
OUT
OUT
IN
IN
OUT
4.
4 times dynamically,
then 4 breaths
each side
OUT
IN
5.
6 times
OUT
IN
6.
6 times dynamically, then
6 breaths arms raised
IN
OUT
7.
rest
8.
6 times dynamically,
then 6 breaths each leg
OUT
IN
9.
6 times
IN
OUT
10.
6 times
OUT
IN
11.
prāṇāyāma:
12 breaths alternate
nostril inhale,
throat exhale

Practice 4

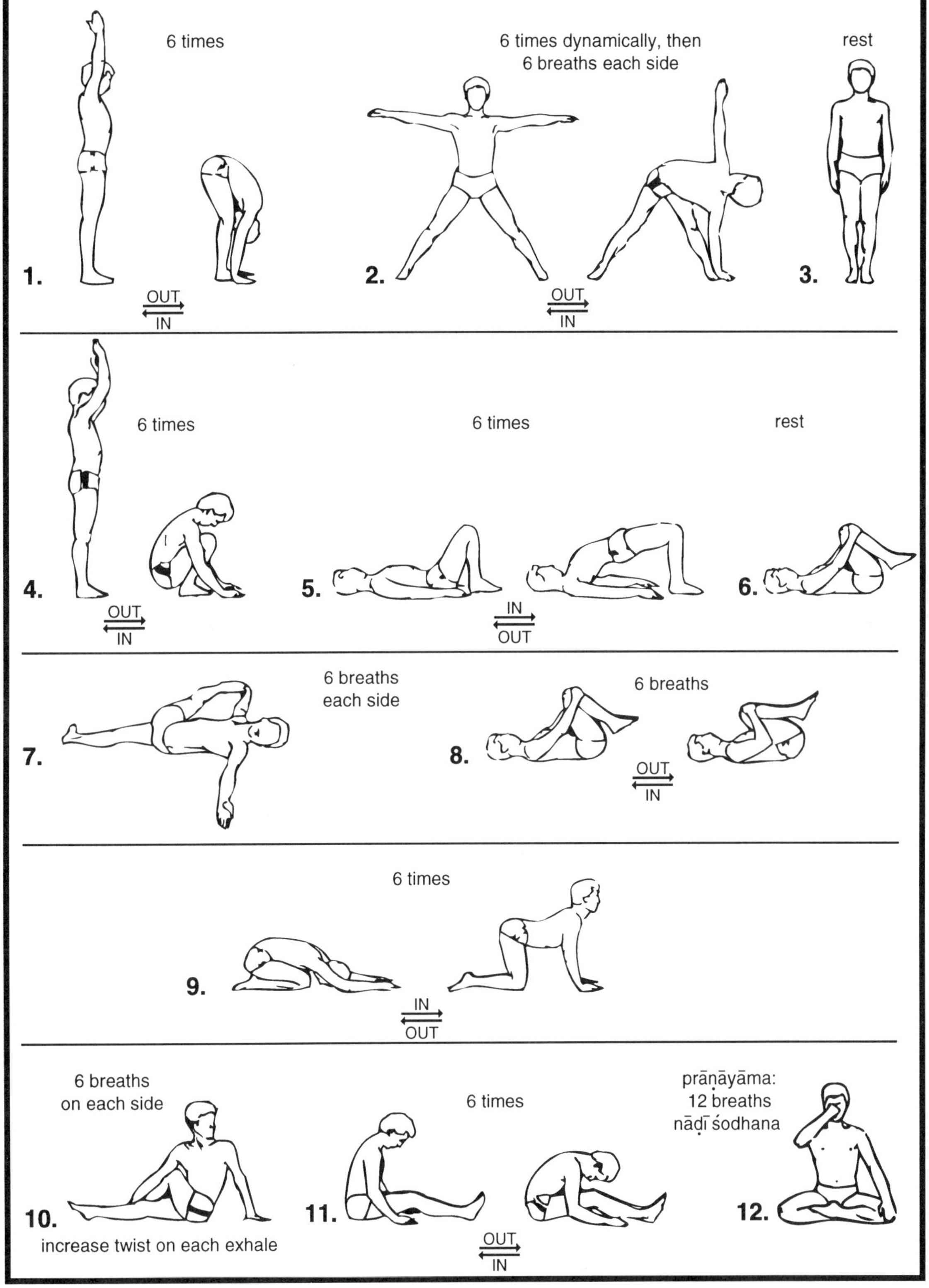
1.
6 times
OUT
IN
2.
6 times dynamically, then
6 breaths each side
OUT
IN
3.
rest
4.
6 times
OUT
IN
5.
6 times
IN
OUT
6.
rest
7.
6 breaths
each side
8.
6 breaths
OUT
IN
9.
6 times
IN
OUT
10.
6 breaths
on each side
increase twist on each exhale
11.
6 times
OUT
IN
12.
prāṇāyāma:
12 breaths
nāḍī śodhana

Glossary

abhiniveśa: the source of fear, attachment to life; one of the kleśas

abhyantara kumbhaka: holding the breath after inhaling

abhyāsa: practice

ācārya: teacher

adhomukha śvānāsana: downward-facing dog pose

advaita: nondualism

agni: fire, one of the bhūtas

agni sāra: a cleansing process using the "fire" of the human body to remove impurities

ahamkāra: the sense of "I"

ahiṁsā: noninjury, consideration, love; one of the yamas

ākāśa: space; one of the bhūtas

ānanda: a state of bliss

ananta: without end

aṅga: a "limb," or aspect, of yoga

antara: within, internal

antaraṅga sādhana: internal practice in referance to Pantañjali's path of concentration (dhāraṇā), meditation (dhyāna), and integration (samādhi)

antarāya: obstacle to a clear and stable mind

anuloma ujjāyī prāṇāyāma: prāṇāyāma where one inhales with a sound in the throat (ujjāyī) and exhales in a regulated way through alternate nostrils

ap: water; one of the bhūtas

apāna: dirt; the center in which bodily waste collects

apāna-vāyu: the aspect of prāṇa responsible for excretion

apānāsana: wind-relieving pose

aparigraha: to receive exactly what is appropriate and no more; one of the yamas

ardha padma paścimatānāsana: forward-bending half-lotus pose

ardha utkaṭāsana: half-squat pose

artha: meaning, purpose

āsana: posture

asmitā: sense of ego; one of the kleśas

asmitā samādhi: the merging of the mind with the object of meditation

aṣṭāṅga: eight limbs. Aṣṭāṅga yoga is the eight limbs of yoga as explained by Patañjali in the second chapter of the *Yoga Sūtra.*

asteya: not coveting what belongs to others; one of the yamas

ātman: the self

avidyā: misapprehension, incorrect knowledge, false understanding; the most important of the kleśas

bahiraṅga: external limb

bahiraṅga sādhana: external practice that includes the first four limbs of aṣṭāṅga yoga

bāhya kumbhaka: holding the breath after exhalation

bandha: to bind or lock

Bhagavad Gītā: a part of the epic ***Mahābhārata*** where Kṛṣṇa teaches yoga to Arjuna

bhakti: devotion

bhakti yoga: yoga in which devotion to God is prominent

bhastrika: bellows

bhastrika prāṇāyāma: bellows breathing through alternate nostrils

bhujaṅgāsana: cobra pose

bhūtas: elements of space, air, light, water, and earth

brahmacarya: one of the yamas. Moving toward the highest modification of the senses, it is the stage of life where the young student studies the sacred texts.

bṛmhaṇa: to expand

buddhi: intellect

cakras: energy centers along the spinal column

cakravākāsana: cat pose

cit: consciousness

citta: mind

citta vṛtti nirodha: mental state devoid of agitation

dana: to give away

darśana: one of the six classical points of view of Indian thought

deśa: place

dhanurāsana: bow pose

dhāraṇā: the state of mind in which the mind is oriented toward one point

dharma: duty, ethical value

dhyāna: meditation

dhyāna mudrā: gesture indicating meditation practice

dhyāta: one who is in the state of dhyāna

draṣṭṛ: the seer, that which sees

dṛśya: that which is seen

duḥkha: feeling of discomfort, pain

dveṣa: dislike, hatred; one of the kleśas

dvipāda pītham: table pose

eka pāda uttānāsana: a standing posture where the torso bends forward and one leg is lifted behind

ekāgratā: single direction, single-mindedness

guṇas: qualities of the mind; qualities of the universe

halāsana: plow pose

hasta mudrā: hand symbol

Haṭha Yoga Pradīpikā: a classical text on haṭha yoga

haṭha yoga: yoga in which the aim is to unify the two energies of ha (the left) and ṭha (the right), and merge them into suṣumṇā in the center of the spine; the merging of prāṇa and apāna into the center of the body, at the heart

iḍā: a nādī that terminates at the left nostril

indriyas: senses

Īśvara: God or Lord

īśvarapraṇidhānā: to surrender and offer all actions to God, without attachment to the fruits of our action; one of the niyamas and a component of kriyā yoga

jālandhara bandha: chin lock

japa: repetition of mantra

jñāna yoga: yoga in which the emphasis is on inquiry

kaivalya: ultimate state of yoga, freedom

kapālabhātī prāṇāyāma: bellows breathing

kāraṇa: cause

karma yoga: yoga in which action is done as duty, without concern for success or failure

kleśa: affliction

kriyā: action

kriyā yoga: yoga of purifying action as taught by Patañjali

kṣipta: agitated mind

kumbhaka prāṇāyāma: breathing exercise in which emphasis is on the retention of the breath

kuṇḍalinī: the obstacle located in the center of the spine that obstructs the movement of prāṇa into suṣumṇā

laṅghana: to reduce

laya: to merge

līlā: the divine play

mahāmudrā: a classic sitting pose

mahat: the great principle

manas: the power behind the senses

mantra: a sacred sound, often used as the object of focus during meditation

matsyendrāsana: half spinal twist

mṛgi mudrā: finger position to control the nostrils during prāṇāyāma

mūdha: dull state of mind

mudrā: symbol

mūla bandha: base-of-trunk lock

nāda: sound

nāḍī: subtle passage in the body through which prāṇa moves

nāḍī śodhana prāṇāyāma: alternate nostril breathing, bringing purification of the nāḍīs

nidrā: dreamless sleep

nimitta kāraṇa: intelligent cause, catalyst

nirodha: restraint, state in which the mind focuses totally on one thing

niyama: personal discipline

om: a representation of Īśvara

padmāsana: lotus pose

pariṇāmaduḥkha: duḥkha arising from change

pariṇāmavāda: the recognition that all we perceive is subject to change

parivṛtti: redirection, reorientation

pārśva uttānāsana: a standing pose with one leg forward and the trunk folded on it

paścimatānāsana: seated forward bend

piṅgalā: nāḍī that terminates at the right nostril

pradhāna: original source

prajñā: clear understanding in the spiritual field

prakṛti: matter

pramāṇa: right perception

prāṇa: life-force energy

prāṇa-vāyu: one of the five main life energies

prāṇava: mystic syllable that represents Īśvara

prāṇāyāma: regulated breathing technique

prasarita pada uttānāsana: standing posture with the torso bent forward between the legs

pratikriyāsana: counterpose

pratyāhāra: withdrawal of the senses

pūraka prāṇāyāma: breathing exercise in which the emphasis is on the inhalation

puruṣa: source of consciousness, perceiver

rāga: attachment or desire; one of the kleśas

rajas: the quality of prakṛti responsible for activity

rāja yoga: yoga in which union with the highest power is the goal; the yoga of Patañjali

recaka prāṇāyāma: breathing exercise in which the emphasis is on the exhalation

ṛta prajñā: perception of a spiritual truth

sādhana: practice

śakti: power

śalabhāsana: locust pose

samādhi: state of meditation in which only the object of meditation is apparent

samāna-vāyu: prāṇa of the central region of the body, responsible for digestion

samavṛtti prāṇāyāma: breathing technique in which different components of breathing are equal

saṃskāra: habitual movement of the mind; habit, conditioning

saṃskāra-duḥkha: duḥkha caused by habits

saṃtoṣa: contentment; one of the niyamas

saṃyama: total continuous concentration on one object

saṃyoga: entanglement or confused identification

sannyāsin: one who has given up everything except God

sarvajña: all-knower, omniscient

sarvāṅgāsana: shoulderstand

sattva: one of the three qualities of prakṛti responsible for clarity and lightness

satvāda: the concept that everything we see, experience, and feel is not illusion, but is true and real

satya: truth, truthfulness; one of the yamas

śauca: cleanliness, purity; one of the niyamas

śavāsana: corpse pose

siddhi: gift; power that is given

śirṣāsana: headstand

śītalī prāṇāyāma: breathing exercise in which one inhales through the mouth, shaping the tongue in a particular way

smṛti: memory

śodhana: purification

sthira: steadiness and alertness

sukha: lightness and comfort; happiness

sukhāsana: simple cross-legged pose

sūrya namaskar: sequence of āsanas collectively called the salute to the sun

suṣumṇā: central nāḍī running through the center of the spine, from the base to the top of the head

svadharma: your own position

svādhyāya: self-inquiry; any study that helps you understand yourself; the study of sacred texts; one of the niyamas and a component of kriyā yoga

tadāsana: mountain pose

tamas: one of the three qualities of prakṛti, responsible for heaviness and stability

tanmātras: the characteristics of sound, touch, form, taste, and smell

tantra: technique

tantra yoga: yoga in which the focus is the elimination of obstacles that block the free movement of prāṇa in suṣumṇā

tanu: mild, feeble

tāpa-duḥkha: pain caused by craving

tapas: process of removing impurities; elimination, purification; one of the niyamas and a component of kriyā yoga

trāṭaka: gazing at a static object to invite meditation

trikonāsana: triangle pose

udāna-vāyu: the aspect of prāṇa responsible for speech and upward movement

uddāyīna bandha: abdominal lock

ujjāyī: breathing technique in which one inhales with a sound in the throat

urdhvamukha śvānāsana: upward-facing dog pose

uṣṭrāsana: camel pose

utkaṭāsana: squatting pose

uttānāsana: standing forward bend

vairāgya: detachment, letting go

vajrāsana: thunderbolt pose

vāyu: air, breath, wind; one of the bhūtas

Vedas: Hindu scriptures that are the basis for all yoga

vicāra: reflection on a subtle object

vidyā: clear understanding, high level of knowledge

vikalpa: imagination

vikṣipta: state in which the mind is moving without any consistent purpose or direction

viloma krama prāṇāyāma: breathing exercise in which one inhales in a regulated way through alternate nostrils and exhales through both nostrils with a sound in the throat

viloma ujjāyī prāṇāyāma: breathing exercise using nostril control for inhalation and exhalation

viṅyāsa krama: a correctly organized course of āsanas progressing appropriately toward a desired goal

viparyaya: false perception

vīrabhadrāsana: warrior pose

vīrāsana: hero pose

viṣamavṛtti prāṇāyāma: breathing technique in which the different components of the breathing are not equal

viśeṣa puruṣa: Īśvara

Viṣṇu: God, one of the Trinity

vitarka: reflecting on a gross object

viveka: discrimination

vyāna-vāyu: prāṇa responsible for distribution of energy throughout the whole body

yama: discipline concerning our dealings with society and the world

yoga sādhana: yoga practice

Yoga Sūtra: Patañjali's classic text on yoga

yogi: someone adept at yoga